Introduction to Cerebral Angiography

Introduction to Cerebral Angiography

Anne G. Osborn, M.D.

Associate Professor of Radiology
University of Utah College of Medicine
Salt Lake City, Utah

with **Julian G. Maack,** M.F.A.
Chief, Medical Illustrations Department

and *BRADLEY R. NELSON, THOMAS C. CASWELL*
Medical Photographers

Cover illustration adapted from drawing by ANNE G. OSBORN

HARPER & ROW, PUBLISHERS

HAGERSTOWN

Cambridge   London
New York   Mexico City
Philadelphia   São Paulo
San Francisco   Sydney

1817

10 9 8 7 6 5 4 3 2

Library of Congress Cataloging in Publication Data

Osborn, Anne G
  Introduction to cerebral angiography.

  Includes index.
  1. Brain – Blood vessels – Radiography.
2. Angiography. I. Title. [DNLM: 1. Cerebral
angiography.   WL141 08li]

RC386.6.A54082   616.8'047572   80-11227
ISBN 0-06-141829-3

*The authors and publisher have exerted every effort to ensure
that drug selection and dosage set forth in this text are in ac-
cord with current recommendations and practice at the time of
publication. However, in view of ongoing research, changes in
government regulations, and the constant flow of information
relating to drug therapy and drug reactions, the reader is urged
to check the package insert for each drug for any change in indications and dosage and for added warnings and precautions.
This is particularly important when the recommended agent is a
new and/or infrequently employed drug.*

To MY PARENTS
You opened all the doors

Contents

Preface

WHILE THE ADVENT of cranial computed tomography (CT) has eliminated the need for angiography in some situations, angiography is still the procedure of choice for delineating lesions of the cerebral vasculature. Angiography also adds important complementary diagnostic information in a variety of other disease processes. Therefore, thorough familiarity with some of the technical aspects of these procedures as well as the normal and pathologic anatomy of the cerebral vasculature remains requisite for the modern neuroangiographer.

Introduction to Cerebral Angiography is designed as a basic text for general angiographers, residents and fellows in the neurosciences, and diagnostic radiology trainees. While several excellent, short introductory monographs and multivolume, multiauthor series have been written on the subject, no relatively comprehensive single volume text is available. It is my hope that Introduction to Cerebral Angiography will fill this gap, providing a moderately detailed yet basic presentation that covers the fundamentals of this important subject.

A. G. O.
Salt Lake City
Utah, 1980

Acknowledgments

I AM INDEBTED to many people for their assistance in making this project possible.

The James A. Picker Foundation provided support for the prototype monographs, initially structured as self-teaching manuals, from which this text was conceived. Paul J. Toscano, Edward E. Green, and John Kerr of the Division of Instructional Research, Development and Evaluation at Brigham Young University provided expert help in the development of the prototype monograph and rendered invaluable editorial assistance with the subsequent text.

My colleagues, Drs. Robert E. Anderson and S. Douglas Wing, reviewed the manuscript, adding helpful suggestions and comments. They were also instrumental in developing the extensive teaching file which was an invaluable resource for many of the angiograms utilized in this text.

Mr. Julian G. Maack and his associates in the Department of Medical Illustrations at the University of Utah provided superb quality drawings and reproductions for what is primarily a visually-oriented text. Our special procedures technicians under the direction of Ms. Kathy Wallin and Mr. David School consistently obtained the high quality angiograms that have been utilized as the illustrations for this text.

Finally, a special note of thanks to Connie Staples, Pat Mavor, and the other secretaries who translated my almost indecipherable handwriting.

A.G.O.

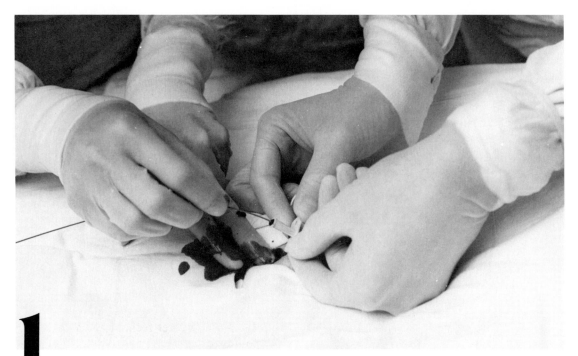

1 Technical Aspects of Cerebral Angiography

As a diagnostic consultant, the neuroradiologist's role is to recommend, perform, and evaluate appropriate diagnostic imaging sequences for the patient with a neurologic disorder. Angiography is only one of a wide variety of techniques that may or may not be appropriate in any given clinical setting. Both a comparison of different imaging modalities and a comprehensive discussion of neuroangiographic techniques are beyond the scope of this text; however, an introduction to the technical aspects is helpful for orientation. The indications for cerebral angiography, the various types of contrast media that are utilized, preparation of the patient for angiography, filming and injection techniques, and some technical aspects of the procedure itself are briefly reviewed, along with the complete angiographic procedure itself.

INDICATIONS AND CONTRAINDICATIONS FOR ANGIOGRAPHY

Indications for Angiography

The advent and nearly universal acceptance of cranial computerized tomography (CT) has altered many of the criteria for angiography. CT has virtually replaced angiography in the evaluation of acute head trauma except when arterial dissection or laceration, pseudoaneurysm, or thrombosis of a major vessel is suspected.[51] Angiography may also be used when the CT scan is normal and isodense or balanced extracerebral fluid collections are suspected.[55] CT has replaced angiography in the evaluation of intracranial metastatic disease as well. In many other disease processes, cerebral angiography often adds important complementary information. For example, the management of subarachnoid hemorrhage secondary to ruptured aneurysm is aided using both procedures. CT can often detect blood in the subarachnoid spaces and distinguish the angiographically avascular mass effect of infarction from an acute intracerebral hematoma. Angiography is necessary to visualize small aneurysms, the configuration and neck of the aneurysm itself, its relationship to adjacent structures, and the presence of vascular spasm.[16]

Large cerebral infarcts or areas of hypertensive hemorrhage can be detected by CT. Most recent studies, however, have shown that this examination results in little demonstrable improvement, in either the cost of care or clinical management of patients with cerebrovascular disease.[4] Angiography is required to demonstrate extra- and intracranial vascular stenoses, occlusions, and ulcerated plaques. Patterns of collateral blood flow are also completely delineated only by angiography. While arteriography is the study of choice in evaluating cerebrovascular disease, it should be used only in those patients whose therapy might be altered if a surgically correctable vascular lesion were to be discovered.[51]

Many contrast–enhancing masses may closely resemble one another in CT scans.[55] Here, angiography is helpful in distinguishing suprasellar aneurysms or vascular tumors from other apparently similar masses (*i.e.*, large pituitary adenomas).[44A, 59B] Arteriography is also employed in defining the precise location of and blood supply to primary intracranial tumors and vascular malformations. One study has reported a progressive decrease in the proportion of normal angiograms since the advent of CT, indicating that CT has made this more invasive neurodiagnostic procedure more efficacious patients with suspected lesions.[36]

In the future, non-invasive techniques (*i.e.*, carotid ultrasound or IV cervico-cerebral angiography with digital video subtraction and computer enhancement or computerized fluoroscopy) may provide alternative methods of studying vascular lesions in cases where intra-arterial catheter techniques may be contraindicated.[11A, 14A, 63A]

Contraindications to Angiography

No absolute contraindications for angiography exist except when it is unnecessary for diagnosis. Some relative contraindications do exist. The delivery of large amounts of hypertonic contrast may precipitate acute tubular necrosis. Caution is advised when deciding to perform cerebral angiography in patients with migraine headache. The apparent increased incidence of vascular spasm may result in an increased risk of serious complications.

Known allergic reaction to iodinated contrast media is not an absolute contraindication to angiography. Intraarterial administration of these agents is less hazardous than the intravenous route.[14, 34] Premedication with steroids may be of some help in these cases.[19]

CONTRAST MEDIA

Physical Characteristics

The development of low toxicity water-soluble contrast media has made safe cerebral angiography possible. Most currently used intravascular agents have both a cationic and an anionic component. While a variety of different preparations are available, pure methylglucamine (cationic portion) salts of diatrizoate, iothalamate, and metrizoate (anionic components) appear to be the best tolerated for cerebral studies.[1] Recently, isosmolar, nonionic contrast media have been introduced and evaluated as possible angiographic agents as well.[26A, 73]

For selective cerebral studies, we use a 60% iothalamate meglucamine concentration (282 mg/ml organically bound iodine),* which gives excellent vascular opacification; a higher concentration is necessary for aortic arch studies (we use a combination of 52% iothalamate meglumine and 26% iothalamate sodium† which yields approximately 400 mg/ml organically bound iodine).

Metabolic Considerations

Most commonly used contrast media are hypertonic under normal conditions.[26A] Following intravascular injection, contrast media are rapidly circulated to the kidneys where they are excreted unchanged by glomerular filtration.

Toxicity

A personal or family history of bronchial asthma or allergy may imply a slightly greater risk of adverse reaction to the use of iodinated intravascular contrast media.[11B] Most contrast reactions are mild and require no therapy (see below). There is a significantly lower incidence of adverse reactions to intraarterial compared to intravenous injection.[14]

Premedication seems to have no significant effect in diminishing the overall incidence of adverse reactions. Routine pretesting with 0.5 to 1 contrast by any route is considered of no significant value. Only 6.6% of all patients with a history of contrast reaction to the same previously performed examination are likely to react adversely if that study is repeated.[34]

PATIENT CARE AND PREPARATION

Optimal preparation of the patient for cerebral angiography follows what are essentially common sense guidelines. First and foremost, the neuroangiographer is a physician — one who must accept complete responsibility for the total welfare of the patient while he is in the radiology department. Although some activities may be delegated to the technician, angiographic nurse, or other paramedical personnel, the angiographer is ultimately responsible for both the quality and safety of the examination.

Ideally, the patient should be visited and briefly examined, and the chart and pertinent radiographs reviewed prior to the angiogram. The physician should establish rapport with the patient and review with him what to expect when he arrives in the angiographic suite. The procedure should be explained including a description of the physical sensations that might be experienced during the study, and any questions or concerns the patient might have should be addressed. The angiographer should outline candidly the hazards and complications together with the likelihood of their occurrence and obtain an informed consent. The explanation can begin in this fashion: "Mr. _____, like many major diagnostic procedures in medicine, a cerebral angiogram is not without a small degree of risk." Follow with a careful explanation of just exactly what those potential complications are.

Patients should be well hydrated prior to any angiographic procedure. Clear liquids up to the time of the study should be encouraged. The patient is asked to void prior to coming to the radiology department. When he arrives in the angiographic suite, the patient's groin is shaved (if a transfemoral approach is to be used). An intravenous infusion may be used if desired. While barbiturate, phenothiazine, and atropine premedication can be given, small increments of intravenous diazepam administered during the procedure itself is usually adequate. Many patients require no sedation at all.

Prior to beginning the procedure, the angiographer should check vital signs and use a felt tip pen to mark the appropriate peripheral pulses on the patient. This will assist both the angiographer and the ward nurses to check the pulses following the angiogram.

---

* Conray 60 (Mallinckrodt Pharmaceuticals)
† Vascoray (Mallinckrodt Pharmaceuticals)

FILMING

Preliminary films (scout films) should be obtained prior to the procedure. This will permit minor adjustments in radiographic technique and patient positioning that determine the difference between an inadequate, adequate, or elegant study.

Radiographic projections of various types are used, depending on the information desired and the anatomic area being studied. Aortic arch studies for cerebrovascular disease should be centered to include the apex of the arch, origins of all the great vessels, and most of the neck. While single plane RPO films are usually obtained, other projections may be required (see Chapter 2).

Selective common carotid angiograms for evaluation of the carotid bifurcation should be obtained in at least two projections: anteroposterior (AP) and lateral. Often an oblique view adds valuable information. Biplane filming techniques will minimize the number of injections into a potentially diseased vessel.

Routine views of the supratentorial intracranial circulation are usually obtained in the AP and lateral projections. Collimated AP views should superimpose the superior rim of the orbits and the petrous ridges (the so-called carotid angle is about +10° to the canthomeatal line). Supplemental views such as a zero degree AP, submentovertex, or Water's projection may be helpful in visualizing certain structures such as the anterior communicating artery. Oblique studies are often used in the evaluation of aneurysms and extra-axial fluid collections. Magnification lateral, zero degree AP, and AP Towne views are standard for most posterior fossa examinations.

Magnification lateral films are frequently helpful in delineating small vessel abnormalities, faint vascular blushes, and so forth.[60] A 0.3-mm focal spot tube and primary geometric air gap magnification are used, usually allowing 20 inches from tube to patient and another 20 inches from patient to film changer. This results in about a 2:1 magnification effect.

Film sequencing varies somewhat according to the clinical setting. In the majority of cases, it is desirable to visualize the intracranial circulation from the early arterial through late venous phase. A standard film sequence is two films every half second for three seconds, then one film every second for 6 seconds. This provides a total of 12 films. If rapid intracranial circulation with arteriovenous shunting is present, the sequence can be speeded up to obtain 3, 4, or even 6 films per second. Conversely, patients with slow intracranial blood flow (as might occur with subarachnoid hemorrhage and resultant vascular spasm) may require a prolonged film sequence. It is important to tailor the films and their sequencing to fit the particular clinical setting.

Subtraction films of cerebral angiograms are particularly useful in visualizing small vessel detail, free of overlapping bony structures. Arterial, capillary, and venous phase subtraction films are often used routinely. The first film of any given sequence is timed so that no contrast is present (Fig. 1-1A). A transparent positive print or "mask" (actually a photographic reversal) is made of the initial film (Fig. 1-1B). A final print is made by photographing the superimposed angiogram and mask (Fig. 1-1C, D). Both must be exactly superimposed; any patient motion during the film sequence seriously degrades the image. Small lesions, virtually undetectable on routine films, are often clearly visible using this technique of photographic subtraction. Subtraction prints have been used almost exclusively in this text.

CATHETER ANGIOGRAPHY

While cerebral angiograms can be performed by either direct puncture of the carotid/vertebral artery or puncture of a remote vessel (such as the brachial artery) with retrograde

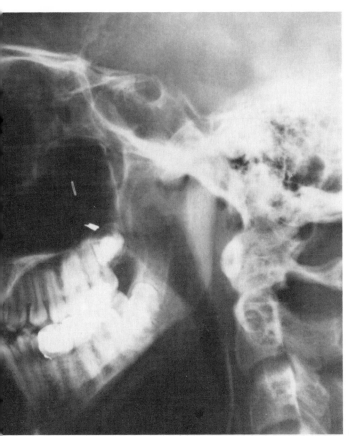

Fig. 1-1. Subtraction prints of cerebral angiograms made by timing the sequence so that no contrast is present on the first film **(A)** of the series. Photographic reversal of this initial film produces a transparent positive print or mask **(B).** When the mask is placed over a later film with contrast **(C),** a final print **(D)** is made by photographing the superimposed mask and angiogram. This process subtracts most of the bone from the angiogram and shows the vessels in detail.

(Fig. 1-1 continued on p. 6)

A
B

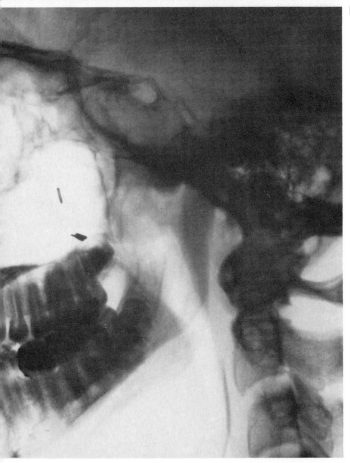

(Fig. 1-1 continued)

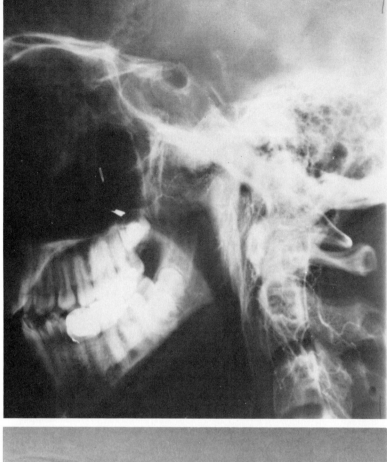

C

D

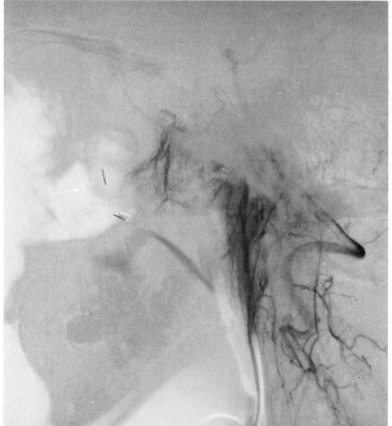

6

injection of a contrast bolus, the vast majority of neuroangiographic procedures are done by the transfemoral catheter technique. The staff of the University of Utah School of Medicine favors this approach for several reasons: (1) only one arterial puncture is needed to evaluate multiple vessels; (2) the arterial puncture is at a site remote from the cerebral vessels and therefore any local arterial complication cannot cause a neurologic complication; (3) because the femoral puncture is generally less traumatic for the patient, less sedation and other premedication are required; general anesthesia is rarely used; (4) with meticulous attention to technique, the complication rate is quite low.

The equipment required for modern, safe cerebral angiography is relatively complex. Image-intensified fluoroscopy and an angiographic table with a movable or free-floating top capable of a wide range of excursion are absolute prerequisites. Rapid-sequence filming capability with, if possible, biplane, magnification, and angiotomographic options is necessary. Small focal spot (0.3 mm) tubes with a three-phase 1200 Ma. generator are required for magnification studies that show sharp, detailed visualization of the smaller intracranial vessels.

The standard angiographic tray is relatively simple (Fig. 1-2). Two different sized sets of glass luer-lock syringes are provided; 20 ml syringes are used for flushing the catheters with heparinized saline and 10 ml syringes for test doses of contrast medium. Separate sterile bowls are used for guidewire storage and as a receptacle for used flushing solutions. A bottle of heparinized saline or 5% dextrose in water with connecting tubing and a three-way stopcock are used for withdrawing all fluid both for rinsing the syringes and flushing the catheters. This type of closed system is necessary, both to prevent accidental contamination of the solutions and to provide particulate-free flushing material.

A plastic syringe, along with a variety of needles, is provided for the local anesthetic.

Sterile drapes and towels, gauze sponges, and a few basic surgical instruments such as mosquito clamp and scalpel with a No. 11 blade are readily available. A ring forceps and sterile glass medicine cups with alcohol and iodine solutions are provided for cleansing the patient's skin. A hollow bore needle with stylet is used for the arterial puncture (see Fig. 1-2).

Catheters for cerebral angiography come in an almost infinite variety of sizes, shapes, and materials (Fig. 1-3). Many angiographers prefer to make the majority of their own catheters themselves, utilizing soft, thin-walled small diameter (5 French) polyethylene tubing and tailor-making each to fit the particular case in question. Complex, curved, larger "head hunter" catheters preformed from stiffer, wire-braided material provide somewhat better torque control and may, on occasion, be required for successful catheterization of tortuous, ectatic brachiocephalic vessels. However, the small flexible catheters are preferred for most selective studies. If the stiffer catheters must be used, they are usually positioned in the proximal portion of the arch vessels.

The tip of each catheter is carefully tapered over the guidewire to be used during the procedure (Fig. 1-4A; the distal end is flared to accommodate a stopcock adapter (Fig. 1-4B, C). There are almost as many different catheter shapes and curves as there are angiographers. Personal preference and experience largely determine which of the highly variable catheter types are selected. One method is to form each catheter so it has three basic curves (Fig. 1-4D, E). The so-called tertiary curve is simply the one already in the catheter (there as a consequence of being coiled in its packaging). This curve lies easily inside the aortic arch. The first or primary curve is formed in a plane with the tertiary curve but in an opposite direction. This segment is at the end of the catheter and is shaped so that the tip will easily engage the brachiocephalic vessel origins. The secondary curve is immediately distal to the primary one and is formed to help keep the catheter tip pointed cephalad.

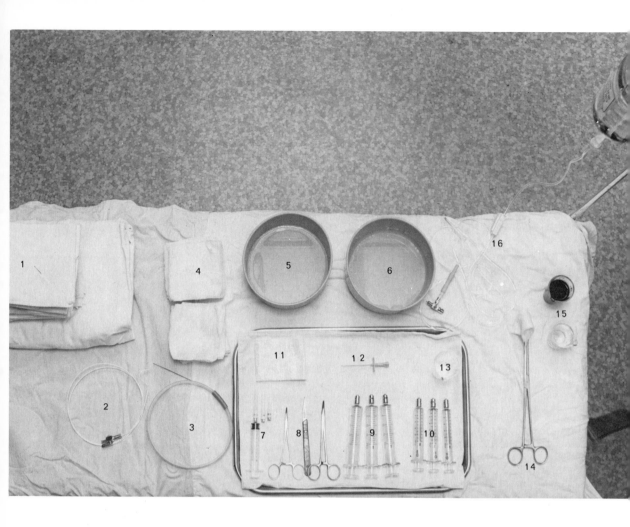

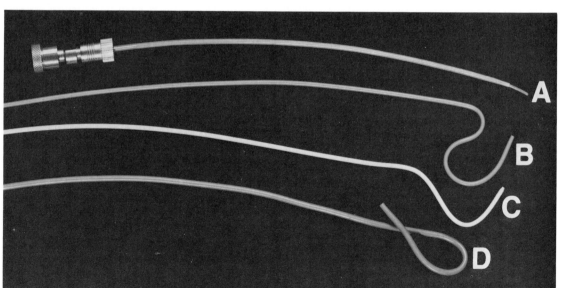

◀ **Fig. 1-2.** Standard angiographic tray. **1.** Sterile towels and drapes. **2.** Catheter. **3.** Guide wire in wire holder. **4.** 4″ × 4″ gauze sponges. **5.** Bowl with heparinized saline for guidewire storage during the procedure. **6.** Receptacle for discarded flushing solution. **7.** Plastic syringe and needles for local anesthetic. **8.** Scalpel and small clamps. **9.** 20 ml glass syringes. **10.** 10 ml glass syringes. **11.** Telfa sponge for wiping guidewire. **12.** 18 gauge Potts-Cournand needle. **13.** Glass medicine cup for contrast. **14.** Ring forceps. **15.** Iodine and alcohol prep. **16.** Heparinized saline with connecting tubing and three-way stopcock for rinsing syringes and flushing catheters.

◀ **Fig. 1-3.** A variety of catheters and cannulae for cerebral angiography. **A.** Davis cannula with interlocking obturator for direct carotid arteriography. **B.** Preformed 5F Mani cerebral catheter. **C.** 5F polyethylene cerebral catheter (As used in Fig. 1-4). **D.** High torque control wire wrapped catheter modified for transaxillary cerebral angiography.

Guidewires. Because of the wide variety of available guidewires the exact choice of guidewire type is largely a matter of personal preference. Guidewires not only permit percutaneous introduction of the catheter into the artery itself but are necessary for safe, accurate selective catheterization. Most modern guidewires are stainless steel with a stiff inner core (either fixed or movable) and an outer coil that may be Teflon- or heparin-coated. Internal safety wires are present to minimize wire breakage. The flexible distal tip is often tapered over a variable distance and may be straight or curved. Guidewires are also available in a variety of lengths, sizes, and degrees of stiffness.[72A] While most manufacturers recommend using the wire only once, many neuroradiologists reuse these wires repeatedly, discarding them only when they are bent or damaged.[52] A recent study has supported the safety of reusing guidewires.[59] Guidewires are reused at the University of Utah College of Medicine with a remarkably low rate of neuroangiographic complications.

Procedural Details

Once the preliminary films have been taken, fluoroscopy checked, and the patient's groin shaved and prepared, the actual procedure can begin. Since cerebral angiography is one of the few radiologic examinations in which simple errors can result in the death or permanent disability of an otherwise healthy patient, meticulous attention to detail is an absolute necessity. As a necessary precaution, the angiographer should slide the guidewire entirely through the arterial needle, dilator, and catheter. He should check for snug fit, making certain the wire is about 30 cm longer than the catheter (Fig. 1-5).

The safe, successful neuroangiographic procedure begins with adequate local anesthesia. This is a prerequisite both for patient comfort and for reduction of arterial spasm. If the patient is not allergic to lidocaine, a 1% solution without epinephrine for local anesthesia is used. The femoral artery (usually the right) is

(Text continued on p. 13)

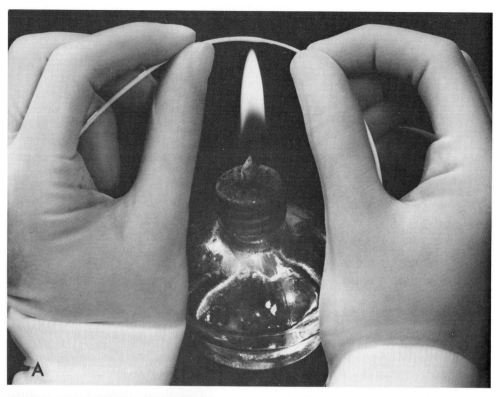

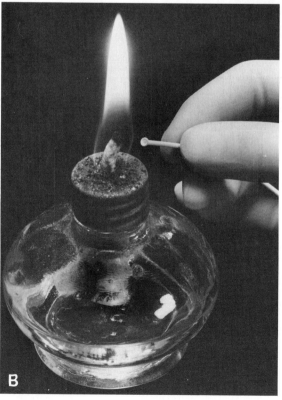

Fig. 1-4. Making a catheter. **A.** Thin-walled 5F polyethylene tubing is tapered over the guide-wire. **B.** The proximal end of the catheter is flared to accommodate a stopcock adapter. **C.** The stopcock adapter is attached. **D.** The distal end of the catheter is shaped over a forming wire. **E.** The catheter curve is fixed over steam; the tip is protected from the steam so it does not loose its taper.

(Fig. 1-4 continued on opposite page)

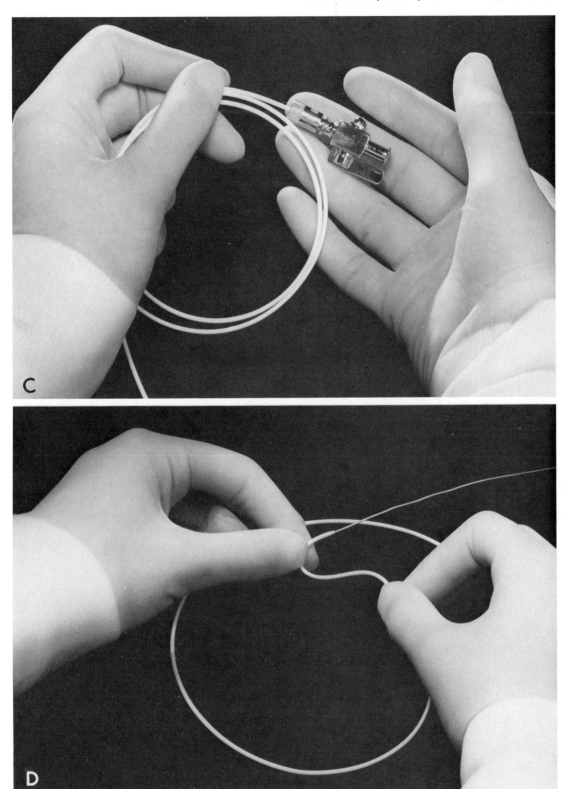

(Fig. 1-4 continued on p. 12)

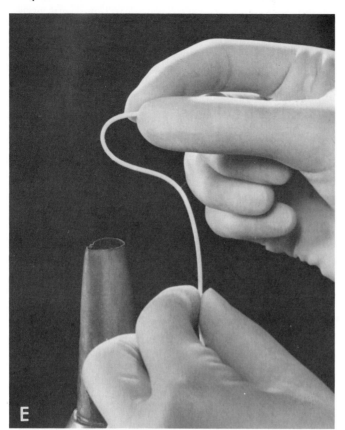

(Fig. 1-4 continued)

Fig. 1-5. Prior to beginning the procedure, the angiographer checks the catheter and guidewire for length and fit. Lead glasses may be worn to protect the cornea from scattered radiation.

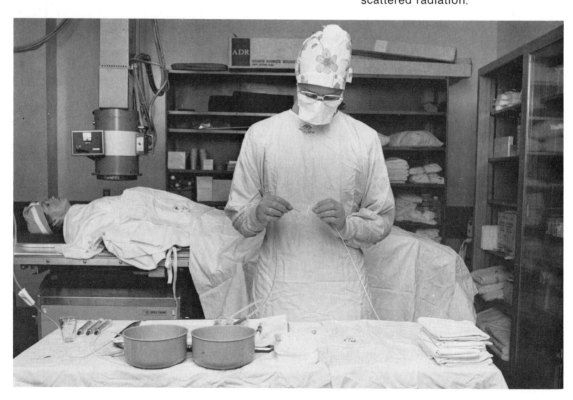

palpated and a skin wheal raised directly above the artery approximately 3 cm below the inguinal ligament (Fig. 1-6A). With satisfactory local anesthesia the patient will feel touch and pressure but should experience no discomfort.

Once the groin is adequately anesthetized and the appropriate catheters and guidewires have been made or selected the angiographer is ready to perform the arterial puncture itself.

Using a scalpel with a No. 11 blade held flat and parallel to the skin, the angiographer makes a small incision over the artery 3 cm distal to the inguinal ligament (Fig. 1-6B). Gently palpating the femoral pulse, he aligns the fingers of the left hand (or right, if a left femoral puncture is to be used) along the course of the artery just above the incision. The percutaneous needle is held between the index and third fingers of the right hand with the thumb resting delicately on the hub. At approximately a 45° angle to the skin, the angiographer gently and slowly advances the needle through the incision and subcutaneous tissue (Fig. 1-6C). When the needle tip is just above the femoral artery, a transmitted pulse is usually felt along the needle to the thumb. The needle is firmly advanced through the artery (Fig. 1-6D). If the needle is in or immediately adjacent to the femoral artery, the hub will usually swing slightly with the arterial pulsations. The stylet is removed and the needle slowly withdrawn. When the tip enters the arterial lumen cleanly, vigorous spurting of blood will occur and the guidewire can be introduced (Fig. 1-6E). If only a weak spurt or dribble is present, the needle is in either the femoral vein or the sidewall of the artery. The guidewire should not be introduced until satisfactory arterial flow is achieved.

If a single wall puncture is desired, a small syringe filled with heparinized saline can be attached to an 18-gauge thin-walled needle and advanced until the ventral wall of the artery is punctured. Blood will spurt back into the syringe. The needle is turned so the bevel faces dorsally, the syringe is removed, and the guidewire introduced.[52] A single wall puncture can also be performed without using an attached syringe. This results in less manipulation of the needle once it is within the vessel.

Once vigorous spurting of blood through the needle cannula is achieved, the guidewire is introduced into the artery through the needle (Fig. 1-6E). Under fluoroscopic control, the guidewire is advanced into the midabdominal aorta. The needle is removed over the wire by maintaining firm pressure on the femoral artery with the last three fingers of the left hand while holding the wire between the thumb and index finger. This maneuver prevents inadvertent removal of the wire from the artery. A wet Telfa sponge dipped in heparinized saline is used to wipe blood from the entire wire (Fig. 1-6F). If an arterial dilator is to be used, it is now passed over the wire and into the artery. The same procedure is used for removing the dilator as was described for the needle. (When pulling the tip for a polyethylene catheter, make a dilator out of the remaining end of the catheter tubing. This simple procedure provides a dilator that fits exactly over the guidewire and is the precise size of the catheter.)

The tip of the catheter is now placed over the wire and advanced to the puncture site (Fig. 1-6G). Enough guidewire should be pulled back through the catheter so that its end is protruding through the catheter's stopcock. With a definite rotary movement, the catheter is pushed into the artery. The end of the guidewire is firmly held and, under fluoroscopy, the catheter is advanced into the abdominal aorta while the wire is slowly withdrawn. The wire is then removed, wiped, coiled, and placed in its basin with the heparinized saline.

A glass syringe filled with a 5 to 10 ml heparinized flush solution is attached to the catheter stopcock and several milliliters of blood withdrawn (Fig. 1-6H). Carefully check for clots. If any are present, another few milliliters should be withdrawn using a second syringe. Another flush-filled syringe is attached to the catheter and, with the tip of the syringe pointed downward the plunger is gently withdrawn. Any air bubbles in the system should float out into the syringe. This is continued until a small amount of blood is

(Text continues on p. 18)

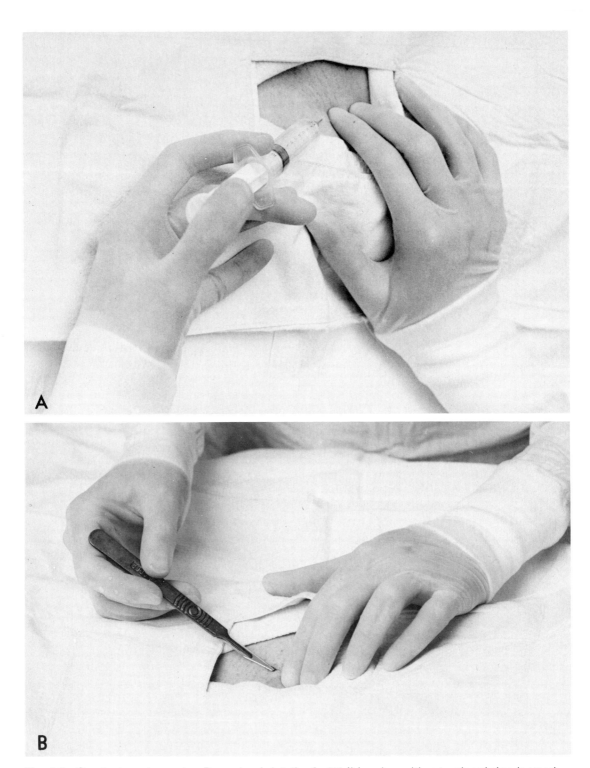

Fig. 1-6. Cerebral angiography: Procedural details. **A.** 1% lidocaine without epinephrine is used to infiltrate the skin and soft tissues around the femoral artery. **B.** The scalpel is held almost parallel to the skin and a 3 to 4 mm incision made about 3 cm below the inguinal ligament above the femoral artery. **C.** The first 2 or 3 fingers of the left hand gently palpate the femoral artery. The needle is slowly introduced through the skin and subcutaneous tissues at a 45° angle until the transmitted femoral pulsations are felt. (This may not be possible in an obese patient or a patient with a weak pulse.) **D.** The needle is advanced firmly through the femoral artery. Here the

(Fig. 1-6 continued on opposite page)

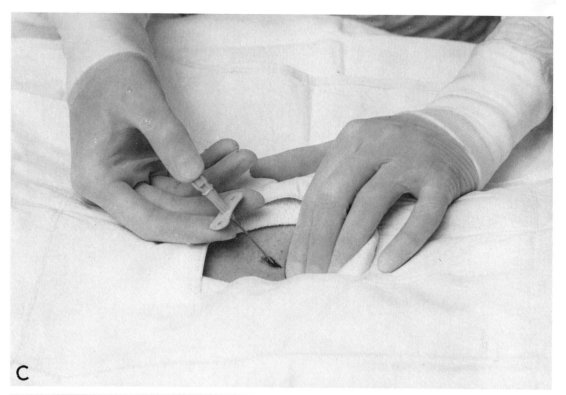

C

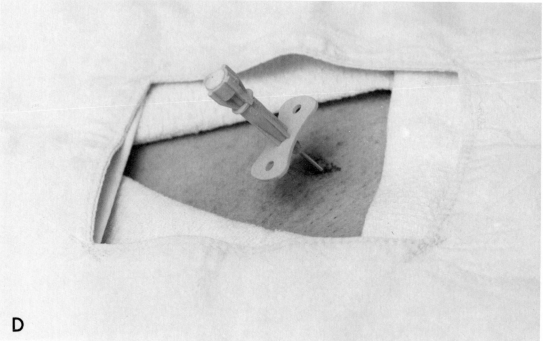

D

needle has pierced both walls of the artery and is embedded in the tissues beneath it. **E.** The stylet is removed and the needle slowly withdrawn until its tip pops into the femoral artery. If strong pulsatile blood flow is achieved, the guidewire can be introduced. **F.** A Telfa sponge dampened with heparinized saline is used to wipe the guidewire before the catheter is introduced. **G.** The catheter is introduced into the femoral artery by sliding it over the guidewire. **H.** The catheter is double flushed with heparinized saline after a small amount of blood has been withdrawn and discarded.

(Fig. 1-6 continued on p. 16)

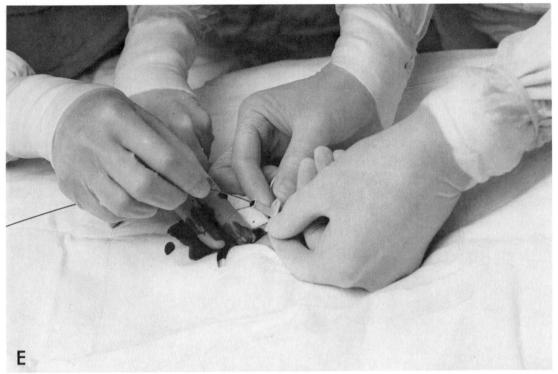

E

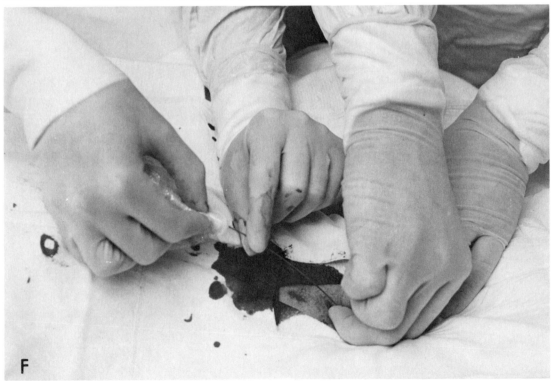

F

(Fig. 1-6 continued on opposite page)

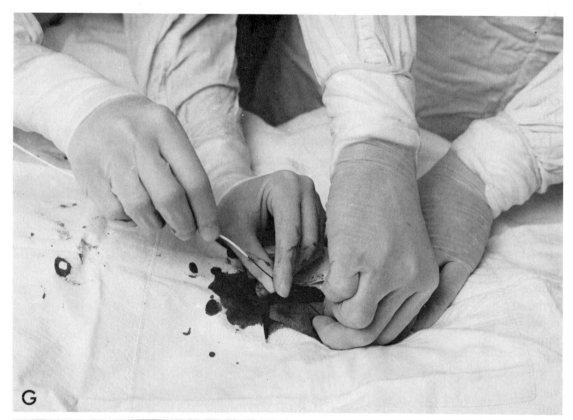

G

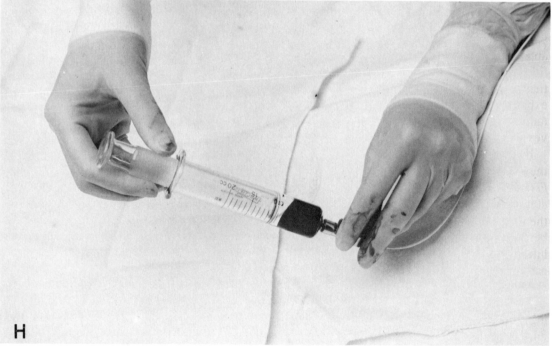

H

withdrawn, then 3 to 5 ml are flushed forward. The stopcock is turned off just before the flush is terminated. This leaves the catheter filled with heparinized solution. This is the so-called double flush technique and should be used meticulously throughout the procedure. The catheter is flushed approximately every 90 to 120 seconds during the angiogram.

Once the catheter has been inserted and properly flushed, one of the syringes is filled with contrast. (The syringes should not be filled with contrast until they are ready to be used. Prolonged waiting may allow contrast to crystallize along the barrel and "freeze" the syringe.) The syringe is attached to the catheter and the plunger withdrawn until all air in the system is removed and a small amount of blood is also withdrawn. With the nose of the syringe pointing downward, under fluoroscopy, a small amount of contrast is injected through the catheter to make certain it is within the aortic lumen.

Still under fluoroscopy, the catheter is advanced over the aortic arch and gently rotated until the tip of the primary curve points cranially. By advancing or withdrawing the catheter the brachiocephalic vessel orifices can be engaged. A small test injection following an appropriate double flush will confirm the location of the catheter tip. At this point, the patient should be reminded what sensations to expect: a feeling of warmth in the face, metallic taste, and so forth, depending on which vessel has been catheterized.

If the catheter tip is in the desired vessel, the guidewire is passed through it (*flexible tip first!*) and advanced into the artery. The catheter can then be advanced over the wire and the wire removed. Again, the catheter is double flushed. If no clots are present, a small test injection of contrast may be made to verify the catheter position.

Once the appropriate vessel is successfully catheterized, contrast is injected during a filming sequence. Hand injections of contrast produce relatively poor intravascular opacification, expose the angiographer to unnecessary radiation, and may be difficult to time properly. Therefore, most institutions use a me-

chanical pressure injector both to keep the rate and volume of contrast injection constant and to provide proper timing with modern rapid sequence film changers.

The injector barrel and connecting tubing should be checked to make certain all air bubbles are expelled.

As soon as the technician has positioned the patient, the catheter is flushed once more and, with the stopcock open, attached to the connecting tubing. The technician slowly backs up fluid from the tubing until the blood-fluid interface is clearly seen. If no air bubbles are present, 1 or 2 ml of contrast medium are flushed forward through the catheter. The injector syringe should be pointed down and arranged so that no kinks or curves are present in the catheter. The volume and rate of injection as well as injector delay are selected. (If biplane films are to be obtained a delay of about 0.2 seconds is usually necessary. This insures a non-contrast film that can be used later to make a subtraction mask.) Typical contrast volumes are 10 ml at 8 ml/second for common carotid injections, 8 ml at 7ml/second for internal carotid studies, and 6 or 7 ml at 5 or 6 ml/second for vertebral artery injections. The volumes and injection rates vary considerably with the size of the catheterized vessel as well as the intracranial flow and should be adjusted accordingly.

The mechanical volume stop on the injector is set, the patient's position quickly checked, all injector settings rechecked, and the catheter stopcock opened. The film programming sequencing and technique settings are quickly checked. The patient is reminded of the sensations and temporary discomfort he is likely to experience. His cooperation in remaining perfectly immobile during the run is again requested.

After the film sequence is completed, the stopcock is closed and the injector is disconnected. The patient's neurological status is quickly assessed. It is usually advisable to withdraw the catheter from the injected vessel and position it in a safe place in the thoracic aorta until the films are checked.

This procedure is repeated until all the requisite vessels have been examined. After the study is completed, the appropriate pulses are checked before and immediately after gently removing the catheter from the artery. Moderate manual pressure over the puncture site should be maintained for 10 to 20 minutes. (The meticulous angiographer holds the artery rather than delegating this task to a nurse or technician.) The local puncture site should be inspected for hematoma and the local and peripheral pulses rechecked. Whenever possible, a follow-up visit later in the day is advisable.

Precautions

A few precautions: Never allow the catheter or guidewire to pass beyond the vertebral artery origin or common carotid artery bifurcation until you have checked for stenoses or plaques with either fluoroscopy or spot films. Do not advance the catheter without the guidewire protruding slightly as this may result in subintimal wedging of the sharp, stiff catheter tip.

DIRECT PUNCTURE TECHNIQUES

With the advent of improved catheter techniques, visualization of the carotid and vertebral arteries by direct percutaneous puncture has diminished in importance. Nevertheless, this technique may be required in certain patients with severe, generalized occlusive vascular disease, extremely tortuous great vessels, or for some therapeutic embolization procedures.[9A]

The patient is placed in the supine position with the shoulders elevated and the neck hyperextended. The point of maximum carotid pulsation is determined and the skin anesthetized with 1% lidocaine (without epinephrine). Infiltration of the subcutaneous and deep tissues is carried down to and on either side of the common carotid artery. Immobilization of the artery with a 20-gauge needle may also be helpful.[24A]

A variety of needle-cannula systems and various stabilization devices have been de-

vised for direct percutaneous carotid puncture. These all employ a thin-walled cannula with a sharp, hollow interlocking stylet and blunt-tipped obturator. The cannula and stylet are introduced through the skin and gently advanced at an angle of 30 to 45° until the carotid pulsations are felt against the needle tip. The cannula is passed into the artery; if it has passed through both walls, the stylet is removed and the cannula slowly withdrawn until vigorous backwards spurts of blood are achieved. The cannula may then be advanced by threading it over a short flexible guidewire or blunt obturator. (Some cannulation sets include a soft polyethylene cannula and locking obturator that can be used in place of the stiff steel needle and do not require continuous irrigation; see Fig. 1-2). Flexible tubing is attached to the cannula and gentle but meticulous flushing of the system with heparinized saline is followed by a small test injection of contrast medium. Rapidly processed regular or Polaroid biplane films are quickly taken to check needle position. If the cannula is satisfactorily positioned and no spasm or intimal damage is present, routine films may then be obtained. Following the procedure, the needle is removed and firm (but not occlusive) pressure applied to the puncture site.[17]

Other direct puncture techniques (*i.e.,* retrograde brachial angiography or direct percutaneous vertebral angiography, are seldom used in most institutions (see below).

MISCELLANEOUS ANGIOGRAPHIC TECHNIQUES

Retrograde Brachial Angiography

Percutaneous catheter angiography has virtually replaced most direct-puncture techniques. However, retrograde injection of contrast medium into the brachial artery may provide a suitable alternative method. Its advantages are its relative safety and simplicity; its distinct drawbacks include the pain produced by the injection itself and local complications (*i.e.,* hematoma, median nerve damage, and vessel thrombosis).[17] The intracranial vasculature is also less than optimally visualized. (If a right retrograde study is performed, the carotid and vertebral arteries are both opacified simultaneously and are superimposed on the AP views.)

The technique resembles that used for direct carotid angiography. The brachial artery is cannulated in a similar manner and, if test injection demonstrates satisfactory intraluminal position of the cannula, a large bolus of contrast medium is injected (30–50 ml in approximately 2 seconds). Rapid sequence biplane films are obtained.

Transaxillary Catheter Angiography

In some instances, transfemoral arteriography may be neither safe nor technically feasible. Severe extracranial vascular disease, the presence of recent arterial grafts, or marked tortuosity of either the iliac or brachiocephalic vessels may preclude a successful transfemoral study. In patients who are not candidates for this approach, a transaxillary approach can often be used safely.

A 5 or 6 French polyethylene catheter is formed with a tight "figure-of-eight" distal curve and is introduced into the right axillary artery with the Seldinger technique (see Fig. 1-2). A 3-mm "J-shaped" guidewire is utilized to position the catheter in the ascending aorta. The curve is reformed and the catheter flushed with heparinized saline (see above). The catheter is withdrawn into the innominate artery and the tip rotated until it engages the orifice of the common carotid artery. Pulling back on the catheter slightly seats the distal curve firmly in the proximal common carotid artery (Fig. 1-7A-C).

The left common carotid and right vertebral arteries can also be successfully studied from an axillary approach. The catheter loop is reformed in the aortic arch and the tip rotated toward the orifice of the appropriate vessel. Again, gently pulling back on the catheter seats the distal curve securely in the artery. If more selective studies are desired, the catheter can often be advanced over the guidewire by utilizing vigorous rotation of the catheter to efface its primary curve.[32, 52]

Complications of axillary arteriotomies include thrombosis, hematoma formation, brachial plexus injury, and neurological deficit.[16] These are unusual and can be minimized by meticulous but rapid performance of the study, application of adequate pressure over the site of arteriotomy when the catheter is removed, and careful postangiographic observation. In most instances, permanent brachial nerve damage from an axillary hematoma can be prevented through early detection and appropriate surgical management.[48]

Angiotomography

Tomography during angiography is not used often. Linear tomography or autotomography may be used to obtain single or serial films during angiography. Multilayer cassettes have also been used with varying success.[32A, 49] These techniques have been a valuable adjunct in the evaluation of small posterior fossa lesions and can be helpful in some cases of aneurysms microangiomas, or pituitary tumor.[58, 61] Occasionally, angiotomography may demonstrate subtle vascular abnormalities that are obscured by more conventional or routine angiographic views.[56]

Stereoscopic Angiography

Stereoscopic angiography can be obtained with two x-ray tubes using short focal-film distance and a rapid film changer. Single tube stereoscopy has also been reported.[65] The utility of such studies has been limited by the advent of multiplanar computed tomography. However, stereoscopic angiography may be useful in delineating the pedicle of intracranial berry aneurysms and the three dimensional relationships of vessels comprising an arteriovenous malformation.

Cross-compression During Angiography

The "cross-circulation test" in carotid angiography is often helpful in evaluating extracerebral hematomas, sellar or suprasellar mass lesions, and intracranial aneurysms.[47] The noninjected carotid artery is temporarily

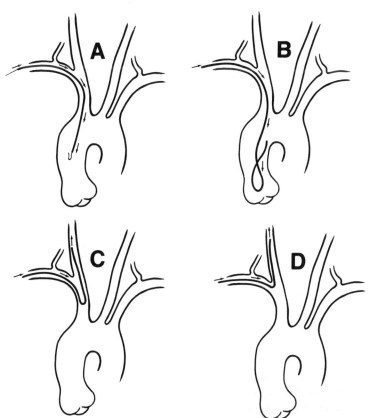

Fig. 1-7. Transaxillary catheter cerebral angiography. **A.** Following percutaneous puncture of the right axillary artery, the guidewire is introduced into the ascending aorta. The specially formed catheter is passed over the guidewire. **B.** The tight figure-of-eight catheter curve is reformed in the ascending aorta. **C.** The catheter is withdrawn into the innominate artery and its tip rotated so it enters the common carotid artery. **D.** Slight withdrawal of the catheter seats it firmly in the carotid artery.

compressed below its bifurcation during injection of contrast into the contralateral carotid artery. This permits contrast to fill the vessels in both hemispheres. Serial films are obtained (usually in the AP oblique or submentovertex projections) that allow minor asymmetries in vascular configuration to be readily assessed. Cross compression should be used with great caution in patients over the age of 60, since atheromatous disease in this age group is common.

COMPLICATIONS OF CEREBRAL ANGIOGRAPHY

General Considerations

Complications of cerebral angiography can be local (related to the puncture site), systemic (hypersensitivity or contrast reactions), or cerebral. A large series recently reported an 0.16% major complication rate (*i.e.,* death, permanent neurologic deficit or femoral thrombosis requiring surgery).[42] Complication rates increase with the elapsed time of the procedure, with inexperience of the angiographer, and, in at least one instance, with increased amount of contrast used.[40, 41] The highest complication rates are also apparently found in patients with occlusive cerebrovascular disease, subarachnoid hemorrhage, and postoperative or post-traumatic conditions.[41] A somewhat higher incidence of major complications has been reported in a large series using direct puncture carotid angiography.[46]

Local Complications

Peripheral complications include hematomas, vessel lacerations, intimal tears, perivascular or subintimal contrast injection, pseudoaneurysm formation, etc. Some authors have reported an 0.6% incidence of intimal tears and subintimal hematomas with femoral-cerebral catheter studies.[68] The vast majority of these problems has been eliminated by using small, soft catheters and highly flexible guidewires.

The reported incidence of hematoma at the site of arteriotomy varies from study to study; one recent report recorded a 25.3% incidence of carotid artery hematomas following direct puncture compared to 15.7% axillary or brachial and 10.7% femoral hematomas.[54] Most hematomas are small and do not require surgical decompression. However, the brachial plexus is particularly vulnerable to severe lasting damage from compression by an axillary hematoma. Permanent deficits as a complication of axillary arteriotomy can usually be prevented through early detection and prompt, proper surgical management.

Systemic Reactions

Fever, sepsis, or other generalized complications of angiography are rare. When performing angiography in infants, dehydration, overhydration, and acidosis are potential complications.[25] In children and adults, mild adverse effects vary from feeling temporary warmth or discomfort to nausea and vomiting. More serious complications range from mild reactions such as urticaria (2-3% of all cases) to bradycardia, laryngospasm, and seizures. Anaphylaxis and angioedema can result in death. The incidence of fatal reactions is about 1:10,000 to 20,000.[63]

The precise mechanism by which adverse contrast reactions occur is unknown. While some authors have suggested a direct-tissue chemotoxic effect, others believe that with the newer contrast agents chemotoxicity is probably a rare cause of complications and is likely to occur only with excessive dosage or specific predisposing conditions (i.e., dehydration, renal failure, or multiple myeloma).[5] Other variables considered include histamine release, activation of the serum complement and coagulation systems, antigen–antibody reactions, aggregation and clumping of blood components resulting in microemboli, and fear or anxiety states (vasovagal reactions).[5, 11C, 14, 34A, 37]

Some preliminary studies report cytogenetic damage both in vitro and in vivo in cells exposed to contrast media. Structural aberrations have included the inhibition of mitosis, induction of micronuclei, and chromosome aberrations.[2, 53] While the clinical implications of these studies are uncertain, it is apparent that at least some contrast agents are capable of inducing cytogenetic damage in tissues apart from any radiation effect.

Most mild adverse contrast reactions can be successfully treated with 25 to 50 mg of diphenhydramine (Benadryl) IM. (Intravenous [IV] administration may result in profound bradycardia and hypertension.) More serious reactions are treated with 0.2 to 0.3 mg of 0.01% epinephrine IV. Atrophine sulfate is the drug of choice in severe vagus nerve-mediated reactions, 0.4 mg IV is given in aliquots; a dose of up to 2 mg may be required in severe cases.[5, 11A]

Cerebral Complications

Contrast media do penetrate the blood-brain barrier as a function of contact time, anions, and dosage.[34A] Either new abnormal central nervous system (CNS) symptoms or the aggravation or exacerbation of previously existing ones are considered as angiograpic complications, regardless of etiology.[54] The majority of CNS complications are transient but fixed deficits following angiography do occur (approximately 1 in 1000 cases).[42] With the presence of persisting neurological deficits, some authors recommend treatment with pressor amines for 3-5 days and, occasionally, high dosage barbiturate therapy.[31] The therapeutic efficacy of this regimen is highly debatable. The incidence of serious complications seems to be less with careful femoral–cerebral catheter angiography than with direct puncture techniques.[46, 54, 68] Others have pointed out that because of improved catheter techniques, reduced procedure times, and careful, meticulous attention to detail, mortality and morbidity rates have continued to decline.[31]

SUPERSELECTIVE AND THERAPEUTIC ANGIOGRAPHY

Superselective angiographic examination of the smaller rami of both the extra- and intracranial vasculature is a relatively recent development. With the perfection of these techniques, catheter occlusion of a broad variety of vascular abnormalities became technically feasible.[50] As these procedures have become increasingly more common, the role of the neuroangiographer has been expanded into the therapeutic realm. Embolic arterial occlusion has been used to control epistaxis, shrink tumor masses, reduce the blood supply to vascular lesions prior to surgery, close arteriovenous fistulae or vascular malformations, and ablate aneurysms.

A wide variety of techniques and materials have been used in superselective angiography and transcatheter arterial occlusive procedures.[10, 11] A brief discussion of the general principles of these techniques is helpful for the modern neuroangiographer.

Superselective Angiography

Ordinary catheters and guidewires cannot normally be directed through the carotid siphon or into the most distal external carotid artery branches. Small, magnetically guided catheters and highly flexible silicone or polyethylene balloon-tipped, flow-directed catheters have been used successfully to visualize even sixth or seventh order arterial branches.[18, 21, 57, 57A, 62] These catheters are introduced either by direct carotid puncture or the Seldinger transfemoral technique. With the latter, a coaxial system is used. A larger, outer catheter is advanced selectively into the appropriate vessel and a small (1 or 2F) balloon catheter is then introduced through its external counterpart. Once past the orifice of the external catheter, the microcatheter is advanced by inflating and deflating the balloon tip with small amounts of contrast medium.[30A] A balloon catheter with a calibrated leak has recently been designed that allows contrast material or occluding agents to escape while the balloon remains intact.[27, 29]

It should be emphasized that these procedures are essentially still experimental and require a high degree of technical expertise. They should be undertaken in appropriate clinical cases, only with the proper equipment, and after considerable practice in the animal laboratory.[31A]

Indications for Therapeutic Angiography

Several factors must be considered in detail when assessing a patient for potential therapeutic embolization: (1) the nature of the primary disease process and whether short- or long-term occlusion is desired; (2) the patient's hematologic status (if clotting factor deficiency or fibrinolytic system activation is present, simple autologous clot should not be used for embolization); (3) which materials and techniques should be used (complete familiarity with the technical aspects of the procedure itself as well as the advantages and drawbacks of each agent is requisite); (4) which vessels are to be embolized as well as their size and configuration (in-depth knowledge of vascular anatomy is necessary, including which adjacent structures are supplied by the vessel to be embolized, actual and potential collateral flow patterns, etc.); (5) whether or not the lesion can be approached satisfactorily by any other less hazardous method. Since the use of some materials such as isobutyl 2-cyanoacrylate (IBC) is still considered experimental and carries the risk of significant complications, this procedure should be undertaken only if the lesion is surgically inaccessible.[29]

Technical Aspects of Therapeutic Neuroangiography

A variety of techniques and agents have been used for transcatheter embolization of vascular lesions.[10, 11] For acute processes (*i.e.*, posttraumatic hemorrhage, intractable epistaxis, or immediate preoperative embolization of vascular tumors), fresh autologous blood clot,

(Text continues on p. 26)

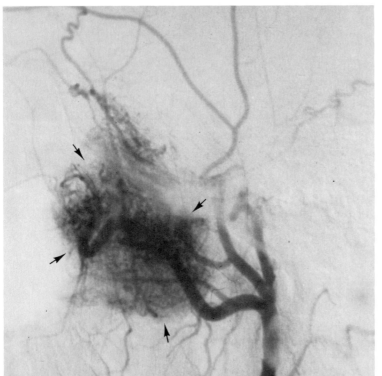

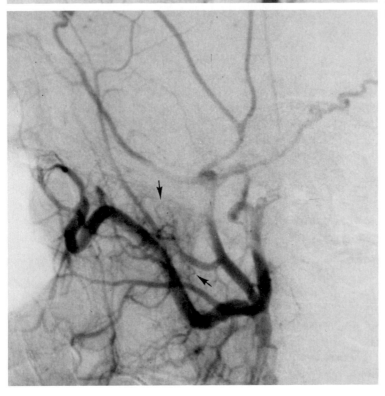

Fig. 1-8. Juvenile nasopharyngeal angiofibroma **(A)** before and **(B)** following preoperative embolization with gelatin sponge particles. Selective distal external carotid angiogram (midarterial phase, lateral view) shows marked reduction in blood supply to this highly vascular tumor.

A

B

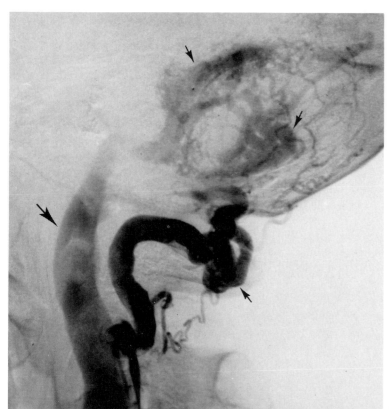

Fig. 1-9. Selective left vertebral angiogram (mid-arterial phase, lateral view) of a large dural arteriovenous malformation **(small arrows).** **(A)** Pre-embolization study shows rapid shunting through the malformation into the internal jugular vein **(large arrow). (B)** Following embolization with isobutyl 2-cyanoacrylate, the malformation has been almost completely obliterated.

A

B

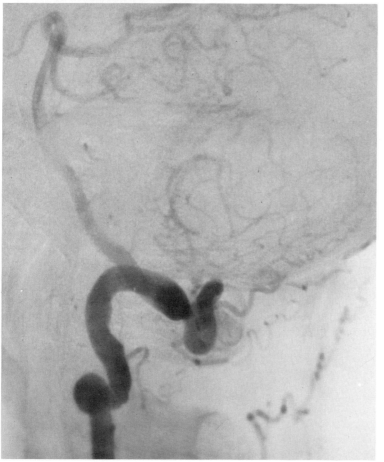

oxidized cellulose, or gelatin sponge particles have usually been the agents of choice (Fig. 1-8A, B).[7] Vessels embolized with these materials have a very high incidence of recanalization. Therefore, these agents are not suitable for lesions requiring permanent vascular occlusion.[8]

Long-term occlusions have been achieved with a broad spectrum of agents. Tissue adhesives such as IBC are initially liquid but polymerize almost immediately on contact with blood, forming a dense plug that extends into large- and medium-sized rami.[29] The advantages of IBC include rapid intra-arterial polymerization which diminishes the chance of its passage through large vascular shunts (Fig. 1-9A, B). A coaxial system with a nonionic solution in the delivery catheter must be used to avoid catheter occlusions and internal gluing of the system. The catheter tip should be lubricated with sterile silicone grease. IBC can be rendered radiopaque with powdered tantalum or iophendylate. The latter substance also permits some control of polymerization time.[15]

Low-viscosity silicone rubber (LVSR) is not a tissue adhesive. This agent produces organized arterial thrombi without associated inflammatory changes. The addition of variable amounts of a cross-linker such as tetra-ethyl-silicate permits the material to polymerize at different time intervals.[9B] Since vulcanization occurs in the capillary bed or interstices of lesions rather than within feeding vessels, LVSR may be the current agent of choice in many vascular malformations (Fig. 1-8A, B).[44] Because LVSR is more viscous than the acrylates, a special delivery system must be used when micro-catheters are employed.[45]

Permanent vascular occlusion has also been achieved with a variety of other materials (*i.e.*, silicone spheres, polyvinyl alcohol sponge, Gianturco–Wallace–Anderson stainless steel coils, wax microemboli, or small nylon bristle brushes).[3, 4, 13, 30, 38, 39, 59A, 64, 69] These agents are used primarily to produce thrombosis of larger vessels. A variety of inflatable and detachable silicone or latex balloons have also

been used for vascular occlusive procedures.[24, 33, 71] Transcatheter electrocoagulation has also been investigated recently as a potential technique for vessel occlusion.[10, 43, 66, 67] The ingenuity of many angiographers will undoubtedly result in continuous introduction of new, improved techniques and materials for therapeutic procedures.

Complications of Therapeutic Angiography

A variety of factors govern the course of emboli during therapeutic procedures.[74] Embolic material straying into unwanted sites may result in potentially disastrous CNS complications. The critical point in any therapeutic embolization occurs when the procedure is nearly complete. The sump effect of the lesion is dramatically reduced and runoff through the feeding vascular bed is sluggish. Introduction of too many additional particles too rapidly may cause reflux into arteries supplying normal structures. If silicone spheres or particulate emboli are to be used, they can be suspended in contrast medium to permit direct monitoring of vessel runoff and progression of the occlusion.[28] Other materials may be mixed with a radiopaque marker such as tantalum powder. Embolic reflux has also been prevented by using balloon catheters to occlude the orifice of the target vessel.[23]

Polymerized acrylics have a high degree of local tissue toxicity. In the experimental animal they provoke significant chronic foreign body-type inflammatory changes with severe intimal disruption in the occluded vessels although initial clinical studies have demonstrated only a mild giant cell foreign body reaction in humans.[20, 44] There is also a potential carcinogenic effect of acrylics, although it is as yet undocumented in humans.[72] In the abdomen, embolization with the tissue adhesive IBC has resulted in sterile biliary cysts, hepatic infarcts, and gastric ulcers. The extensive vascular plugs formed by such materials (particularly if they are too forcefully injected) can preclude the development of collateral blood flow and result in a high rate of ischemic

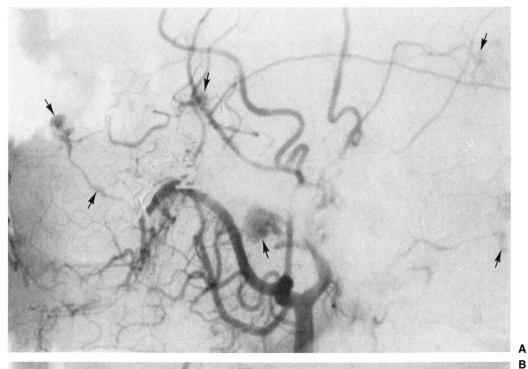

A
B

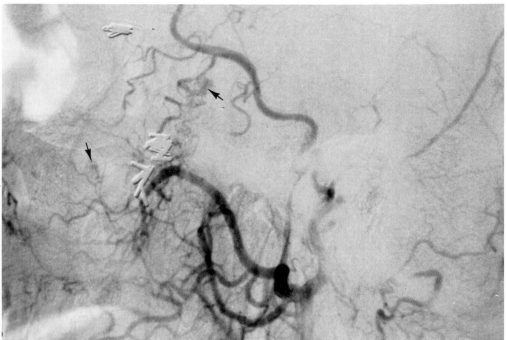

Fig. 1-10. Selective left external carotid angiogram (mid-arterial phase, lateral view) of Osler-Weber-Rendu disease and recurrent severe epistaxis despite multiple ligation of the maxillary and ethmoidal arteries. **(A)** Pre-embolization study disclosed numerous small capillary telangiectasies **(arrows). (B)** After embolization with low viscosity silicone rubber, most of the vascular niduses have been obliterated. Only two small lesions **(arrows)** remain.

complications.[72] The extremely rapid intravascular polymerization of acrylics has also resulted in inadvertent gluing of the catheter within the embolized vessel.

LVSR produces permanent vascular occlusions without inciting significant inflammatory reaction. However, this agent can vulcanize in small end arteries, producing adjacent tissue ischemia and necrosis.[12, 44] Improper control of the polymerization can also result in passage of the material through arteriovenous shunts, resulting in pulmonary embolus.

Polyvinyl alcohol sponge, stainless steel coils, or nylon bristle brushes all produce permanent vascular occlusions. Varying degrees of inflammatory reaction in the walls of the embolized vessels have been reported with all these agents although long-term tissue damage is apparently less than with the acrylics.[13, 22, 72]

Recanalization of vessels occluded with fresh autologous blood clot or gelatin sponge particles occurs in a significant percentage of cases. Fibrinogen degradation products are elevated in patients embolized with these materials. Although no consistent bleeding diathesis has been attributed to this abnormality, one episode of disseminated intravascular coagulation following therapeutic gelatin sponge particulate embolization has been reported.[6]

There is a risk of deflation when using the inflatable, releasable balloons for embolization. Subsequent distal migration, balloon leak or rupture with subsequent spillage of the inflating material, or failure of the balloon to detach properly can also occur.[24] Progressive osmotic balloon enlargement can also take place when undiluted contrast is used as the inflating material. In addition to producing a decrease in opacity, balloon rupture occurs if osmotic growth exceeds the maximum inflatable volume. Recently, balloons have been successfully inflated with isosmolar metrizamide and these problems circumvented.[9]

REFERENCES

1. **Abrams HL:** Angiographic agents: Clinical application. In Miller RE, Skucas J (eds): Radiographic Contrast Agents, pp 337–363. Baltimore, University Park Press, 1977
2. **Adams FH, Norman A, Renata S et al:** Effect of radiation and contrast media on chromosomes. Radiology 124:823–826, 1977
3. **Anderson JH, Wallace S, Gianturco C:** Transcatheter intravascular coil occlusion of experimental arteriovenous fistulas. Am J Roentgenol 129:795–798, 1977
4. **Anderson JH, Wallace S, Gianturco C et al:** "Mini" Gianturco stainless steel coils for transcatheter vascular occlusion. Radiology 132:301–303, 1979
5. **Andews EJ Jr:** The vagus reaction as a possible cause of severe complications of radiological procedures. Radiology 121:1–4, 1976
6. **Ansell JE, Widrich WC, Johnson WC et al:** Gelfoam and autologous clot embolization: effect on coagulation. Invest Radiol 13:115–120, 1978
7. **Bank WO, Kerber CW:** Gelfoam embolization: a simplified technique. Am J Roentgenol 132:299–301, 1979
8. **Barth KH, Strandberg JD, White RI Jr:** Long term follow-up of transcatheter embolization with autologous clot, Oxycel, and Gelfoam in domestic swine. Invest Radiol 12:273–280, 1977
9. **Barth KH, White RI Jr, Kaufman SL et al:** Metrizamide, the ideal radiopaque filling material for detachable silicone balloon embolization. Invest Radiol 14:35–40, 1979
9A. **Bauer J, Salazar JL, Sugar O et al:** Direct percutaneous cerebral angiography in neurosurgical practice. J Neurosurg 52:525–528, 1980
9B. **Berenstein A:** Flow-controlled silicone fluid embolization. Am J Neuroradiol 1:161–166, 1980
10. **Berenstein A, Kricheff II:** Catheter and material selection for transarterial embolization: technical considerations. I. Catheters. Radiology 132:619–630, 1979
11. **Berenstein A, Kricheff II:** Catheter and material selection for transarterial embolization: technical considerations. II. Materials. Radiology 132:631–639, 1979
11A. **Brody WR, Enzmann D et al:** IV carotid arteriography using scanned projection radiography. Presented at the Association of University Radiologists, 28th annual meeting, Tucson, Arizona, March 25–28, 1980
11B. **Brash, RC:** Allergic reactions to contrast media: Accumulated evidence. Am J Roentgenol 134:797–801, 1980

11C. **Bush, WH Jr, Mullarkey MF, Webb DR:** Adverse reactions to radiographic contrast material. West J Med 132:95–98, 1980

12. **Calcaterra TC, Riard RW, Bentson JR:** Ischemic paralysis of the facial nerve: a possible etiologic factor in Bell's palsy. Laryngoscope 86:92–97, 1976

13. **Castaneda-Zuniga, Sanchez R, Amplatz K:** Experimental observations on short and long-term effects of arterial occlusion with Ivalon. Radiology 126:783–785, 1978

14. **Cho KJ, Thornbury JR:** Severe reactions to contrast material by three consecutive routes: intravenous, subcutaneous and intra-arterial. Am J Roentgenol 131:509–510, 1978

14A. **Cristenson PC, Ovitt TW et al:** IV cervicocerebrovascular angiography utilizing a digital video subtraction system. Presented at the American Society of Neuroradiologists, 18th annual meeting, Los Angeles, California, March 16–21, 1980

15. **Cromwell LD, Kerber CW:** Modification of cyanoacrylate for therapeutic embolization: preliminary experience. Am J Roentgenol 132:799–801, 1979

16. **Davis KR, Poletti CE, Robersen GH et al:** Complementary role of computed tomography and other neuroradiologic procedures. Surg Neurol 8:437–447, 1977

17. **Deck MDF:** Direct puncture techniques for cerebral angiography. In Newton TH, Potts DG (eds): Radiology of the Skull and Brain, Vol 2, pp 908–919. St. Louis, CV Mosby, 1974

18. **Djindjian R:** Superselective internal carotid arteriography and embolization. Neuroradiology 9:145–156, 1975

19. **Fischer HW:** Contrast media. In Newton TH, Potts DG (ed): Radiology of the Skull and Brain, Vol 2, pp 893–907. St. Louis, CV Mosby, 1974

20. **Freeny PC, Mennemeyer R, Kidd CR et al:** Long-term radiographic-pathologic follow-up of patients treated with visceral transcatheter occlusion using isobutyl 2-cyanoacrylate (Bucrylate). Radiology 132:51–60, 1979

21. **Gacs G:** Catheterization and superselective angiography of the cerebral vessels. Neuroradiology 12:237–241, 1977

22. **Gomes AS, Rysavy JA, Spadaccini CA et al:** The use of the bristle brush for transcatheter embolization. Radiology 129:345–350, 1978

23. **Greenfield AJ, Athanasoulis CA, Waltman AC et al:** Transcatheter embolization: prevention of embolic reflex using balloon catheters. Am J Roentgenol 131:651–655, 1978

24. **Guillaume J, Roulleau J:** Experimental embolization with inflatable and releasable balloons in dogs. Neuroradiology 14:85–88, 1977

24A. **Guinto FC Jr:** Needle immobilization of a carotid puncture site. Am J Roentgenol 134:403, 1980

25. **Harwood-Nash DC, Fitz CR:** Neuroradiology in Infants and Children, p 340. St. Louis, CV Mosby, 1976

26. **Huckman MS, Shenk GI, Neems RL et al:** Transfemoral cerebral arteriography versus direct percutaneous carotid and brachial arteriography: a comparison of complication rates. Radiology 132:93–97, 1979

26A. **Ingstrup HM, Anderson A:** Clinical testing of Conray meglumine and Amipaque in cerebral angiography. Neuroradiology 18:235–238, 1979

27. **Kerber CW:** Balloon catheter with a calibrated leak. Radiology 120:547–550, 1976

28. **Kerber CW:** Catheter therapy: fluoroscopic monitoring of deliberate embolic occlusion. Radiology 125:538–540, 1977

29. **Kerber CW, Bank WO, Cromwell LD:** Calibrated leak balloon microcatheter: a device for arterial exploration and occlusive therapy. Am J Roentgenol 132:207–212, 1979

30. **Kerber CW, Bank WO, Horton JA:** Polyvinyl alcohol foam: prepackaged emboli for therapeutic embolization. Am J Roentgenol 130:1193–1194, 1978

30A. **Kerber CW, Bank WO, Manelse C:** Control and placement of intracranial microcatheters. Am J Neuroradiol 1:157–159, 1980

31. **Kerber CW, Cromwell LD, Drayer BP et al:** Cerebral ischemia. I. Current angiographic techniques, complications, and safety. Am J Roentgenol 130:1097–1103, 1978

31A. **Kerber CW, Flaherty LW:** A teaching and research simulator for therapeutic embolization. Am J Neuroradiol 1:167–169, 1980

32. **Kerber CW, Mani RL, Bank WO et al:** Selective cerebral angiography through the axillary artery. Neuroradiology 10:131–135, 1975

32A. **Kobayashi M, Masuzawa H, Wakamatu O:** A new method of simultaneous multisectioned tomography with cerebral angiography. Radiology 135:225–227, 1980

33. **Laitinen L, Servo A:** Embolization of cerebral vessels with inflatable and detachable balloons. J Neurosurg 48:307–308, 1978

34. **Lang EK:** Clinical evaluation of side effects of radiopaque contrast media administered via intravenous and intra-arterial routes in the same patient. Radiology 85:666–669, 1965

34A. **Lalli AF:** Contrast media reactions: Data analysis and hypothesis. Radiology 134:1–12, 1980

35. **Larson EB, Omenn GS, Loop JW:** Computed tomography in patients with cerebravascular disease: impact of a new technology in patient care. Am J Roentgenol 131:39–40, 1978

36. **Larson EB, Omenn GS, Margolis MT et al:** Impact of computed tomography on utilization of cerebral angiograms. Am J Roentgenol 129:1–3, 1977

37. **Lasser EC, Slivka J, Lang JH et al:** Complement and coagulation: causative nonsiderations in contrast catastrophies. Am J Roentgenol 132:171–176, 1979

38. **Latchaw RE, Gold LHA:** Polyvinyl foam embolization of vascular and neoplastic lesions of the head, neck, and spine. Radiology 131:669–679, 1979

39. **Layne TA, Finck EJ, Boswell WD:** Transcatheter occlusion of the arterial supply to arteriovenous fistulas with Gianturco coils. Am J Roentgenol 131:1027–1030, 1978

40. **Mani RL, Eisenberg RL:** Complications of catheter cerebral arteriography: analysis of 5,000 procedures. II. Relation of complication rates to clinical and arteriographic diagnosis. Am J Roentgenol 131:867–86, 1978

41. **Mani RL, Eisenberg RL:** Complications of catheter cerebral arteriography. Analysis of 4,000 procedures. III. Assessment of arteries injected, contrast medium used, duration of procedure and age of patient. Am J Roentgenol 131:871–874, 1978

42. **Mani RL, Eisenberg RL, McDonald EJ Jr et al:** Complications of catheter cerebral angiography: analysis of 5,000 procedures. I. Criteria and incidence. Am J Roentgenol 131:861–865, 1978

43. **McAlister DS, Johnsrude I, Miller MM et al:** Occlusion of acquired renal arteriovenous fistula with transcatheter electrocoagulation. Am J Roentgenol 132:998–1000, 1979

44. **Miller FJ Jr, Rankin RS, Gliedman JB:** Experimental internal iliac artery embolization: evaluation of low viscosity silicone rubber, isobutyl 2-cyanoacrylate, and carbon microspheres. Radiology 129:51–58, 1978

44A. **Miller JH, Peña AM, Segall HD:** Radiological investigation of sellar region masses in children. Radiol 134:81–87, 1980

45. **Miller FJ Jr, Nakashima EN, Mineau DE, Osborn AG:** Delivery systems for low viscosity silicone rubber through small co-axial catheters. Radiology 131:538, 1979

46. **Miller JDR, Grace MG, Russel DR et al:** Complications of cerebral angiography and pneumography. Radiology 124:741–744, 1977

47. **Moller A, Ericson K:** Some aspects of contralateral compression in carotid angiography. Radiology 125:725–729, 1977

48. **Molnar W, Paul DJ:** Complications of axillary arteriotomies. Radiology 104:269–276, 1972

49. **Morris JL, Wylie I:** Cerebral angiotomography. Radiology 120:105–109, 1976

50. **Moseley I:** Therapeutic embolization of the carotid arteries: a review. Head Neck Surg 1:519–532, 1979

51. **Naidich TP, Solomon S, Leeds NE:** Computerized tomography in neurological evaluations. JAMA 240:565–568, 1978

52. **Newton TH, Kerber CW:** Techniques of catheter cerebral angiography. In Newton TH, Potts DG (eds): Radiology of the Skull and Brain, Vol 2, pp 920–938. St. Louis, CV Mosby, 1974

53. **Norman A, Adams FH, Rile RF:** Cytogenetic effects of contrast media and triiodobenzoic acid derivatives in human lymphocytes. Radiology 129:199–203, 1978

54. **Olivecrona H:** Complications of cerebral angiography. Neuroradiology 14:175–181, 1977

55. **Osborn AG:** Cranial computed tomography in neurological diagnosis. Annu Rev Med 30:189–198, 1979

56. **Osborn AG, Pode GJ:** Angiographic signs of corpus callisal tumors: a reappraisal. Radiology 115:97–102, 1975

57. **Pevsner PH:** Micro-balloon catheter for superselective angiography and therapeutic occlusion. Am J Roentgenol 128:225–230, 1977

57A. **Pevsner PH, Doppman JL:** Therapeutic embolization with a microballoon catheter system. Am J Neuroradiol 1:171–180, 1980

58. **Poole GJ, Potts DG, Newton TH:** Angiotomography. In Newton TH, Potts DG (eds): Radiology of the Skull and Brain, Vol 2, pp 981–1001. St. Louis, CV Mosby, 1974

59. **Ravin CE, Koehler PR:** Reuse of disposable catheters and guide wires. Radiology 122:577–579, 1977

59A. **Raziel A, Puisieux F, Terracol D et al:** Wax microemboli tailored for therapeutic embolization. Am J Roentgenol 134:404–405, 1980

59B. **Richmond IL, Newton TH, Wilson CB:** Indications for angiography in the preoperative evaluation of patients with prolactin-secreting pituitary adenomas. J Neurosurg 52:378–380, 1980

60. **Sandor T, Adams DF:** Minimum blood vessel diameter measured by magnification angiography. Am J Roentgenol 132:433–436, 1979

61. **Sartor K, Nadjimi M:** Angiotomography for aneurysms and arterioyenous malformations of the head and neck. Neuroradiology 18:89–100, 1979

62. **Serbinenko FA:** Balloon catheterization and occlusion of major cerebral vessels. J Neurosurg 41:125–145, 1974

63. **Shehadi WH:** Adverse reactions to intravascularly administered contrast media: a comprehensive study based on a prospective survey. Am J Roentgenol 124:145–152, 1975

63A. **Strother CM, Sackett JF et al:** IV angiography of the carotid artery using computerized fluoroscopy. Presented at the American Society of Neuroradiologists, 18th annual meeting, Los Angeles, California, March 16–21, 1980

64. **Tadavarthy SM, Moller JH, Amplatz K:** Polyvinyl alcohol (Ivalon): a new embolic material. Am J Roentgenol 125:609–616, 1975

65. **Takahashi M, Tamakawa Y, Goto K et al:** Serial cerebral angiography in stereoscopic magnification. Am J Roentgenol 126:1211–1218, 1976

66. **Thompson WM, Johnsrude IS, Jackson DC et al:** Vessel occlusion with transcatheter electrocoagulation: initial clinical experience. Radiology 133:335–340, 1979

67. **Thompson WM, Mcalister DS, Miller M et al:** Transcatheter electrocoagulation: experimental evaluation of the anode. Invest Radiol 14:41–47, 1979

68. **Vitek JJ, Powell DF, Anderson RD:** Damage of the brachiocephalic vessels due to catheterization. Neuroradiology 9:63–67, 1975

69. **Wallace S, Gianturco C, Anderson JH et al:** Therapeutic vascular occlusion utilizing steel coil technique: clinical applications. Am J Roentgenol 127:381–387, 1976

70. **Westcott JL, Taylor PT:** Transaxillary selective four-vessel arteriography. Radiology 104:277–281, 1977

71. **White RI Jr, Kaufman SL, Barth KH et al:** Embolotherapy with detachable silicone balloons. Radiology 131:619–627, 1979

72. **White RI Jr, Strandberg JV, Gross GS et al:** Therapeutic embolization with long-term occluding agents and their effects on embolized tissues. Radiology 125:667–687, 1977

72A. **Willson JKV:** A new technique for cerebral angiography: The variable stiffness guidewire. Radiology 134:427–430, 1980

73. **Wilmink JT, Van der Berg W, Kramer HJ et al:** Comparative evaluation of metrizamide and meglumine ioxithalamate in angiography of the vessels of the head and neck. Neuroradiology 15:267–272, 1978

74. **Wolpert SM, Stein BM:** Factors governing the course of emboli in the therapeutic embolization of cerebral arteriovenous malformations. Radiology 131:125–131, 1979

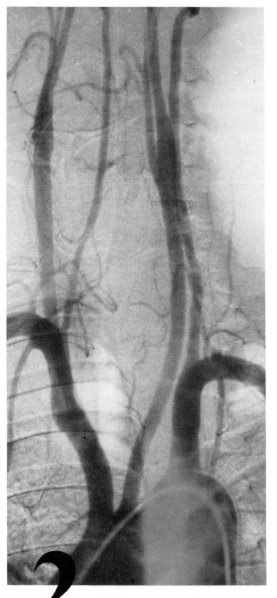

2 *The Aortic Arch and its Branches*

A thorough understanding of the normal aortic arch and its major branches as well as their common anatomic variants is necessary for safe, successful transfemoral catheterization of the cerebral vessels. In addition, a variety of disease processes primarily affecting the aortic arch may produce significant intracranial symptomatology. Therefore, a consideration of neuroangiographic anatomy begins with the aortic arch.

NORMAL GROSS AND ANGIOGRAPHIC ANATOMY OF THE AORTIC ARCH

Gross Anatomy

The normal aortic arch lies in the superior mediastinum and gradually courses from right to left in front of the trachea. The aorta curves posteroinferiorly above the left mainstem bronchus, descending to the left of the trachea and esophagus.

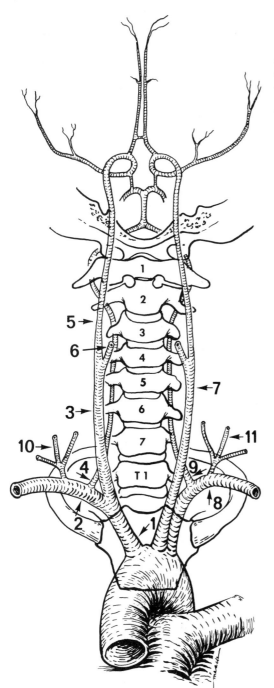

Fig. 2-1. Diagrammatic sketch of the aortic arch and its major branches (anteroposterior view). **1.** Innominate artery (brachiocephalic trunk). **2.** Right subclavian artery. **3.** Right common carotid artery. **4.** Right vertebral artery. **5.** Right internal carotid artery. **6.** Right external carotid artery. **7.** Left common carotid artery. **8.** Left subclavian artery. **9.** Left vertebral artery. **10.** Right thyrocervical trunk. **11.** Left thyrocervical trunk.

The first branch arising from the aortic arch is normally the innominate artery, which is also termed the brachiocephalic trunk (Figs. 2-1 and 2-2, arrow 1). Shortly after its origin, the innominate artery divides into its two major branches—the right subclavian artery (arrow 2) and right common carotid artery (arrow 3). The right vertebral artery (arrow 4) arises from the right subclavian artery, then courses posteromedially and enters the foramen transversarium of C6. (In 5 percent of all cases, the vertebral artery enters the foramen transversarium at other cervical levels.)

The second major branch of the brachiocephalic trunk is the right common carotid artery, which bifurcates into the internal (arrow 5), and external (arrow 6) carotid arteries at the mid-cervical level (about C3 or C4). However, the common carotid bifurcation may be as high as C1 or occasionally as low as T2.

A small, inconstant branch, the arteria thyroidea ima, arises from the aorta or proximal brachiocephalic trunk and supplies the inferior part of the thyroid gland. Unless the other thyroid vessels are congenitally deficient or the thyroidea ima becomes enlarged as a source of collateral blood flow, it is rarely seen on aortic arch angiograms (Fig. 2-15).

The second major branch of the aortic arch is the left common carotid artery. In approximately 75 percent of all cases the left common carotid artery (arrow 7) arises slightly to the left of the innominate artery. The bifurcation of the left common carotid artery is also usually at the C3 or C4 level although it too may be as high as C1 or as low as T2.

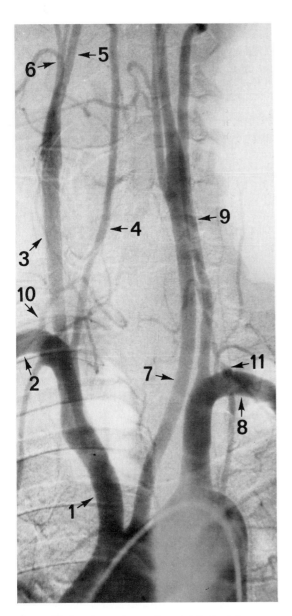

Fig. 2-2. Aortic arch angiogram (arterial phase, right posterior oblique view). **1.** Innominate artery (brachiocephalic trunk). **2.** Right subclavian artery. **3.** Right common carotid artery. **4.** Right vertebral artery. **5.** Right internal carotid artery. **6.** Right external carotid artery. **7.** Left common carotid artery. **8.** Left subclavian artery. **9.** Left vertebral artery. **10.** Right thyrocervical trunk. **11.** Left thyrocervical trunk.

The last branch to arise from the aortic arch is the left subclavian artery (arrow 8). The first branch of this vessel is the left vertebral artery (arrow 9), which usually originates near the superior portion of the left subclavian artery and enters the foramen transversarium of C6. Occasionally the vertebral artery may arise from the proximal subclavian trunk (Fig. 2-11). In 75 percent of all cases the left vertebral artery is the same size as or larger than the right vertebral artery. This anatomic fact is of importance in performing selective vertebral angiography for posterior fossa studies. In 75 percent of all cases, catheterization of the left vertebral artery is satisfactory since this vessel is either dominant or at least equal in size to the right vertebral artery.

The right (arrow 10) and left (arrow 11) thyrocervical trunks arise from their respective subclavian arteries distal to the vertebral artery origin.

Radiographic Anatomy

On anteroposterior angiograms, extensive overlapping of the aorta and its branches is evident. When a patient is placed in either the right (Fig. 2-3A) or left (Fig. 2-3B) posterior oblique position, a profile of the ascending aorta and its great vessels is seen. Some overlap of the arch vessels is often seen in a single oblique view; hence, a small lesion at the origin of the obscured vessel could be overlooked. Both right and left posterior oblique views are often necessary to delineate the course and origin of each of the aortic arch branches clearly.

AORTIC ARCH ANOMALIES

True Anomalies of the Aortic Arch

The most common true anomaly of the arch vessels is an aberrant right subclavian artery (Fig. 2-4, black arrows), which occurs in about 0.5 to 1.0 percent of all cases.[8] When present, the aberrant right subclavian artery is the last instead of the first brachiocephalic vessel to arise from the aortic arch. The aberrant artery

(Text continues on p. 37)

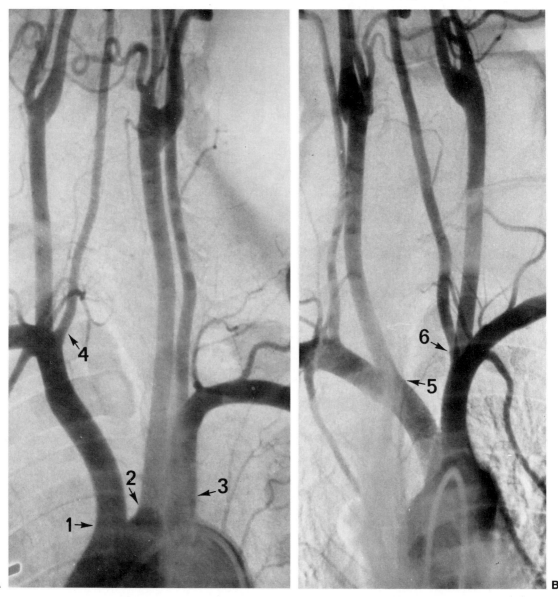

Fig. 2-3. Aortic arch angiogram (arterial phase). **A.** Right posterior oblique view (RPO). **B.** Left posterior oblique view (LPO). In the RPO view, the origins of the innominate **(arrow 1),** left common carotid **(arrow 2),** left subclavian **(arrow 3)** and right vertebral **(arrow 4)** arteries are clearly seen. The origins of the right common carotid and left vertebral arteries are obscured because the arch vessels overlap.

On the LPO view, the origins of the right common carotid **(arrow 5)** and left vertebral **(arrow 6)** arteries are clearly visible.

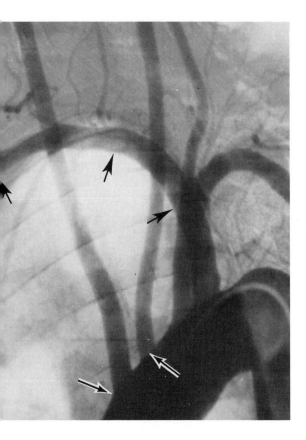

Fig. 2-4. Aortic arch angiogram (arterial phase, right posterior oblique view). This illustrates an aberrant right subclavian artery **(black arrows).** Both common carotid arteries arise as separate branches **(outlined arrows)** from the aortic arch.

Normal Variants

Although not technically a true anomaly, the left common carotid and innominate arteries frequently arise from the aortic arch together forming a "V" (Fig. 2-8, arrow). The left common carotid artery originates directly from the innominate artery in approximately 10 percent of all cases (Fig. 2-9). In rare cases, both carotid arteries may arise from a common trunk or separately from the aortic arch.[3]

The right vertebral artery is normally the first branch of the right subclavian artery. Occasionally it may arise:

1. from either the right common or internal carotid artery,
2. directly from the aortic arch itself, or
3. from the right subclavian artery distal to the thyrocervical trunk (Fig. 2-10, white arrow).[14]

The right vertebral artery is larger than the left in approximately 25 percent of all cases.

The left vertebral artery originates directly from the aortic arch in 5 percent of all cases (Fig. 2-10, outlined arrow). On occasion, the vertebral origin may be very low on the subclavian artery instead of near its apex (Fig. 2-11). The vertebral artery may also share a common origin with other anomalous vessels.[15A]

These various anomalies of the aortic arch may make transfemoral catheterization of the cerebral vessels more difficult. When the preangiogram chest film suggests a possible anomaly, an initial aortic arch study may be helpful in facilitating successful selective angiography.

courses superolaterally from left to right, passing behind the esophagus. Both the right and left common carotid arteries usually arise from the aortic arch as separate branches (Fig. 2-4, outlined arrows). Rarely the subclavian artery may arise as the first branch of the aortic arch. In these cases, the innominate artery is absent and the carotid arteries share a common trunk.[2]

A right aortic arch with mirror image branching of the arch vessels (Fig. 2-5) is a less common anomaly and is usually associated with cyanotic congenital heart disease (*e.g.*, Tetralogy of Fallot), unless situs inversus is present. In this instance, associated cardiac malformations are present in 5 percent of all cases.[16] A right aortic arch can also occur with an aberrant left subclavian artery (Fig. 2-6).

Rare anomalies include a double aortic arch, a cervical aortic arch, and a type of right aortic arch that occurs with isolation of the left subclavian artery.[6] When a cervical aortic arch occurs, it is associated with multiple anomalous origins of the arch vessels (Fig. 2-7).

(Text continues on p. 41)

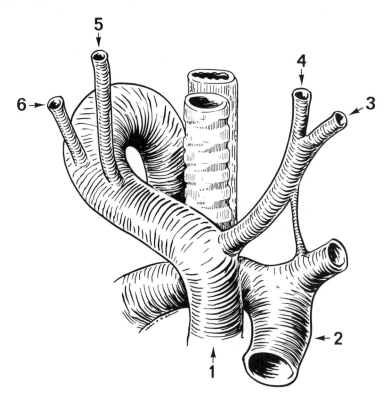

Fig. 2-5. Anatomic sketch of a right aortic arch with mirror image branching of the arch vessels. **1.** Aorta. **2.** Pulmonary trunk. **3.** Left subclavian artery. **4.** Left common carotid artery. **5.** Right common carotid artery. **6.** Right subclavian artery. *(Modified from Shuford WH, et al.: The three types of right aortic arch. Am J Roentgenol 109:67, 1970)*

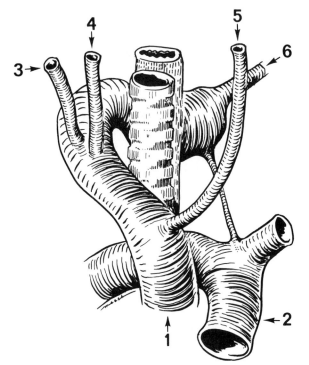

Fig. 2-6. Anatomic sketch of a right aortic arch with an aberrant left subclavian artery. **1.** Aorta. **2.** Pulmonary trunk. **3.** Right subclavian artery. **4.** Right common carotid artery. **5.** Left common carotid artery. **6.** Left subclavian artery. *(Modified from Shuford, WH, et al.: The three types of right aortic arch. Am J Roentgenol 109:67, 1970)*

Fig. 2-7. Aortic arch angiogram (arterial phase, right posterior oblique view). This illustrates a left cervical aortic arch and right descending thoracic aorta. Note the anomalous origins of the arch vessels.

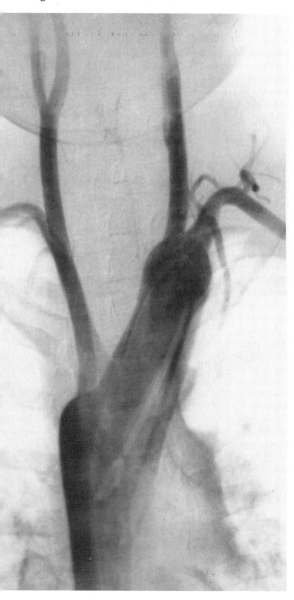

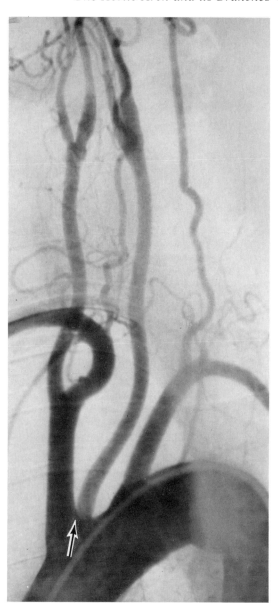

Fig. 2-8. Aortic arch angiogram (arterial phase, right posterior oblique view). This illustrates a common origin of both the left common carotid and innominate arteries **(arrow)**.

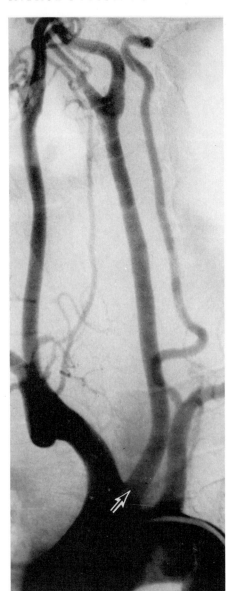

Fig. 2-9. Aortic arch angiogram (arterial phase, right posterior oblique view). This illustrates origin of the left common carotid artery from the innominate artery **(arrow).**

Fig. 2-10. Aortic arch angiogram (arterial phase, right posterior oblique view). The right vertebral artery **(white arrow)** arises from the subclavian artery distal to the thyrocervical trunk **(black arrow).** The left vertebral artery originates directly from the aortic arch **(outlined arrow)** and is smaller than the right vertebral artery.

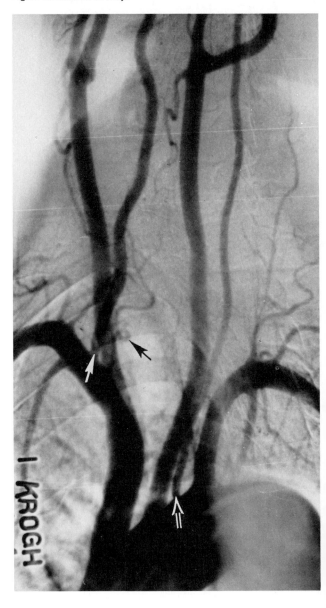

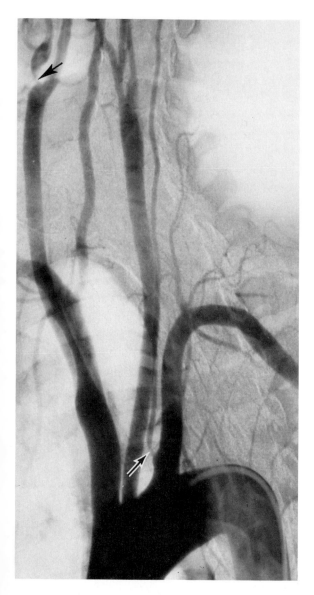

Fig. 2-11. Aortic arch angiogram (arterial phase, right posterior oblique view). The left vertebral artery **(outlined arrow)** is small and has a low origin from the proximal subclavian artery. Some atherosclerotic narrowing of the right carotid artery is incidentally noted **(black arrow).**

and tortuousity (Fig. 2-12). When filled with contrast, the walls of the affected vessels may appear irregular with areas of actual ulceration (Figs. 2-13, 2-14). With progression of the disease, the arterial lumen narrows and may eventually become occluded (Figs. 2-14, 2-15, 2-16). Stenosis becomes hemodynamically significant when the cross sectional area of the lumen is decreased by 75 percent. Angiographically, this is represented by a 50 percent decrease in transverse diameter of the opacified vessel. In descending order of frequency, the most common sites of significant extracranial stenosis of the arch vessels are:

1. the proximal internal carotid artery,
2. the proximal vertebral artery, and
3. the proximal subclavian artery.

In the presence of hemodynamically significant occlusive vascular disease, collateral blood flow from other vessels may develop. For example, when a vertebral artery is occluded or stenotic, collateral blood flow may develop via the muscular branches of the external carotid artery (Fig. 2-16A, arrow 3), the contralateral vertebral artery (Fig. 2-16A, arrow 2), or thyrocervical and intercostal collaterals (Figs. 2-14, 2-16A, arrow 5).

In classical subclavian steal (numbered arrows, Figure 2-16A, B), the low pressure in the subclavian artery distal to the site of occlusion (arrow 1) attracts collateral blood flow from the contralateral vertebral artery (arrow 2) via the basilar artery (arrow 3), and then, in retrograde fashion, down the ipsilateral vertebral artery (arrow 4) to the distal subclavian artery (arrows 5, 6). The resultant decrease in cerebral blood flow may result in ischemic attacks. This is termed the *subclavian steal* syndrome.

It should be noted that aortic arch studies alone are inadequate for complete evaluation

(Text continues on p. 45)

ABNORMALITIES OF THE AORTIC ARCH AND ITS BRANCHES

Atherosclerosis is the most common of all arterial diseases. The distribution of atherosclerotic plaques is quite variable, but tends to be greatest near the origins of the arch vessels and their major branches.

The radiographic findings in atherosclerotic disease include arterial calcification, ectasia,

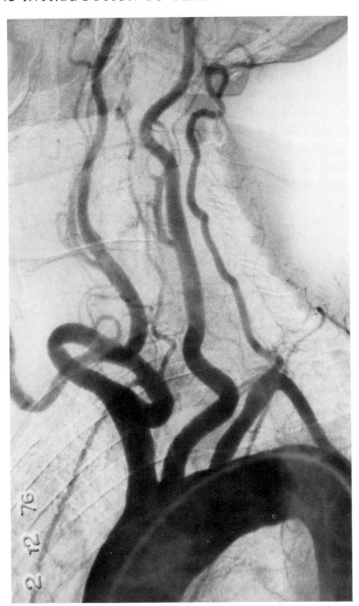

Fig. 2-12. Aortic arch angiogram (arterial phase, right posterior oblique view). Note the marked ectasia and tortuousity of the arch vessels and their major branches.

Fig. 2-13. Aortic angiogram (arterial phase, right posterior oblique view). Severe ulcerative atherosclerotic disease is present **(arrows).**

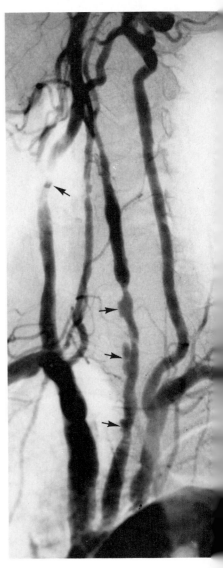

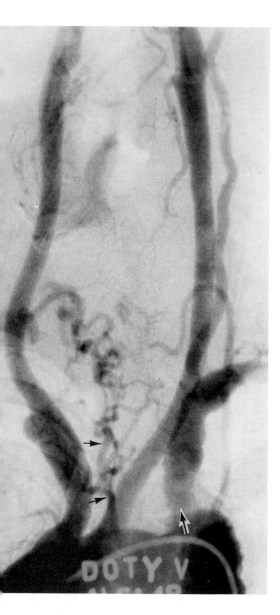

Fig. 2-14. Aortic arch angiogram (arterial phase, right posterior oblique view). The right subclavian artery is completely occluded. A stenotic, ulcerating plaque is present at the origin of the left subclavian artery **(outlined arrow)**. An enlarged arteria thyroidea ima **(black arrows)** supplies blood flow to the occluded right subclavian artery via thyrocervical collaterals.

Fig. 2-15. Aortic arch angiogram (arterial phase, right posterior oblique view). The left common carotid artery **(large arrow)** is occluded. The right vertebral artery is dominant. A tiny left vertebral artery **(outlined arrow)** arises directly from the aortic arch between the innominate and left common carotid artery origins.

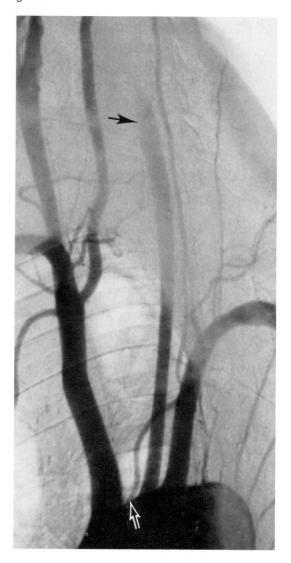

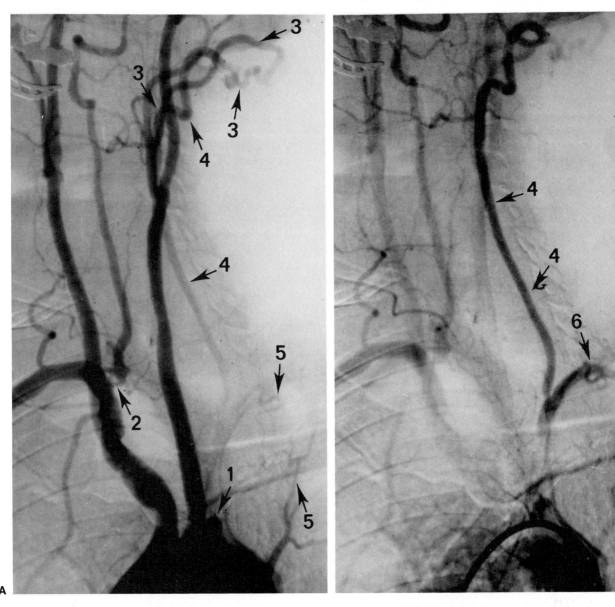

Fig. 2-16. Aortic arch angiogram (right posterior oblique view). This early arterial phase **(A)** demonstrates total occlusion of the left subclavian artery **(arrow 1).** Marked stenosis is present at the origin of the right vertebral artery **(arrow 2),** and enlarged occipital branches **(arrow 3)** of the left external carotid artery provide collateral blood flow to the left vertebral artery **(arrow 4).** The proximal left vertebral and left subclavian arteries are faintly visible. Intercostal collaterals are indicated by **arrow 5.**

This late arterial phase **(B)** demonstrates opacification of the left vertebral **(arrow 4)** and subclavian **(arrow 6)** arteries from the right vertebral artery and the occipital branches of the left external carotid artery.

Fig. 2-17. Aortic arch angiogram (arterial phase, right posterior oblique view). This patient has severe Takayasu's arteritis affecting the aortic arch and all its major branches. Note the multiple areas of long, smooth, fusiform stenosis **(arrows).** An extensive network of collateral vessels has developed.

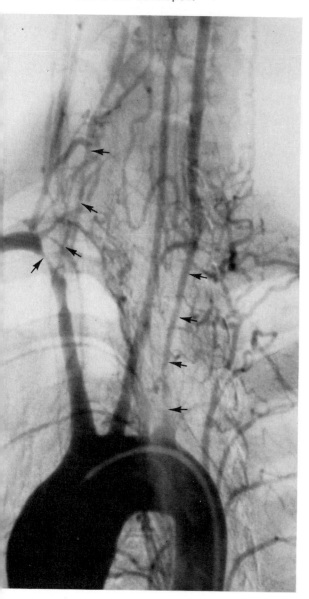

of the patient with atherosclerotic disease and cerebral ischemia. Visualization of the intracranial circulation is necessary to identify branch occlusions, patterns of collateral blood flow, and the presence of other lesions such as aneurysms, arteriovenous malformations, or neoplasms that may present with symptoms of cerebral ischemia. Some neuroangiographers obtain an aortic arch study only:

1. if the patient's symptoms remain unexplained by routine selective studies;
2. if a significant arterial blood pressure differential is present and of clinical concern;
3. if subclavian steal syndrome is suspected;
4. if the chest film suggests the possibility of aberrant great vessel origins.[12]

Nevertheless, since atherosclerosis is usually a multifocal disease process, we have on occasion found arch arteriography helpful in examining the patient with cerebrovascular disease.[11]

Arteritis of the cerebral vessels can result from a variety of causes: viral, mycotic, and bacterial agents, necrotizing angiitis, and autoimmune disorders. Arteritis affecting the aortic arch vessels classically produces either long-segment stenosis or proximal occlusion of its major branches. In either instance, the distal portions of the vessels are usually spared.

Smooth, long-segment, fusiform stenosis of the proximal arch vessels is the classic angiographic finding in Takayasu's arteritis (Fig. 2-17). In severe cases, progressive stenosis may result in complete occlusion of one or more arch vessels. Any single arch branch or any combination of the arch branches may be affected, but in 80 percent of all cases, two or more vessels will be involved. In decreasing order of frequency, lesions are found in: the left subclavian artery (90 percent are located proximal to the vertebral artery origin), the left common carotid artery, and the right subclavian artery. The majority of right subclavian arterial lesions occur distal to the origin of the vertebral artery. Patterns of collateral blood flow are similar to those found in occlusive disease from other etiologies. A saccular, fusiform aneurysm of the aortic arch itself is frequently associated with Takayasu's arteritis.[5, 13]

The radiographic findings in this disease may have some resemblance to atherosclerotic occlusive disease. However, Takayasu's arteritis most commonly affects young females, producing lesions which are often long and smoothly symmetrical, while those of atherosclerosis are more irregular and predominantly affect older individuals of both sexes.

Other arteridities such as giant cell (temporal) arteritis may affect the extracranial vessels. While this disease usually involves the superficial cranial vessels, large- and medium-sized arteries such as the subclavian artery may also be affected. The most common angiographic finding are multiple segmental stenoses. The differential diagnosis includes Takayasu's disease, arteriosclerosis, thoracic outlet syndrome and ergotism.[17]

Aneurysms have a variety of causes. While most lesions involving the thoracic aorta are arteriosclerotic in origin, others may be traumatic, leutic, mycotic, congenital, or secondary to medionecrosis or arteritis.[9] Dissecting thoracic aneurysms may involve the aortic arch and great vessels (Figs. 2-18A, B). Angiographically, three patterns of thoracic aortic dissections are recognized. Type I dissections are the most common; these begin in the ascending aorta and extend beyond the arch vessels, often as distally as the iliac arteries. Type II dissections are limited to the ascending aorta and are most commonly seen in Marfan's syndrome. Type III dissections begin in the thoracic aorta distal to the left subclavian artery and extend for a variable distance.[18]

While the typical clinical picture and plain film chest roentgenogram are often suggestive of dissecting aneurysm, aortography is essential to demonstrate the site of primary tear, the

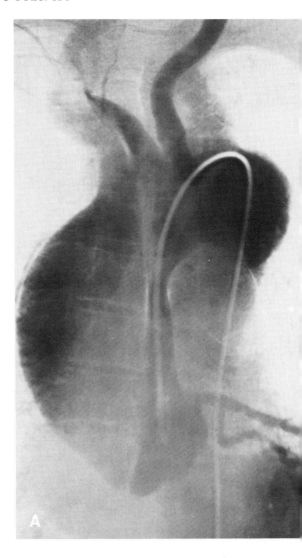

Fig. 2-18. 65 year old hypertensive female with a murmur of aortic regurgitation developed back and shoulder pain radiating throughout the chest. Chest x-ray demonstrated left ventricular enlargement and dilatation of the thoracic aorta. Aortography demonstrated a dissecting aneurysm extending from the aortic root to the midthoracic level. Early arterial films **(A)** with injection into the true lumen

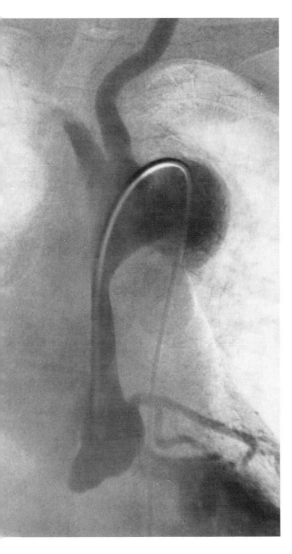

extent of dissection, and the relationship of the aneurysm to other vessels such as the coronary arteries or arch vessels. The angiographic diagnosis is based on the demonstration of two channels, identified either by the presence of a linear radiolucency separating the two lumens or by differences in flow that present as delayed opacification or delayed washout.[10] Failure to visualize main branches of the aorta may be due to their involvement in the dissecting process or to extreme reduction in pressure distal to a severe compression of the main lumen (Fig. 2-18).

Approximately 95 percent of all traumatic aortic ruptures occur in the region of the aortic isthmus at the site of the ligamentum arteriosum. However, the remaining 5 percent originate immediately above the aortic valve and therefore may involve the great vessels.[15] Of all aortic dissections, regardless of etiology, 10 percent are chronic. These typically arise distal to the left subclavian artery and usually do not involve the arch vessels.[1]

Recent studies have shown that many patients with aortic dissections who underwent surgery to abolish flow in the false lumen continued to harbor patent distal false channels. Some developed neurologic deficits while others were asymptomatic or complained only of recurrent pain in the chest, flank, back, or abdomen.[7]

show eccentric aortic valvular insufficiency. A large intimal flap extends from the right sinus of Valsalva superiorly into the innominate artery. The true lumen supplies the left coronary and left common carotid arteries. Later films **(B)** show opacification of the false lumen supplying the right coronary, innominate, right common carotid and left subclavian arteries.

REFERENCES

1. **Ambos MA, Rothberg M, Lefleur RS et al:** Unsuspected aortic dissection: the chronic "healed" dissection. Am J Roentgenol 132:221–225, 1979
2. **Boechat MI, Gilsanz V, Fellows KE:** Subclavian artery as the first branch of the aortic arch: a normal variant in two patients. Am J Roentgenol 131:721–722, 1978
3. **Bryan RN, Drewyer RG, Gee W:** Separate origins of the left internal and external carotid arteries from the aorta. Am J Roentgenol 130:362–365, 1978
4. **DeBakey ME, Henly WS, Cooley DA et al:** Surgical management of dissecting aneurysms of the aorta. J Thorac Cardiovasc Surg 49:130–149, 1965
5. **Deutsch V, Wexler L, Deutsch H:** Takayasu's arteritis. Am J Roentgenol 122:13–28, 1974
6. **Garti IJ, Aygen MM, Levy MJ:** Double aortic arch anomalies: diagnosis by countercurrent right brachial arteriography. Am J Roentgenol 133:251–256, 1979
7. **Guthaner DF, Miller C, Silverman JF et al:** Fate of the false lumen following surgical repair of aortic dissections: an angiographic study. Radiology 133:1–8, 1979
8. **Haughton VM, Rosenbaum AE:** The normal and anomalous aortic arch and brachiocephalic arteries. In Newton TH, Potts DG (eds): Radiology of the Skull and Brain, Vol 2. pp 1145–1163. St. Louis. CV Mosby, 1974
9. **Heitzman ER, McAfee JG:** Aneurysms of the thoracic aorta and its branches. In Abrams HL (ed): Angiography, pp 366–381. Boston, Little, Brown, 1971
10. **Itzchak Y, Rosenthal T, Adar R et al:** Dissecting aneurysm of thoracic aorta: reappraisal of radiologic diagnosis. Am J Roentgenol 125:559–570, 1975
11. **Kadir S, Roberson GH:** Brachiocephalic atherosclerosis: a cause of amaurosis fugax. Radiology 130:171–173, 1979
12. **Kerber CW, Cromwell LD, Drayer BP et al:** Cerebral ischemia. I. Current angiographic techniques, complications, and safety. Am J Roentgenol 130:1097–1103, 1978
13. **Lande A, Rossi P:** The value of total aortography in the diagnosis of Takayasu's arteritis. Radiology 114:287–297, 1975
14. **Moore TS, Morris JL:** Aortic arch vessel anomalies associated with persistent trigeminal artery. Am J Roentgenol 133:309–311, 1979
15. **Sanborn JC, Heitzmann ER, Markarian B:** Traumatic rupture of the thoracic aorta. Radiology 95:293–298, 1970
15A. **Sartor K, Freckmann N, Böker D-K:** Related anomalies of origin of left vertebral and left anterior thyroid arteries. Neuroradiology 19:27–30, 1980
16. **Shuford WH, Sybers RG, Edwards FK:** The three types of right aortic arch. Am J Roentgenol 109:67–74, 1970
17. **Stanson AW, Klein RG, Hunder GG:** Extracranial angiographic findings in giant cell (temporal) arteritis. Am J Roentgenol 127:957–963, 1976
18. **Weinberger G, Randall PA, Parker FB et al:** Involvement of an aberrant right subclavian artery in dissection of the thoracic aorta: diagnostic and therapeutic implications. Am J Roentgenol 129:653–655, 1977

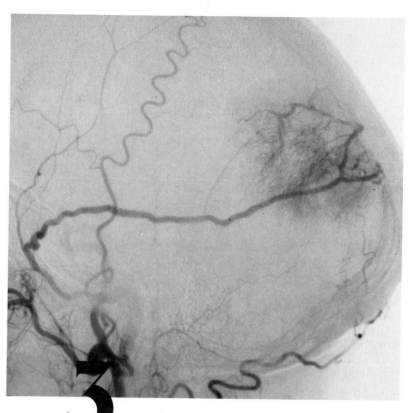

3 *The External Carotid Artery*

Advances in selective catheterization and magnification-subtraction techniques have recently permitted exquisitely detailed study of the external carotid artery (ECA) and its distal branches. Radiographic examination of these rami has proved very helpful in determining the nature, location, and extent of deep facial lesions. With the recent advent of interventional angiography, superselective catheterization of distal ECA branches is also used in the embolization of vascular lesions. In addition, angiographic visualization of the ECA and its branches is often necessary for complete evaluation of intracranial vascular lesions since they may derive part or all of their blood supply from the external carotid circulation. Hence, comprehensive understanding of both the normal and pathologic radioanatomy of the ECA is a prerequisite for modern neuroangiography.

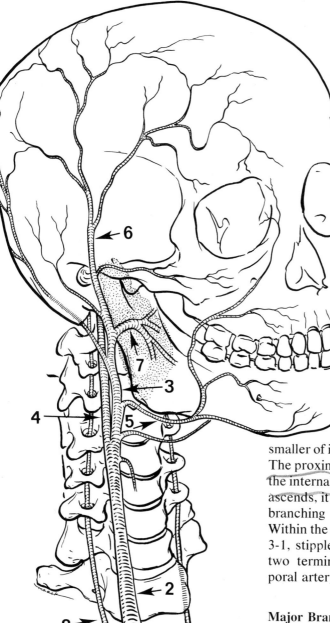

Fig. 3-1. Anatomic sketch of the innominate artery and its major branches (oblique view). The parotid gland is indicated by the stippled area. **1.** Innominate artery (brachiocephalic trunk). **2.** Right common carotid artery. **3.** External carotid artery. **4.** Internal carotid artery. **5.** Facial artery. **6.** Superficial temporal artery. **7.** Maxillary artery. **8.** Right vertebral artery.

NORMAL GROSS ANATOMY

Anatomic Relationships of the External Carotid Artery

The ECA originates from the common carotid artery at the mid-cervical level and is the smaller of its two terminal branches (Fig. 3-1). The proximal ECA is initially anteromedial to the internal carotid artery (ICA). As the ECA ascends, it gradually courses posterolaterally, branching to supply the facial structures. Within the substance of the parotid gland (Fig. 3-1, stippled area), the ECA divides into its two terminal branches, the superficial temporal artery and the maxillary artery.[30]

Major Branches of the External Carotid Artery

The superior thyroid artery (Fig. 3-2, arrow 1) is the first anterior branch of the ECA. It courses anteroinferiorly to supply the larynx and superior pole of the thyroid gland.

The Ascending Pharyngeal Artery (Fig. 3-2, arrow 2) is a small branch arising from either the common carotid bifurcation or the posterior aspect of the proximal ECA. The ascending pharyngeal artery courses superiorly between the ICA and posterolateral wall of the pharynx. Along its extracranial course it gives rise to paravertebral and pharyngeal rami. It also supplies branches to the meninges and middle ear as well as the lower cranial and upper cervical nerves.[11A, 11B, 12] Within the roof of the posterior nasopharynx, the ascending pharyngeal artery anastomoses with other rami of the ECA (*i.e.,* the accessory meningeal, ascending palatine, and vidian arteries). It also anastomoses with intracavernous branches of the ICA and meningeal branches of the vertebral artery (Fig. 4-2).[13] This rich anastomotic system may serve as an important source of collateral blood flow as well as represent a theoretical hazard during therapeutic embolization of extracranial vascular lesions.

The Lingual Artery (Fig. 3-2, arrow 3) arises from the anterior aspect of the ECA, at first coursing superomedially and then turning inferolaterally. It supplies branches to the pharynx and hyoid musculature as well as the submandibular gland and tongue.

The Facial Artery (Fig. 3-2, arrow 4) originates from the anterior aspect of the ECA. It frequently arises from a common trunk with the lingual artery. The facial artery ascends, then passes forward across the cheek and superiorly to the nose where it anastomoses with branches of the ophthalmic artery (a branch of the ICA). This anastomosis between branches of the external and internal carotid arteries is an important potential pathway for collateral blood flow in the event of internal carotid occlusion. The facial artery also has numerous branches that anastomose with other ECA rami to supply the face, palate, and pharynx.[11]

The Occipital Artery (Fig. 3-2, arrow 5) originates at a variable level from the posterior aspect of the ECA and courses posterosuperiorly between the occipital bone and the first cervical vertebra. Its terminal branches supply the musculocutaneous structures of the neck and scalp and also provide meningeal rami to the posterior fossa. Numerous anastomoses are present between its muscular branches and those of the vertebral and ascending cervical arteries, scalp rami of other ECA branches, and other posterior

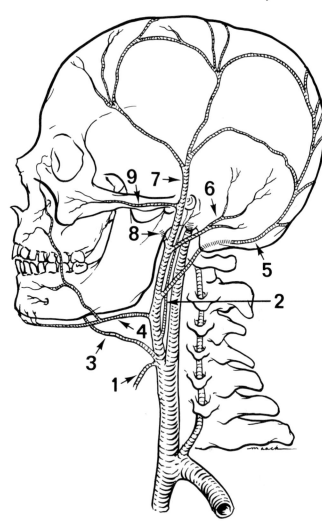

Fig. 3-2. Anatomic sketch of the external carotid artery (ECA) and its major branches (lateral view). **1.** Superior thyroid artery. **2.** Ascending pharyngeal artery. **3.** Lingual artery. **4.** Facial artery. **5.** Occipital artery. **6.** Posterior auricular artery. **7.** Superficial temporal artery. **8.** Maxillary artery. **9.** Transverse facial artery.

fossa meningeal branches. The occipital artery may also have sizeable direct anastomoses with the vertebral artery itself.[2A, 4, 14]

The Posterior Auricular Artery (Fig. 3-2, arrow 6) arises from the posterior aspect of the ACA above the origin of the occipital artery. It courses posterosuperiorly to supply the parotid gland, scalp, pinna, and tympanic cavity.

The Superficial Temporal Artery (Fig. 3-2, arrow 7) is the smaller terminal branch of the ECA and is essentially a cutaneous artery, supplying the anterior two-thirds of the scalp and part of the face.[4] The transverse facial artery (Fig. 3-2, arrow 9), one of the major branches of the ECA, arises near the origin of the superficial temporal artery and courses horizontally, parallel to the zygoma. Branches of the transverse facial artery anastomose with those of the facial artery to supply the buccal area. Other branches of the superficial temporal artery supply the parotid gland, temporomandibular joint, ear, and scalp.[4]

The Maxillary Artery (Fig. 3-2 arrow 8) arises behind the neck of the mandible and is the larger terminal branch of the ECA. It lies initially within the parotid gland, then runs obliquely forward and anteromedially in the infratemporal fossa. It courses either superficially or deep to the lateral pterygoid muscle. The first or mandibular portion of the maxillary artery (Fig. 3-3A, B, solid lines) courses along the inferior aspect of the lateral pterygoid muscle. Its major branches are the deep auricular (arrow 1) and anterior tympanic arteries (arrow 2), the middle meningeal artery (arrow 3), the accessory meningeal artery (arrow 3), the accessory meningeal artery (arrow 9), and the inferior alveolar artery (arrow 4).

The second or pterygoid portion of the maxillary artery (Fig. 3-3A, B, open lines) runs anterosuperiorly and medially through the infratemporal fossa. Its buccal and masseteric branches (arrows 7 and 8) supply the muscles of mastication. The middle (arrow 5) and anterior (arrow 6) deep temporal arteries supply the temporalis muscle. The anterior deep temporal artery has numerous anastomoses with

the intraorbital vessels and may therefore supply vascular lesions in the orbit as well as provide a source of collateral flow through the ophthalmic artery when the ICA is occluded.

Distal Branches of the Maxillary Artery

The third or pterygopalatine portion of the maxillary artery branches within the pterygopalatine fossa. Each branch of the maxillary artery leaves this fossa by passing through a bony canal or foramen (Fig. 3-4). In fact, the branches and their corresponding foramina or fissures share the same name.[1]

Posterior Branches. Three, small posterior branches of the distal maxillary artery course dorsally from the pterygopalatine fossa through their respective openings in the sphenoid bone.[27] The **artery of the foramen rotundum,** the most lateral of the three posteriorly directed branches, passes posterosuperiorly through its canal to anastomose with the artery of the inferior cavernous sinus (Fig. 3-4, arrow 3). The **artery of the pterygoid canal** (vidian artery) runs posteriorly through the pterygoid canal towards the foramen lacerum (Fig. 3-4, arrow 4). Within the roof of the oropharynx it may anastomose with branches of the accessory meningeal and ascending pharyngeal arteries. It may also continue posteriorly to join the petrous segment of the ICA (Fig. 4-2).[27A]

The most medial of the three posteriorly directed branches is the **pharyngeal artery** (Fig. 3-4, arrow 5). This vessel supplies part of the choanae, pharynx, and eustachian tube. It anastomoses with the ascending pharyngeal artery, vidian artery, and cavernous branches of the ICA.

Anterior Branches. The anterior branches of the distal maxillary artery essentially outline the maxillary sinus. These branches are shown diagrammatically in Figure 3-5.

The **posterior superior alveolar artery** (Fig. 3-5, arrow 1) courses along the posterior and lateral walls of the maxillary sinus. It supplies the mucosa of the check, the buccinator muscle, the maxillary antrum, alveolar ridge, and teeth.[4]

Fig. 3-3. Anatomic sketch of the first and second portions of the maxillary artery. The first, or mandibular portion, is indicated by solid lines and the second, or pterygoid portion, is indicated by open lines. **A.** Anteroposterior view. **B.** Lateral view. **1.** Deep auricular artery. **2.** Anterior tympanic artery. **3.** Middle meningeal artery. **4.** Inferior alveolar artery. **5.** Posterior deep temporal artery. **6.** Anterior deep temporal artery. **7.** Masseteric artery. **8.** Buccinator artery. **9.** Accessory meningeal artery.

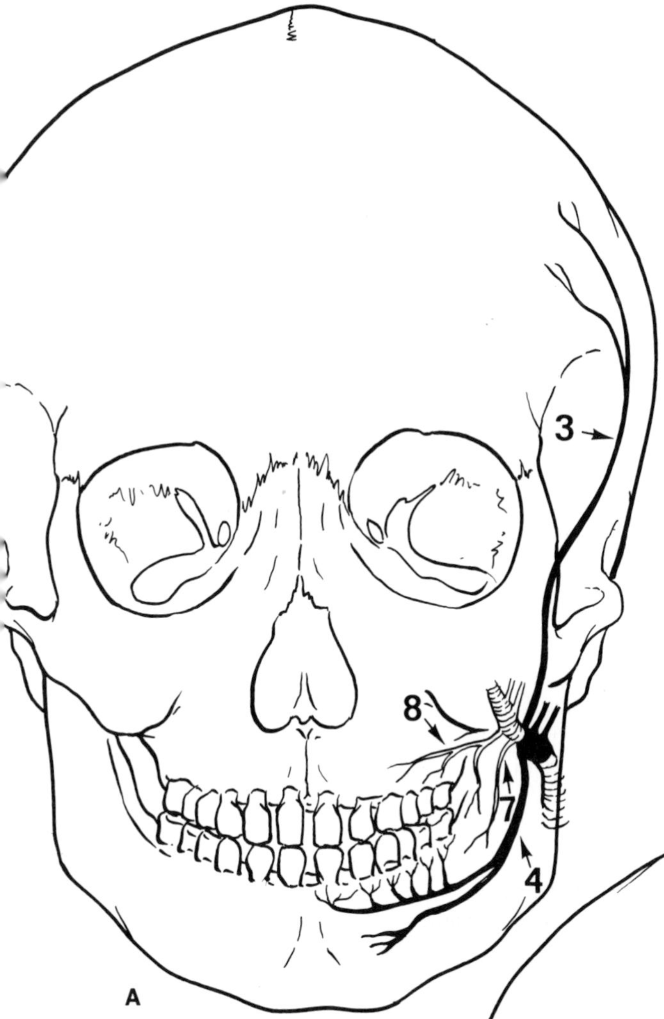

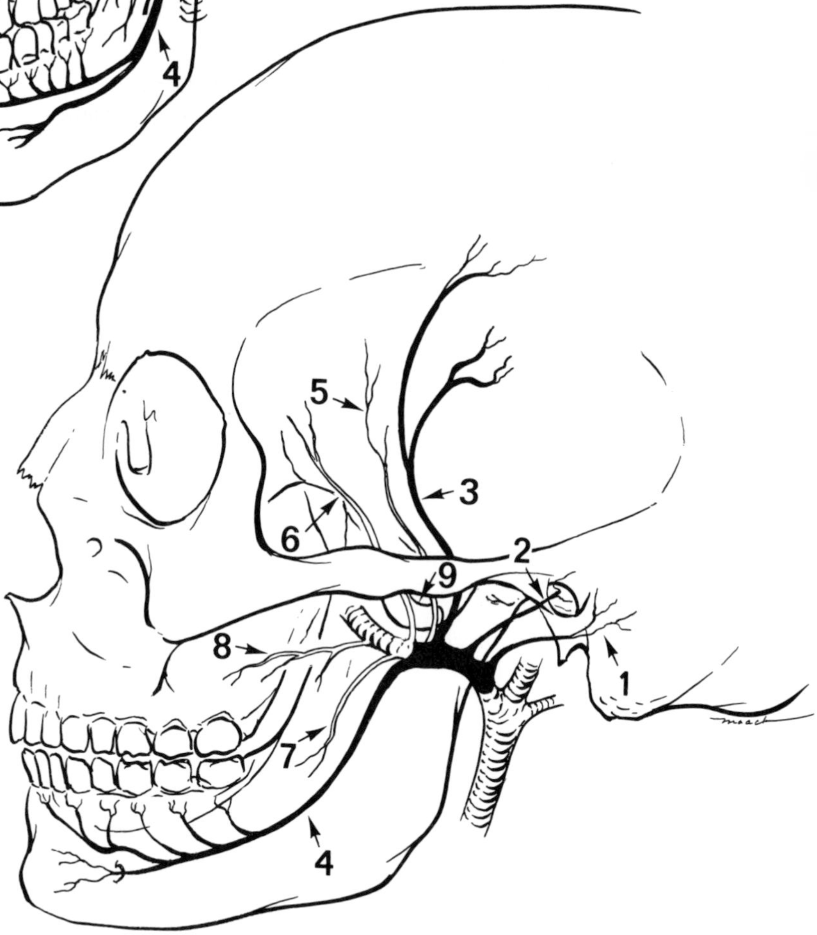

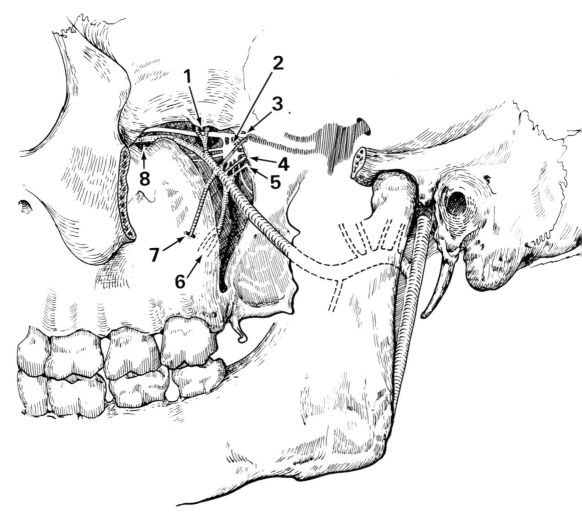

Fig. 3-4. Diagrammatic sketch of the distal maxillary artery as it branches within the pterygopalatine fossa. **1.** Sphenopalatine artery. **2.** Sphenopalatine ganglion. **3.** Maxillary nerve (V₂) and the artery of the foramen rotundum. **4.** Vidian artery. **5.** Pharyngeal artery. **6.** Descending palatine artery. **7.** Posterior superior alveolar artery. **8.** Infraorbital artery.

The **infraorbital artery** (Fig. 3-5, arrow 2) runs anteriorly along the roof of the maxillary sinus, delineating its superior and anterior walls. It is a major source of blood to the orbit and maxilla. The infraorbital artery has extensive anastomoses with branches of the facial and ophthalmic arteries.

The **greater palatine artery** (Fig. 3-5, arrow 3) descends in the pterygopalatine canal and defines the posterior and inferior aspects of the maxillary sinus. It anastomoses with other ECA branches to supply the hard palate.

Branches of the **sphenopalatine artery** (Fig. 3-5, arrow 4), the terminal branch of the maxillary artery, delineate the nasal fossa and medial wall of the maxillary sinus. They supply the nasal turbinates and septum. They also assist in supplying the maxillary, ethmoid, and sphenoid sinuses.[25]

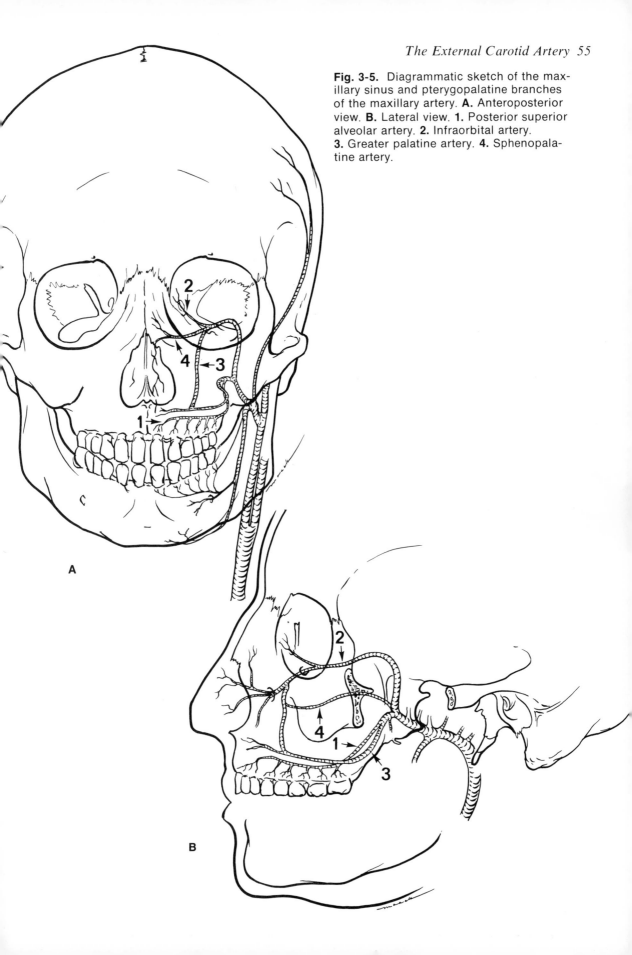

Fig. 3-5. Diagrammatic sketch of the maxillary sinus and pterygopalatine branches of the maxillary artery. **A.** Anteroposterior view. **B.** Lateral view. **1.** Posterior superior alveolar artery. **2.** Infraorbital artery. **3.** Greater palatine artery. **4.** Sphenopalatine artery.

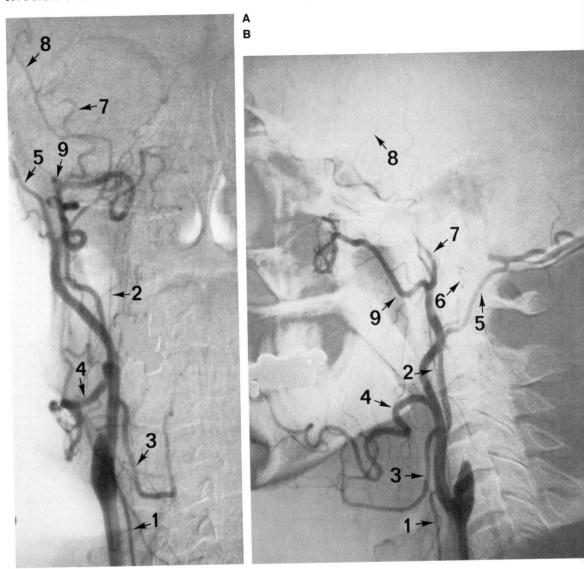

Fig. 3-6. Right common carotid angiogram (arterial phase). Complete occlusion of the internal carotid artery permits an unobstructed view of the entire external carotid artery and all its major branches. **A.** Anteroposterior view. **B.** Lateral view. **1.** Superior thyroid artery. **2.** Ascending pharyngeal artery. **3.** Lingual artery. **4.** Facial artery. **5.** Occipital artery. **6.** Posterior auricular artery. **7.** Superficial temporal artery. **8.** Middle meningeal artery. **9.** Maxillary artery.

NORMAL RADIOGRAPHIC ANATOMY

Major Branches of the External Carotid Artery

On routine angiograms, like the one shown in Figure 3-6A, B, the ECA usually lies anterior and medial to the ICA. Its first branch, the **superior thyroid artery** (arrow 1), courses inferiorly, lying parallel and anterior to the common carotid artery.

The second branch of the ECA, the **ascending pharyngeal artery** (arrow 2), is a small branch that ascends behind the main trunk of the ECA and courses between the external and internal carotid arteries.

The **lingual artery** (arrow 3) has a characteristic "U" appearance on both AP and lateral views. It arises from the ECA just below the facial artery.

The **facial artery** (arrow 4) initially courses inferiorly but then runs superolaterally across the face towards the nose.

The **occipital artery** (arrow 5) follows a serpentine course posterosuperiorly to the occiput.

The **posterior auricular artery** (arrow 6) is usually a small branch and frequently difficult to delineate on unsubstracted, non-magnified films. It courses superiorly and then posteriorly towards the ear. A curvilinear vascular blush representing the pinna can some-

Fig. 3-7. Left external carotid angiogram (arterial phase, lateral view) of a small cribriform plate meningioma **(large arrow). 1.** Superficial temporal artery. **2.** Middle meningeal artery. **3.** Occipital artery. **4.** Posterior auricular artery.

(Note the prominent but normal vascular blush representing the pinna **[small arrows].**)

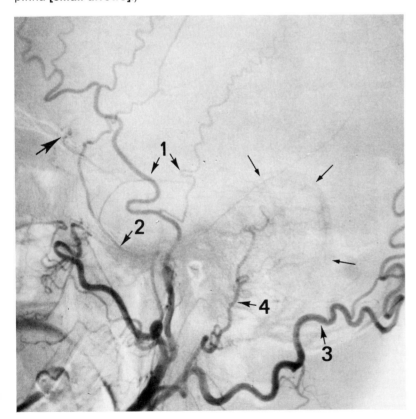

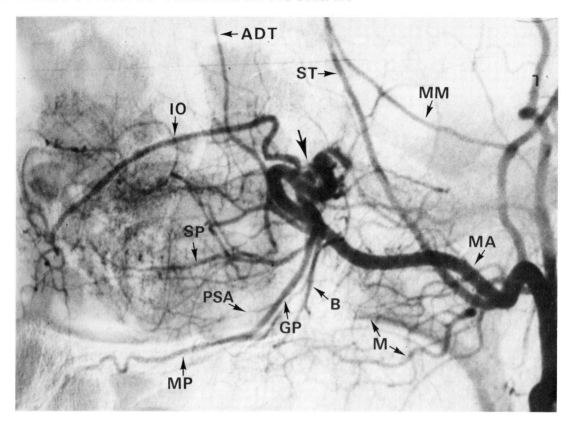

Fig. 3-8. Selective left external carotid angiogram (arterial phase, lateral view). The patient's nose is to the left. Maxillary artery **(MA).** Superficial temporal artery **(ST).** Middle meningeal artery **(MM).** Major palatine artery **(MP).**

times be identified on subtracted ECA angiograms and should not be mistaken for a lesion (Fig. 3-7, small arrows).

The distal ECA finally bifurcates into the **superficial temporal artery** (arrow 7) and **maxillary artery** (arrow 9).

Terminal branches of the superficial temporal artery ramify over the scalp and have a corkscrew appearance (Fig. 3-7, arrow 1). The largest branch of the maxillary artery is the **middle meningeal artery** (Fig. 3-6B, arrow 8 and Fig. 3-7, arrow 2). This artery follows a somewhat straighter course than that of the superficial temporal artery and can usually be identified by its path in the meningeal groove on the inner table of the skull.

Branches of the Distal Maxillary Artery

The distal maxillary artery divides within the pterygopalatine fossa (Figs. 3-5, 3-8). Its terminal branches ramify around the maxillary sinus and delineate its somewhat boxlike structure (Figs. 3-8 and 3-9). A definite nasal mucosal vascular blush is sometimes present and may become pronounced in patients with acute rhinitis (Fig. 3-10). This too should not be mistaken for a vascular malformation or neoplasm.[25]

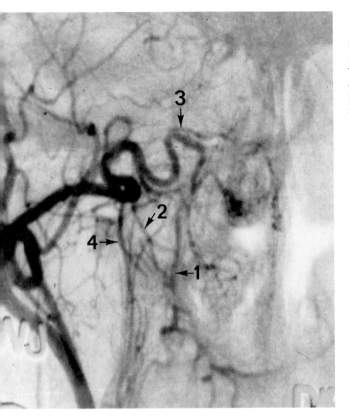

Fig. 3-9. Selective right external carotid angiogram (midarterial phase, AP view **1.** Greater (descending) palatine artery. **2.** Infraorbital artery. **3.** Sphenopalatine artery. **4.** Posterior superior alveolar artery.

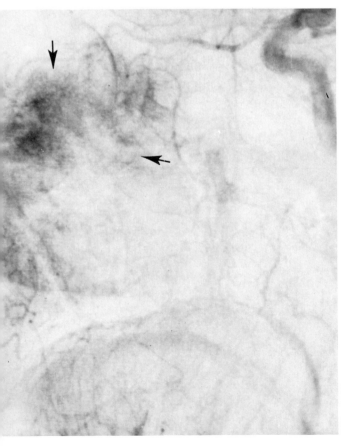

Fig. 3-10. Left common carotid angiogram (late arterial phase, lateral view) of acute rhinitis. There is a prominent nasal mucosal vascular blush **(arrows)**.

ABNORMALITIES OF THE EXTERNAL CAROTID ARTERY

Vascular Malformations and Fistulae

Vascular malformations may take a variety of forms and have been classified into capillary telangiectasias, cavernous angiomas, arteriovenous malformations, and venous malformations.[29] Angiographic abnormalities involving the ECA and its branches are primarily seen with arteriovenous malformations and capillary telangiectasias. Malformations with very slow flow (*i.e.,* venous angiomas) are the most difficult to recognize at angiography. Hyperselective catheterization with slow, prolonged injection of contrast may allow the prominent venous lakes to be identified when non-selective studies fail to demonstrate the abnormality.[4]

Arteriovenous Malformations (AVMs) of the face and scalp are comparatively rare (Fig. 3-11). Congenital AVMs are usually intracranial and most are pure pial malformations (see Chapter 8). Supply from meningeal vessels to intracranial malformations is found with mixed pial-dural (Fig. 3-12) or pure dural AVMs (Fig. 3-13).[6A]

The majority of dural AVMs deriving blood from the ECA are found in the posterior fossa. Supratentorial dural AVMs are rare. The most common vessels contributing to dural AVMs are the occipital artery and meningeal branches of the ECA (Fig. 3-13). Tentorial and small dural branches of the internal carotid and vertebral arteries are also frequent sources of blood supply (see Figs. 5-23, 5-24). It should be noted that angiographically enlarged dural vessels are rare in lesions other than vascular malformations or neoplasms but have been reported in unusual cases of inflammatory disease involving the dura and meninges.

Capillary Telangiectasias are usually solitary and asymptomatic but can be both familial and symptomatic. Osler-Weber-Rendu disease (hereditary hemorrhagic telangiectasia) is a congenital disorder characterized by small arteriovenous fistulae or capillary telangiectasias involving the skin, mucous membranes, and viscera. This disorder is a rare cause of epistaxis. In these cases, selective external carotid angiography may disclose multiple small arteriovenous foci in the mucosa of the nasal fossa and nasopharynx (Fig. 3-14A, B).

Cavernous Sinus Fistulas are abnormal communications between the carotid artery and cavernous sinus. Such fistulous communications may be divided into several types:

1. those between meningeal branches of the ECA and the cavernous sinus,
2. those between meningeal branches of the ICA and cavernous sinus, and
3. direct fistulas between the ICA itself and the cavernous sinus.[28]

Mixed types with contributions from both carotid systems have also been reported. Differentiation between the different kinds of fistulous communications is important for therapeutic considerations. (Types two and three are discussed in Chapter 5.)

Most external carotid-cavernous sinus communications (type 1) are probably based on the pre-existence of an arteriovenous malformation connecting meningeal branches and dural veins in the cavernous sinus. Spontaneous opening of these abnormal communications may occur. However, hypertension, atherosclerosis, trauma, etc., have also been considered as contributing factors.[17]

When the dural fistula involves the ECA, dilated afferent vessels (usually rami of the middle or accessory meningeal arteries, ascending pharyngeal artery, or the posteriorly directed pterygopalatine branches of the maxillary artery) can be easily identified on selective magnification-subtraction studies (Fig. 3-15). These shunts have been successfully occluded using superselective catheterization and subsequent embolization.[7]

Epistaxis

Epistaxis results primarily from atrophic rhinitis, hypertension and aging, or atherosclerotic

(Text continues on p. 65)

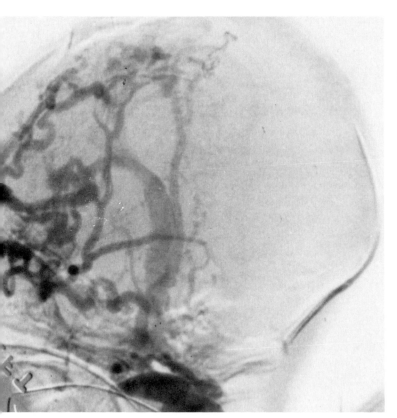

Fig. 3-11. Common carotid angiogram (arterial phase, lateral view) in a newborn child with a huge scalp AVM. *(Courtesy of R. Jaffe, M.D.)*

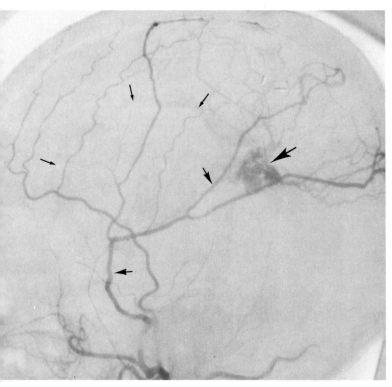

Fig. 3-12. Left external carotid angiogram (arterial phase, lateral view) of a large mixed pial-dural AVM of the parietal lobe. An enlarged middle meningeal artery **(medium arrows)** supplies a portion of the AVM **(outlined arrow)**. Note the faint opacification of the ipsilateral anterior cerebral artery **(small arrows).**

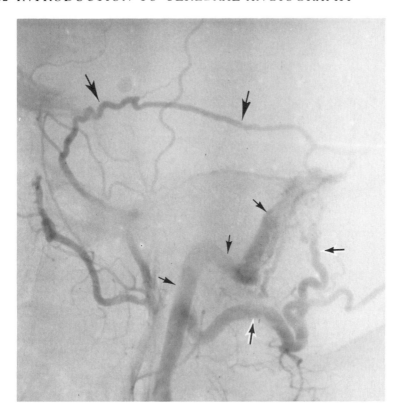

Fig. 3-13. Left external carotid angiogram (arterial phase, lateral view) of an infratentorial dural AVM. The AVM is supplied by enlarged meningeal and dural arteries **(large black arrows)** as well as by dural branches from an enlarged occipital artery **(outlined arrows).** Note the simultaneous opacification of the sigmoid sinus and internal jugular vein **(small black arrows)** draining the AVM.

Fig. 3-14. Selective left external carotid angiogram (arterial phase) of Rendu-Osler- ▶ Weber disease. Multiple small arteriovenous fistulate or telangiectasias **(arrows)** are present. Multiple lesions are also present in the small bowel mucosa. **A.** AP view. **B.** Lateral view. *(Courtesy of T. H. Newton, M.D.)*

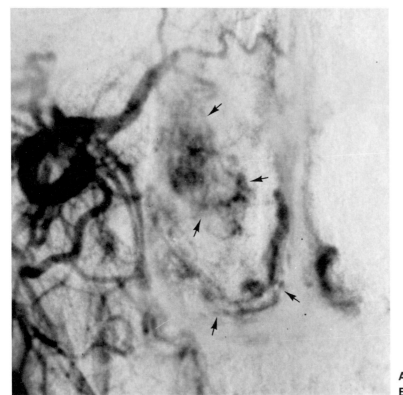

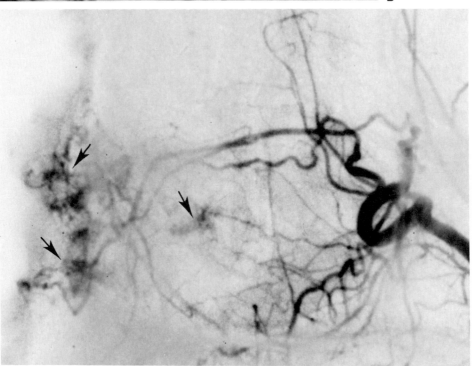

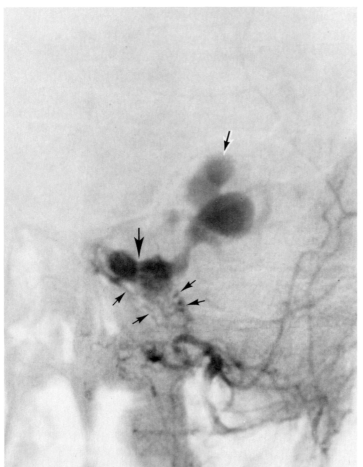

Fig. 3-15. Selective left external carotid angiogram (arterial phase) of pulsatile ex-ophthalmos. **A.** AP view. **B.** Lateral view. Note the carotid-cavernous fistula **(large arrows)** draining into a dilated superior ophthalmic vein **(outlined arrow).** Enlarged arteries of the vidian canal and foramen rotundum **(small arrows)** as well as ethmoidal branches of the sphenopalatine artery supply the lesion.

A

B

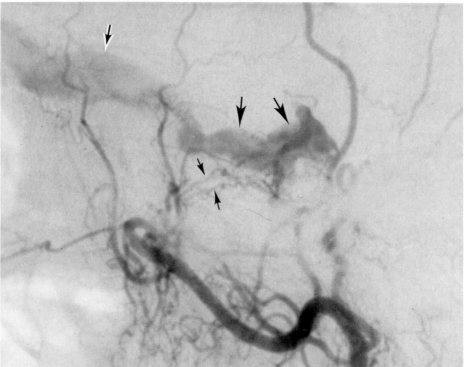

disease involving the sphenopalatine artery.[25] Vascular malformations and neoplasms are less common causes. Some investigators have advocated angiographic evaluation of the maxillary and ethmoidal arteries in difficult cases, particularly posterior epistaxis. More recently, selective embolization procedures have been used in the treatment of recurrent or intractable epistaxis.[28A]

Atherosclerosis

Occasionally, atherosclerotic disease may affect the proximal ECA (Fig. 3-16). Hemodynamically significant lesions are frequently accompanied by severe atherosclerotic disease of the common carotid bifurcation or proximal ICA. As with atherosclerotic disease elsewhere (see Chapter 2), ulcerative lesions may be demonstrated as irregular accumulations of contrast extending into the atheromatous plaque. Stenosis may progress to complete occlusion of the ECA (Fig. 3-17) while leaving the internal carotid origin relatively intact. In such cases, collateral flow from the contralateral external carotid artery or the ipsilateral vertebral artery may supply the ECA (Fig. 3-18). Petrous or cavernous branches of the ICA rarely provides collateral flow to the distal maxillary artery (Fig. 3-19).

Trauma

With the advent of computed tomography, angiography is no longer utilized as the primary diagnostic modality in acute trauma. However, angiography is necessary in order to delineate vessel lacerations, traumatic arteriovenous fistulae, or aneurysms.[26] Blunt head injury occasionally results in traumatic scalp arteriovenous fistulae or in aneurysms of the superficial temporal artery (Fig. 3-20). Aneurysms and fistulae of other external carotid branches are usually the result of penetrating injuries (Fig. 3-21).

Acute head trauma may also result in formation of a subdural or epidural hematoma (see Chapter 9). The epidural space is normally only a potential space between the dura

(Text continues on p. 69)

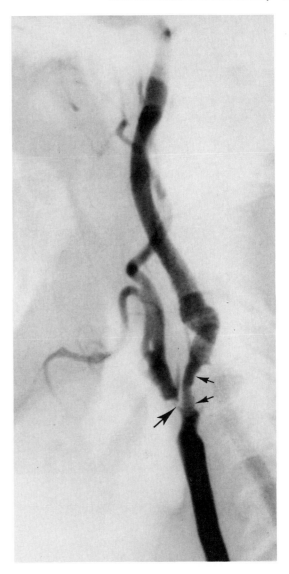

Fig. 3-16. Left common carotid angiogram (arterial phase, lateral view). Near-total occlusion of the external carotid artery **(large arrow)** is shown. An ulcerating, stenotic lesion of the proximal internal carotid artery **(small arrows)** is indicated.

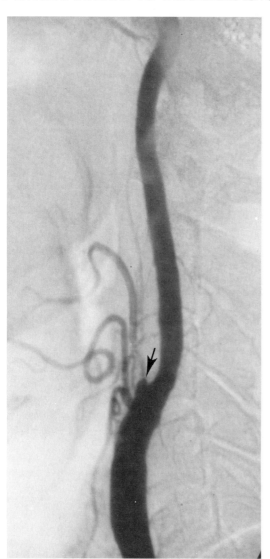

Fig. 3-17. Left common carotid angiogram (arterial phase, lateral view). The external carotid artery is totally occluded **(arrow)** above the origin of the superior thyroid, ascending pharyngeal, lingual, and facial arteries.

Fig. 3-18. Selective left vertebral angiogram (arterial phase, lateral view) showing complete occlusion of the external carotid artery **(large arrow).** The ECA is reconstituted via anastomoses **(small arrows)** between cervical muscular branches of the vertebral and occipital arteries.

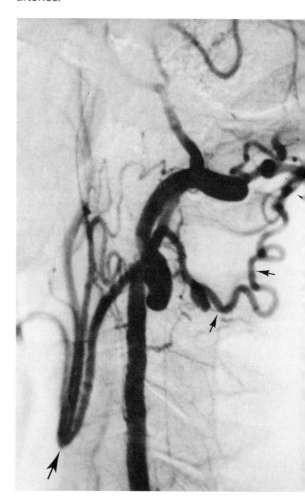

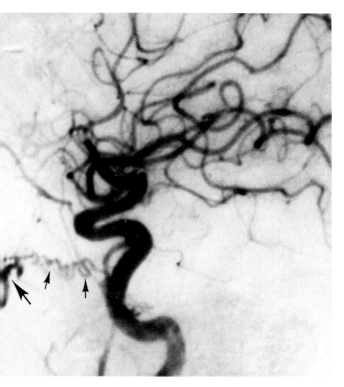

Fig. 3-19. Common carotid angiogram (arterial phase, lateral view). The maxillary artery has been surgically occluded. An enlarged cavernous branch of the internal carotid artery, the artery of the foramen rotundum **(small arrows)**, provides collateral flow to the distal maxillary artery **(large arrow).**

Fig. 3-20. Left external carotid angiogram (late arterial phase, lateral view) of a traumatic aneurysm **(arrow)** arising from the superficial temporal artery. *(Courtesy of F. M. Schroeder, M.D.)*

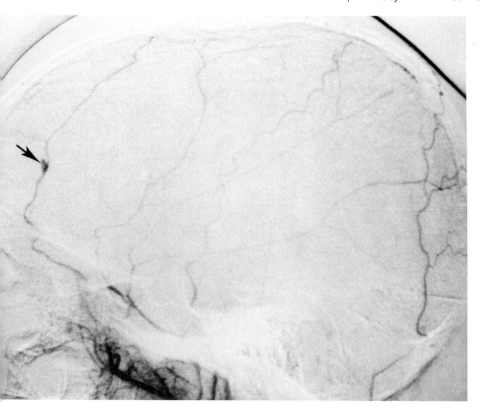

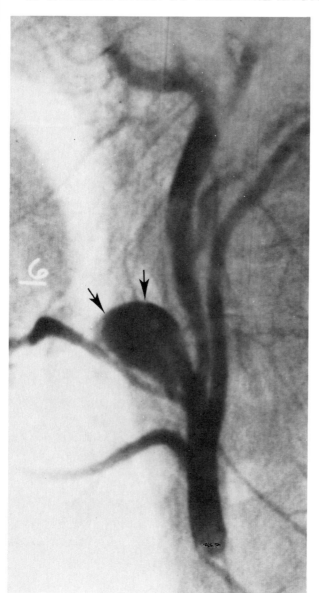

Fig. 3-21. Selective left external carotid angiogram (arterial phase, lateral view) of a posttraumatic pseudoaneurysm **(arrows)** of the ECA. *(Courtesy of B. McIff, M.D.)*

Fig. 3-22. Left common carotid angiogram (arterial phase, anteroposterior view) of a large convexity epidural hematoma. Note the medially displaced middle meningeal artery **(small arrows).** Extravasated contrast medium **(large arrow)** is indicated lying in the epidural space.

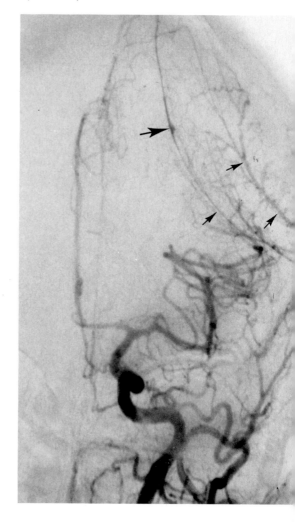

and inner table of the skull. The meningeal arteries lie between the dura and inner table. With forceful injury, blood may extravasate from the middle meningeal artery or from a dural sinus into the epidural space, stripping the dura from the inner table of the skull.

The most common angiographic finding with an epidural hematoma is an extra-axial lenticular or biconvex-shaped avascular zone. Although chronic subdural hematomas may also have a lenticular conformation, the clinical history should permit differentiation of an acute epidural from a chronic subdural hematoma.[5A]

The middle meningeal artery may be displaced medially from the inner table of the skull (Fig. 3-22, small arrows). Amputation of the middle meningeal artery or actual extravasation of contrast from the lacerated vessel may also be seen.[31] Extravasated contrast material may appear in the epidural or diploic space (Fig. 3-22, large arrows), in fracture lines, or under the subgaleal fascia.[6] A traumatic meningeal arteriovenous fistula may be formed with simultaneous opacification of both the meningeal arteries and veins, giving a "railroad track" appearance (Fig. 3-23, small arrows). An ancillary finding with epidural hematoma is displacement of dural sinuses

from the inner table of the skull (see Chapter 11).

Tumors of the Head and Neck Involving the External Carotid Artery

Many tumors of the head and neck affect the ECA either by displacing otherwise normal branches or by deriving abnormal vascular supply from them. A comprehensive discussion of all tumors that can involve the ECA and its branches is beyond the scope of this text. Representative lesions that will be presented and discussed are: paragangliomas (chemodectomas), angiofibromas, meningiomas, miscellaneous vascular tumors, and avascular carcinomas. These have been selected for discussion here as some of the more common lesions involving the ECA and its branches.

Paragangliomas (formerly termed chemodectomas or glomus tumors) arising from extra-adrenal portions of the paraganglion system may be located in numerous sites.[8] They are closely associated with branchial arch mesodermal derivatives such as the carotid arteries and aortic arch.[5] Paragangliomas occur more commonly in females and are multiple in ap-

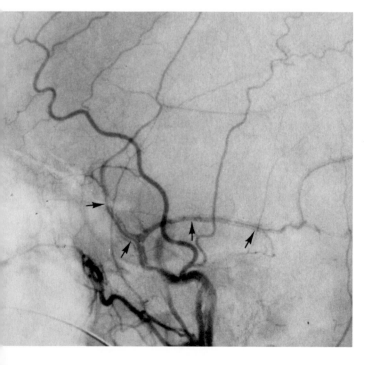

Fig. 3-23. Left external carotid angiogram (arterial phase, lateral view) of an epidural hematoma. Note the traumatic arteriovenous fistulae **(arrows)** involving the middle meningeal artery and paired middle meningeal veins.

proximately five percent of sporadic cases. Studies reporting several kindreds have suggested that familial paragangliomas exhibit a strong tendency toward multicentricity (25 to 33% multiplicity) and are often found in unusual locations in affected family members.[18]

Paragangliomas from various sites are histologically similar. The most common sites of origin in the head and neck are adjacent to the carotid artery bifurcation, within the middle ear, or along the vagus nerve. Less commonly reported locations include the larynx, orbit, nose, and aortic arch.[5]

Meticulous angiography is essential for the diagnosis and complete preoperative evaluation of paragangliomas of the head and neck. The complete vascular supply, size and extent of tumor, possible multiplicity of lesions, and the potential for collateral blood flow in case a major vessel must be ligated at surgery should be assessed.[9]

Carotid body paragangliomas characteristically displace the common carotid bifurcation laterally, splaying or separating the ICA and ECA. A typical carotid body tumor is illustrated in Fig. 3-24. The ICA and ECA are bowed around the tumor. The mass shows a well-defined, reticulated vascular network and a late, dense tumor stain. Although the major blood supply is usually from the proximal ECA, the lesions can also be supplied by small adventitial vessels from both the external and internal branches. While a neurogenic tumor can occasionally mimic a paraganglioma, these tumors are usually much less vascular.[5]

Paragangliomas may also arise from the tympanic branch of the glossopharyngeal nerve (Fig. 3-25) and are the most common neoplasm involving the middle ear. The tympanic branch of the ascending pharyngeal artery is usually the major source of blood supply. Since the ascending pharyngeal artery arises near the common carotid bifurcation, a catheter placed selectively in the ECA may lie beyond its origin. If only selective internal and external angiograms are performed, the lesion may be missed. Hence, a common carotid or selective ascending pharyngeal angiogram

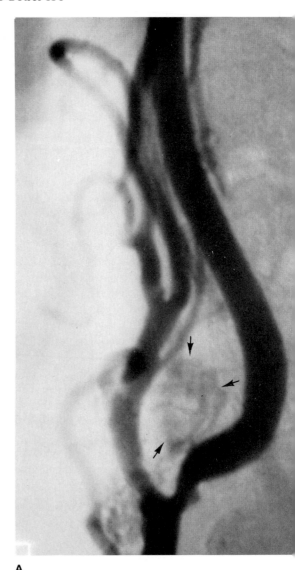

A

Fig. 3-24. Right common carotid angiogram (lateral view). **A.** Early arterial phase. **B.** Late arterial phase. Note the prolonged, densely reticulated vascular stain. A carotid body tumor **(arrows)** is indicated, the internal and external carotid arteries are bowed around the tumor.

(Fig. 3-24 continued on opposite page)

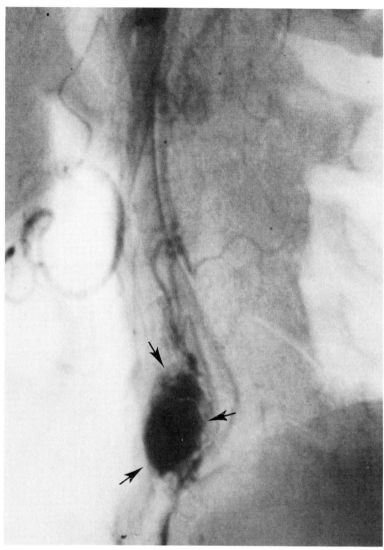

B

should be obtained in all cases of suspected middle ear paragangliomas. Since the bone of the petrous ridge may obscure these lesions, they are best delineated by combined magnification and subtraction technique.

Other vascular lesions that may present in the middle ear and hence can clinically mimic a paraganglioma are an aberrant ICA (see Chapter 4) and an abnormally high jugular bulb (see Chapter 11).

Paragangliomas of the vagus nerve or jugular fossa are highly vascular lesions located above the carotid bifurcation and near the skull base respectively (Fig. 3-26).[20A] As with paragangliomas elsewhere, dense reticular accumulation of contrast medium is a characteristic angiographic finding. Early draining veins are occasionally seen. The vascular supply is predominantly from the ECA although the vertebral artery, ICA, and ascending cervical branches may also supply these lesions. Therefore, thorough cervicocerebral angiography is necessary in such cases.[9]

(Text continues on p. 73)

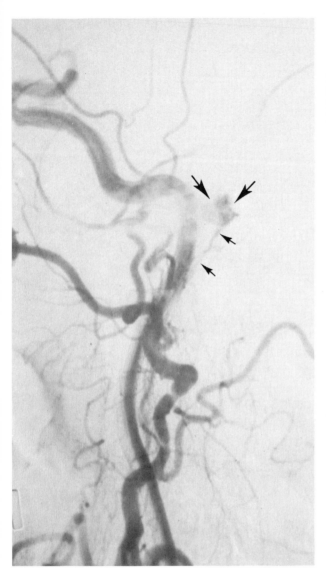

Fig. 3-25. Left common carotid angiogram (arterial phase, lateral view). A middle ear paraganglioma (glomus tympanicum tumor) is identified **(large arrows)**. An enlarged tympanic branch of the ascending pharyngeal artery **(small arrows)** supplies the lesion.

Fig. 3-26. Right external carotid angiogram (arterial phase, lateral view). A jugular fossa paraganglioma **(large arrows)** is indicated. Note the presence of a second lesion, a glomus vagale tumor **(small arrows).**

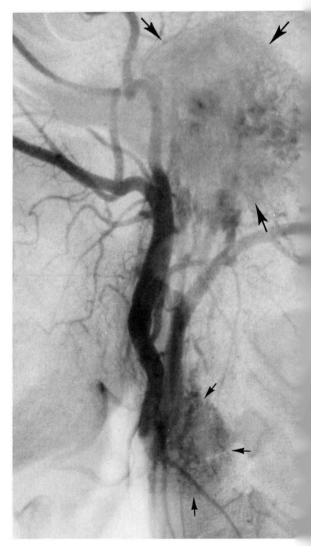

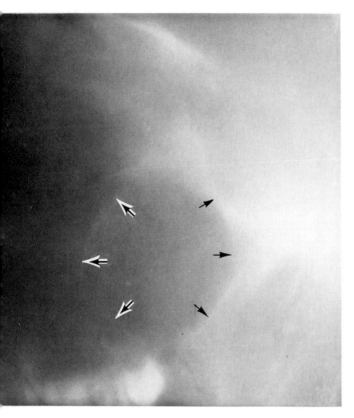

Fig. 3-27. Lateral hypocycloidal to-mogram in a patient with juvenile nasopharyngeal angiofibroma. The posterior wall of the maxillary sinus **(outlined arrows)** is bowed anteriorly while the pterygoid plates **(black arrows)** show pressure erosion of their anterior aspect. This marked enlargement of the pterygopalatine fossa was produced by the slowly expanding tumor.

Angiofibroma (juvenile nasopharyngeal angiofibroma) is a benign vascular nasopharyngeal tumor occurring in adolescent males. The tumor expands the pterygopalatine fossa, bowing the pterygoid plates posteriorly and displacing the posterior wall of the maxillary sinus anteriorly (Fig. 3-27).

An angiofibroma initially derives its blood from the maxillary artery and its pterygopalatine branches. As it extends along natural foramina and fissures, numerous other vessels may contribute to its vascular supply (Fig. 3-28). Extension into the skull base, orbit, and intracranial vault is not uncommon.[9A] Even the vertebral artery may contribute to the vascular supply in advanced cases. Hence, bilateral external and internal carotid angiograms are necessary for complete delineation of tumor extension. Superselective studies and therapeutic embolization may be appropriate in selected patients.[14A]

Angiofibromas characteristically show dense vascular staining with accumulation of contrast medium persisting late into the capillary phase. Early draining veins are uncommon.[33, 35] A typical angiofibroma is shown in Fig. 3-28 (small arrows). Note the stretching of the maxillary artery accompanied by anterior displacement of its pterygopalatine portion (large arrow). While the angiographic appearance of angiofibroma is considered quite characteristic, other lesions such as lymphoepithelioma and fibrous dysplasia may mimic these tumors.[32]

Meningiomas comprise approximately 15 to 20% of all brain tumors and are the most common type of intracranial extracerebral neoplasm. Of all primary intracranial tumors, meningiomas are second in frequency only to gliomas.

Meningiomas are usually attached to the

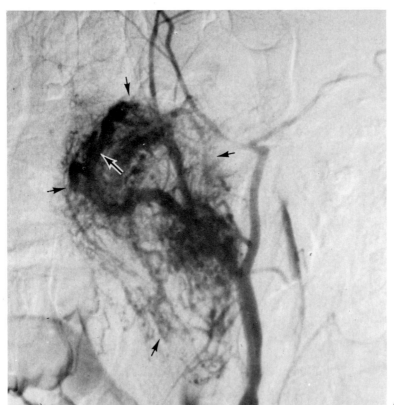

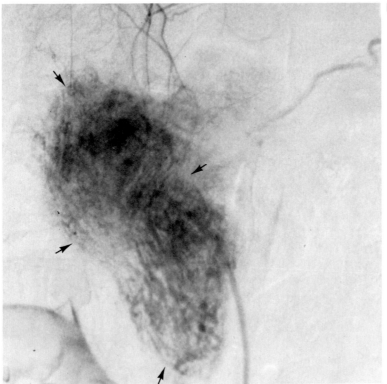

Fig. 3-28. Selective left maxillary angiogram in a patient with juvenile nasopharyngeal angiofibroma. Early arterial **(A)** and capillary phase **(B)** films demonstrate the highly vascular tumor **(small arrows).** The third or pterygopalatine portion of the maxillary artery is displaced anteriorly **(outlined arrow).**

A

B

dura and, more specifically, are considered to arise in this structure from the included arachnoid villi. Thus, incidence and sites of the tumors correspond roughly to the location and relative number of arachnoid villi along the dural sinuses. (The rare intraventricular meningioma probably arises from leptomeningeal rests that formed along with the developing tela choroidea and stroma of the choroid plexuses.[29])

Approximately 90% of all meningiomas are supratentorial. One-third to one-half are found in the parasagittal area, the single most frequent site. In decreasing order of approximate frequency they are found: adjacent to the convexity, sphenoid wing, olfactory groove, tuberculum sellae, petrous ridge, foramen magnum, middle fossa, torcular Herophili, falx, and ventricles.[15]

Meningiomas are most often detected in the middle decades of life. There is a higher incidence in women. These tumors are uncommon in childhood or adolescence, comprising only three to four percent of all intracranial neoplasms in this age group. Meningiomas detected within the first two decades of life are often in an unusual location (such as the posterior fossa or within the ventricles), are frequently associated with neurofibromatosis, and more often prove to be malignant.[21]

Initially a meningioma is supplied entirely by meningeal vessels. As it grows to involve the leptomeninges, it may acquire a dual blood supply by parasitizing adjacent cerebral vessels. Therefore, the central portion of the neoplasm is usually supplied by meningeal vessels while its periphery is vascularized by leptomeningeal branches of the anterior, middle, or posterior cerebral arteries. The rare intraventricular meningioma is supplied primarily by branches of the choroidal arteries (see Fig. 7-7).[24]

The angiographic appearance of a meningioma can often be readily diagnosed although other lesions such as Paget's disease or fibrous dysplasia may appear similar. A typical convexity meningioma is shown in Fig. 3-29. Here, an enlarged middle meningeal artery supplies the central portion of the neoplasm in a radial or "sunburst" pattern. The periphery or surface of the tumor is supplied by small branches of the middle cerebral artery. Dense, homogeneous contrast accumulation is typically seen late into the venous phase of the angiogram (Fig. 3-30), although meningiomas with rapid arteriovenous shunting and early draining veins are not uncommon.[10] Occasionally, a meningioma may appear to be completely avascular, particularly with nonselective, nonmagnification subtraction techniques.

Frontal meningiomas that originate from the cribriform plate, falx, or orbital roof often receive their dominant blood supply from the anterior falx artery which arises from the anterior ethmoidal branch of the ophthalmic artery (an ICA branch). The anterior falx artery may supply falx meningiomas as far posteriorly as the bregma. Hypertrophied dural perforating vessels from external carotid branches such as the superficial temporal artery may also supply frontal meningiomas.

Meningiomas that arise from structures at the base of the skull, such as the tuberculum sellae, planum sphenoidale, sphenoid ridge, or olfactory groove, may also receive their blood supply from both the ICA and ECA. Small meningeal branches from the accessory meningeal artery, anterior deep temporal artery, and branches of the pterygopalatine portion of the maxillary artery frequently supply meningiomas in these locations. Rarely, such tumors grow almost entirely extracranially (Fig. 3-31).

Meningiomas of the torcular herophili, posterior fossa, and occipital area often receive multiple vascular contributions (see Chapter 12). The major blood supply to the dura of the occiput and posterior fossa is usually derived from the posterior meningeal artery (a branch of the middle meningeal or ascending pharyngeal artery). In the presence of an occipital meningioma, this branch may become

(Text continues on p. 78)

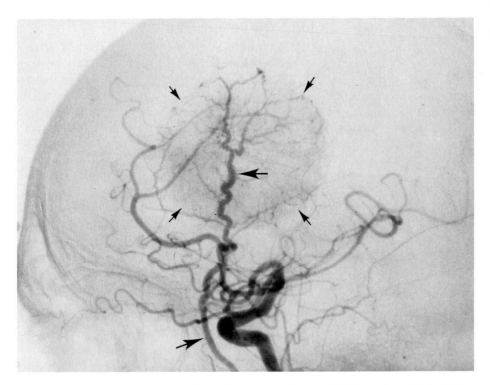

Fig. 3-29. Right common carotid angiogram (early arterial phase, lateral view). An enlarged middle meningeal artery **(large arrows)** supplies a large convexity meningioma **(small arrows).**

Fig. 3-30. Right internal carotid angiogram (venous phase, lateral view). A small falx meningioma is present. Note the prolonged vascular stain persisting into the venous phase of the angiogram **(arrows).**

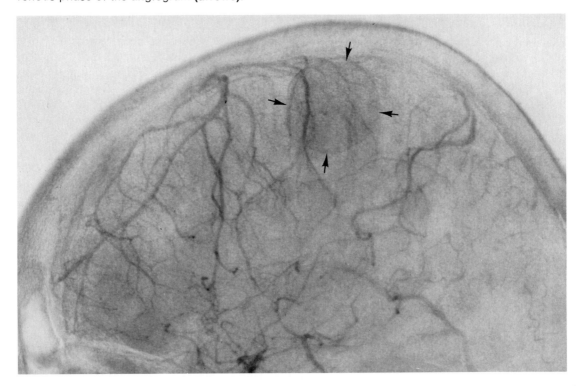

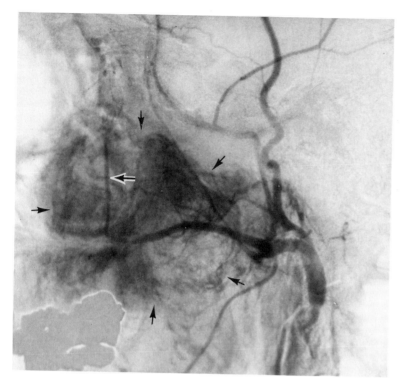

Fig. 3-31. Left external carotid angiogram (arterial phase, lateral view). A sphenoid wing meningioma **(small arrows)** that is almost entirely extracranial is present. Note anteroinferior displacement of the maxillary artery **(outlined arrow)**.

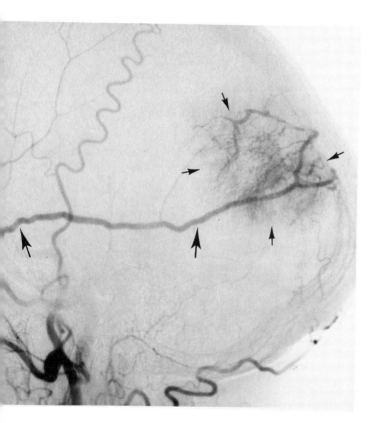

Fig. 3-32. Left external carotid angiogram (arterial phase, lateral view) of a large occipital meningioma that involved the torcular Herophili and the left transverse sinus. A markedly enlarged posterior branch of the middle meningeal artery supplies the lesion.

massively enlarged (Fig. 3-32). Other vessels often involved in supplying meningiomas in these locations are the anterior and posterior meningeal branches of the vertebral artery.

Miscellaneous Vascular Tumors. Although most carcinomas metastatic to the face and neck are avascular (see below), on occasion nonepidermoid metastases may show significant neovascularity. Carcinoma of the paranasal sinuses with intracranial extension may occasionally resemble meningioma on angiographic studies.[3]

Intracerebral tumors that invade the meninges may also acquire some external carotid blood supply. Meningeal invasion has been reported in a variety of both primary and secondary intracranial neoplasms including astrocytoma, melanoma, glioblastoma multiforme, disseminated metastatic carcinoma, medulloblastoma, sarcomas, and tumors of vascular origin. Cerebral angiograms in meningeal sarcomatosis and carcinomatosis may show no definite abnormality. Minimal peripheral vascular irregularities may be present along with varying degrees of narrowing of the major vessels at the base of the brain, particularly the supraclinoid portions of the ICA and the proximal portions of the anterior and middle cerebral arteries. Vascular supply from the ECA is rarely detected.

Occasionally, acoustic neurinomas will derive part or most of their blood supply from meningeal branches of the ECA, usually the middle meningeal or ascending pharyngeal arteries (Figs. 3-33A, B). The angiographic findings in such cases may be virtually indistinguishable from those of a cerebellopontine angle meningioma.[19, 34]

Orbital neoplasms are discussed in detail in Chapter 5. Spread of primarily intraorbital tumors such as hemangioma (Fig. 3-34) and rhabdomyosarcoma (Fig. 3-35) may parasitize vascular supply from the external carotid system.

Lesions of the thyroid gland (*i.e.,* diffuse goiter with thyrotoxicosis or benign adenoma) may, if sufficiently large, produce stretching and bowing of the inferior (a branch of the thyrocervical trunk) and superior thyroidal arteries. Occasionally a dense, rather homogeneous vascular stain may be present (Fig-3-36).

Non-neoplastic masses may occasionally involve the ECA and its branches, although vascularity in these lesions is usually sparse. Fibrous dysplasia, Paget's disease, and metastatic skull lesions may all acquire significant ECA supply (Fig. 3-37).

Avascular Carcinomas. Avascular tumors affecting the ECA are detected only if they encase or displace otherwise normal branches. Tumors usually displaying sparse or no abnormal vascularity include nasopharyngeal carcinomas, primary neurogenic tumors, most metastatic tumors, and clivus chordomas with nasopharyngeal extension.[2]

A typical avascular tumor is the squamous cell carcinoma (Fig. 3-38). This widely invasive mass has involved the floor of the mouth, the tonsils, and has extended posteriorly to involve the cervical lymph nodes and soft tissues of the posterior cervical triangle. Note the encasement, stretching, and draping of the lingual, facial, and occipital branches around the mass.

Arteritis

Involvement of the ECA in cranial arteritis is usually limited to abnormalities affecting the superficial temporal artery. The classic angiographic finding is the appearance of alternating areas of narrowing, beading, and dilatation.[23]

Collateral Blood Flow and the External Carotid Artery

With either occlusion or hemodynamically significant stenosis of the proximal ICA (see Chapter 4), branches of the ECA form an important source of potential collateral blood flow.

While a wide variety of ECA-ICA anastomoses can be identified, several patterns of collateral blood flow are more commonly seen.

(Text continues on p. 85)

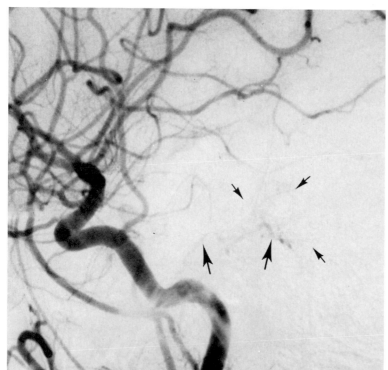

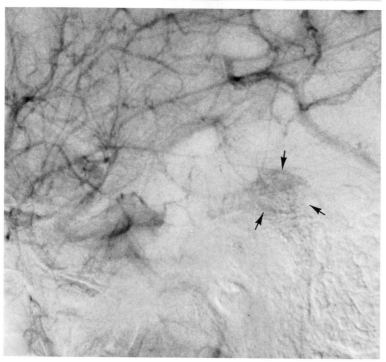

Fig. 3-33. Left common carotid angiogram (lateral view) of a large acoustic neurinoma. **A.** Mid-arterial phase. **B.** Late arterial phase. An enlarged dural branch **(large arrow)** from the external carotid artery supplies the lesion **(small arrows).**

A

B

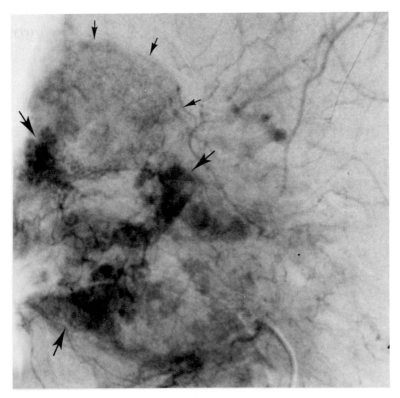

Fig. 3-34. Left common carotid angiograms in a 2-month-old child with a capillary or racemose hemangioma of the orbit **(small arrows)** and face **(large arrows)**. The lesion was supplied by the ophthalmic artery and branches of the external carotid artery.

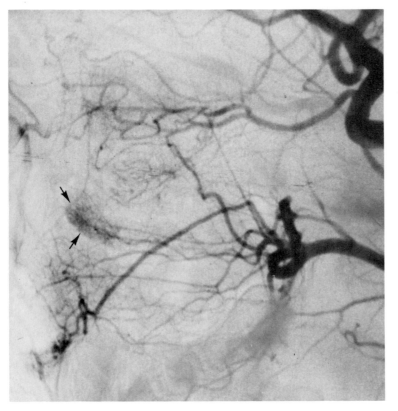

Fig. 3-35. Left common carotid angiogram in a 3-year-old boy with an orbital rhabdomyosarcoma. Enlarged branches of the sphenopalatine artery assist in supplying the tumor **(arrows).**

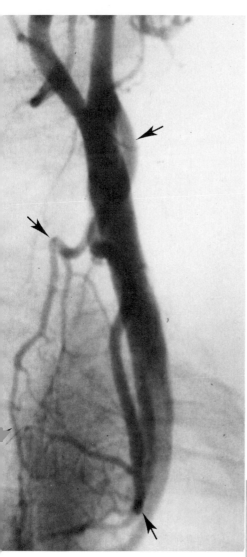

Fig. 3-36. Left common carotid angiogram (AP view) of a large thyroid adenoma. Hypertrophied superior thyroidal branches **(arrows)** of the ECA supply the vascular lesion.

Fig. 3-37. Selective left maxillary angiogram (AP view) of a fibrous dysplasia of the nasal turbinates. Note the sparse, abnormal vascularity **(arrows).**

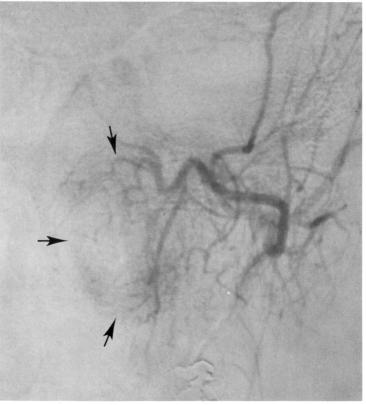

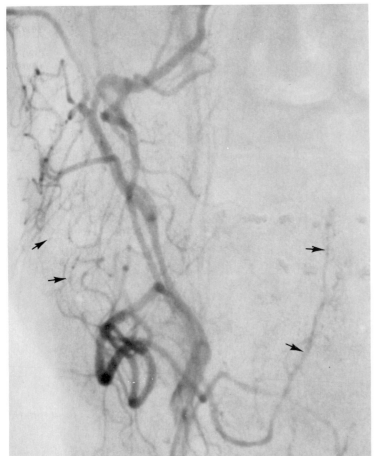

Fig. 3-38. Left common carotid angiogram (mid-arterial phase) of large cervical lymph node metastases from squamous cell carcinoma of the tonsils. **A.** AP view. **B.** Lateral view. The internal carotid artery is bowed posteriorly and branches of the lingual, facial, and occipital arteries **(arrows)** are stretched around the avascular mass. Note medial displacement of the distal lingual artery on the AP view.

A
B

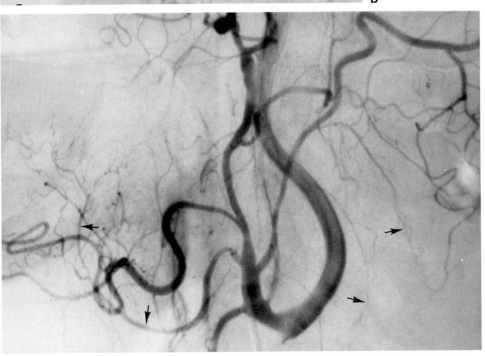

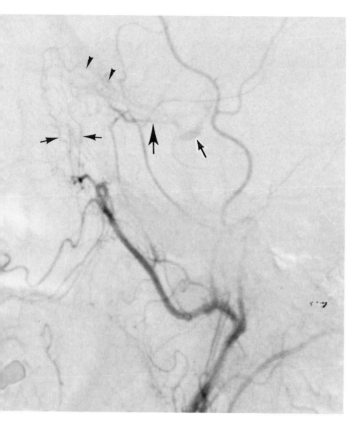

Fig. 3-39. Left common carotid angiogram (arterial phase, lateral view). Complete occlusion of the internal carotid artery is present. Ethmoidal branches **(small black arrows)** of the maxillary artery anastomose with ethmoidal branches of the ophthalmic artery **(arrowheads).** The internal carotid artery **(outlined arrow)** is opacified by retrograde flow through the ophthalmic artery **(large black arrow).**

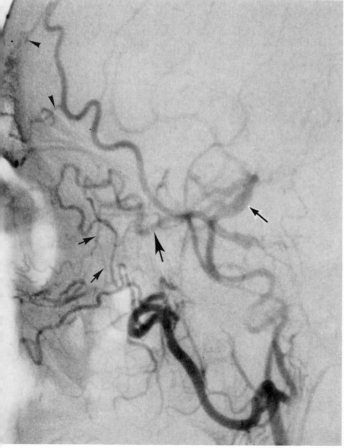

Fig. 3-40. Left common carotid angiogram (arterial phase, lateral view). The internal carotid artery was occluded at its origin. Collateral flow from the external carotid artery is provided by numerous anastomoses through the orbit. Anterior branches of the superficial temporal artery **(small arrowheads)** and ethmoidal branches of the maxillary artery **(small black arrows)** anastomose with orbital branches of the ophthalmic artery **(large black arrow).** The internal carotid artery **(outlined arrow)** is opacified by retrograde flow through the ophthalmic artery.

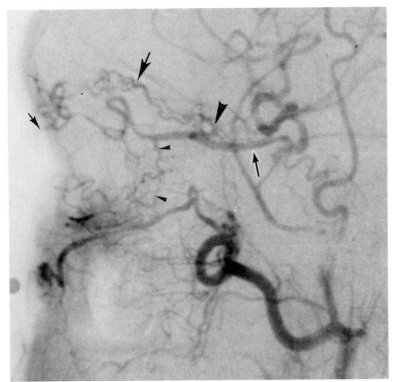

Fig. 3-41. Left common carotid angiogram (arterial phase, lateral view). The internal carotid artery is occluded. Orbital branches **(large black arrow)** of the ophthalmic artery **(outlined arrow)** are opacified by flow from the angular branch of the facial artery **(small black arrow),** ethmoidal branches of the maxillary artery **(small arrowheads),** and branches of the middle meningeal artery **(large arrowhead).**

Fig. 3-42. Right common carotid angiogram (late arterial phase, lateral view). The internal carotid artery is completely occluded. The carotid siphon **(large arrow)** has been reconstituted via collaterals to the artery of the cavernous sinus **(small arrows)** and the lacrimal branches of the ophthalmic artery **(outlined arrow).**

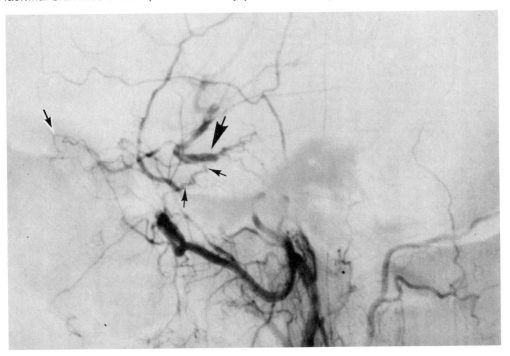

In the most frequent pattern (Figs. 3-39, 3-40), blood flows from the pterygopalatine branches of the maxillary artery to ethmoidal branches of the ophthalmic artery and then to the supraclinoid ICA.[2, 20, 22]

In another common pattern (Fig. 3-40), blood flows from the anterior branch of the superficial temporal artery and then to the carotid artery. Less commonly, anastomoses between branches of the middle meningeal artery and lacrimal branches of the ophthalmic artery may provide significant collateral flow. The angular branch of the facial artery is another source of potential ECA-ICA blood flow through its orbital anastomoses (Fig. 3-41). The artery of the foramen rotundum can also contribute collateral flow via its anastomoses with cavernous branches (inferolateral trunk) of the ICA (Fig. 3-42).

When collateral circulation is inadequate, surgical anastomosis of the superficial temporal artery to an opercular branch of the middle cerebral artery may provide an additional pathway for collateral blood flow (see Chapter 4).[14B, 16]

With basal telangiectasia (see Chapter 5) some collateral blood flow may be derived from anastomoses between numerous perforating meningeal branches of the ECA and ICA (Fig. 5-20).

REFERENCES

1. **Allen WE III, Kier EL, Rothman SLG:** The maxillary artery: normal arteriographic anatomy. Am J Roentgenol 118:517–527, 1973
2. **Allen WE III, Kier EL, Rothman SLG:** The maxillary artery in craniofacial pathology. Am J Roentgenol 121:124–138, 1974
2A. **Ahn HS, Kerber CW, Deeb ZL:** Extra- to intracranial arterial anastomoses in therapeutic embolization: Recognition and role. Am J Neuroradiol 1:71–75, 1980
3. **Banna M, Molot M, Grove J, Schatz S:** Tumor blush with intracranial extension of carcinoma of the paranasal sinuses. Neuroradiology 14:143–145, 1977
4. **Djindjian R, Merland J-J:** Super-selective Arteriography of the External Carotid Artery. New York, Springer-Verlag, 1978
5. **Duncan AW, Lack EE, Deek MF:** Radiological evaluation of paragangliomas of the head and neck. Radiology 132:99–105, 1979
5A. **Ericson K, Bergstrand G, Levander B:** Angiographic findings in subdural hematoma correlated with CT attenuation values. J Comp Asst Tomogr 3:789–794, 1979
6. **Ericson K, Hakansson S, Lofgren J et al:** Extravasation and arteriovenous shunting after epidural bleeding—a radiological study. Neuroradiology 17:239–244, 1979
6A. **Faria MA, Fleischer AS:** Dual cerebral and meningeal supply to giant arteriovenous malformations of the posterior cerebral hemisphere, J Neurosurg 52:153–161, 1980
7. **Gerlock AJ Jr:** Embolization of the external carotid artery in the treatment of carotid cavernous sinus fistulae. Clin Radiol 30:111–116, 1979

8. **Glenner GG, Grimley PM:** Tumors of the extraadrenal paraganglion system (including chemoreceptors). In Atlas of Tumor Pathology, 2nd series, Fascicle 9, p 41. Washington DC, Armed Forces Institute of Pathology, 1974
9. **Handel SF, Miller MH, Wallace S et al:** Angiographic observations on chemodectomas of the head and neck. Am J Roentgenol 129:447–480, 1977
9A. **Jafek BW, Krekorian EA, Kirsch WM et al:** Juvenile nasopharyngeal angiofibroma: Management of intracranial extension. Head and Neck Surg 2:119–128, 1979
10. **Kieffer SA, Larson DA, Gold LHA et al:** Rapid circulation in intracranial meningiomas. Radiology 106:575–580, 1973
11. **Lasjaunias P, Berenstein D, Doyon D:** Normal functional anatomy of the facial artery for superselective angiography. Radiology 133:631–638 (1979)
11A. **Lasjaunias P, Manelfe C:** Arterial supply for the upper cervical nerves and the cervicocarotid anastomotic channels. Neuroradiol 18:125–131, 1979
11B. **Lasjaunias P, Manelfe C et al:** Lower cranial and upper cervical nerves: Radioanatomy and pathological angiographic aspects. Presented at the American Society of Neuroradiology, 18th Annual Meeting, Los Angeles, California, Mar 16–21, 1980
12. **Lasjaunias P, Moret J:** The ascending pharyngeal artery: normal and pathological radioanatomy. Neuroradiology 11:77–82, 1976
13. **Lasjaunias P, Moret J:** Hyperselective angiography in the study of the nasopharynx. J Neuroradiol 5:103–112, 1978

14. **Lasjaunias P, Théron J, Moret J:** The occipital artery. Neuroradiology 15:31–37, 1978

14A. **Lasjaunias P:** Therapeutic embolization of juvenile nasopharyngeal angiofibroma. Radiology, 1980 (in press)

14B. **Latchaw RE, Ausman JI, Lee MC:** Superficial temporal-middle cerebral artery bypass. J Neurosurg 51:455–465, 1979

15. **Lee KF, Lin SR, Whiteley WH et al:** Angiographic findings in recurrent meningioma. Radiology 119:131–139, 1976

16. **Lee MC, Ausman JI, Geiger JD et al:** Superficial temporal to middle cerebral artery anastomosis. Arch Neurol 36:1–4, 1979

17. **Lobato RD, Escudero L, Lamas E:** Bilateral dural arteriovenous fistula in the region of the cavernous sinus. Neuroradiology 15:39–43, 1978

18. **Lotz PR, Bogdasarian RS, Thompson NW et al:** Paragangliomas of the head, neck, urinary bladder, and pelvis in a hypertensive woman. Am J Roentgenol 132:1001–1004, 1979

19. **Moscow NP, Newton TH:** Angiographic features of hypervascular neurinomas of the head and neck. Radiology 114:635–640, 1975

20. **Margolis MT, Newton TH:** Collateral pathways between the cavernous portion of the internal carotid and external carotid arteries. Radiology 93:834–836, 1969

20A. **Marsman JWP:** Tumors of the glomus jugulare complex (chemodectomas) demonstrated by cranial computed tomography. J Comp Asst Tomogr 3:795–799, 1979

21. **Merten DF, Gooding CA, Newton TH et al:** Meningiomas of childhood and adolescence. J Pediatr 84:696–700, 1974

22. **Mishkin MM, Schreiber MN:** Collateral circulation. In Newton TH, Potts DG (eds): Radiology of the Skull and Brain, Vol 2, pp 2344–2374. St. Louis, CV Mosby, 1974

23. **Moncada R, Baker D, Rubeinstein H et al:** Selective temporal arteriography and biopsy in giant cell arteritis: polymyalgia rheumatica. Am J Roentgenol 122:580–585, 1974

24. **Newton TH:** The abnormal external carotid artery. In Newton TH, Potts DG (eds): Radiology of the Skull and Brain, Vol 2, pp 1275–1332. St. Louis, CV Mosby, 1974

25. **Osborn AG:** The nasal arteries. Am J Roentgenol 130:89–97, 1978

26. **Osborn AG:** Computed tomography in neurologic diagnosis. Ann Rev Med 30:189–198, 1979

27. **Osborn AG:** Radiology of the pterygoid plates and pterygopalatine fossa. Am J Roentgenol 132:389–394, 1979

27A. **Osborn AG:** The vidian artery: Normal and pathologic anatomy. Radiology, 1980 (in press)

28. **Peeters FLM Kröger R:** Dural and direct cavernous sinus fistulas. Am J Roentgenol 132:599–606, 1979

28A. **Roberson GH, Reardon EJ:** Angiography and embolization of the internal maxillary artery for posterior epistaxis. Arch Otolaryngol 105:333–337, 1979

29. **Russell DS, Rubenstein LJ:** Pathology of Tumors of the Nervous System, pp 48–65. Baltimore, Williams & Wilkins, 1972

30. **Salamon G, Fauré J, Raybaud C et al:** The external carotid artery. I. Normal external carotid artery. In Newton TH, Potts DG (eds): Radiology of the Skull and Brain, Vol 2, pp 1246–1274. St. Louis, CV Mosby, 1974

31. **Schechter MM, Gutstein RA:** Aneurysms and arteriovenous fistulas of the superficial temporal vessels. Radiology 97:549–557, 1970

32. **Shaffer K, Haughton V, Farley G et al:** Pitfalls in the radiographic diagnosis of angiofibroma. Radiology 127:425–428, 1978

33. **Sinha PP, Aziz HI:** Juvenile nasopharyngeal angiofibroma. Radiology 127:501–505, 1978

34. **Theron J, Lasjaunias P:** Participation of the external and internal carotid arteries in the blood supply of acoustic neurinomas. Radiology 118:83–88, 1976

35. **Wilson GH, Hanafee WN:** Angiographic findings in 16 patients with juvenile nasopharyngeal angiofibroma. Radiology 92:279–284, 1969

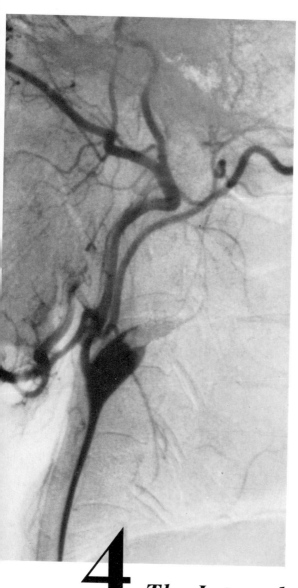

4 The Internal Carotid Artery: Cervical and Petrous Portions

The paired internal carotid arteries, two of the four major arteries supplying the brain, provide most of the blood flow to the frontal, temporal, and parietal lobes. Small branches of these vessels also supply many important structures at the base of the brain.

Because of its important vascular distribution, and its susceptibility to atherosclerotic vascular disease and other abnormalities, the normal and pathological cervical and petrous portions of the internal carotid artery (ICA) will first be carefully studied. A consideration of the cavernous and supraclinoid segments of the ICA begins in Chapter 5.

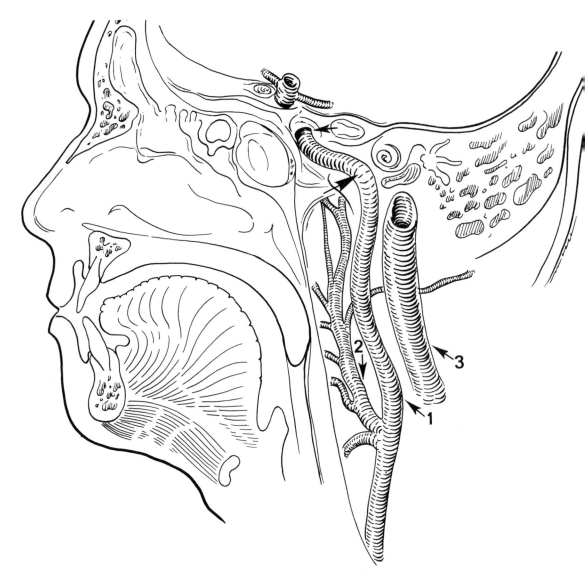

Fig. 4-1. Diagrammatic sketch of the internal carotid artery (ICA) and its adjacent structures. The petrous temporal bone has been dissected to show the entire course of the ICA. The ICA **(1)** initially lies posterolateral to the external carotid artery **(2)** and anterior to the internal jugular vein **(3).** The carotid genu **(large black arrow)** is just in front of the cochlea. The ICA exits from the carotid canal near the petrous apex where it enters the cavernous sinus **(small black arrow).**

Fig. 4-2. Diagrammatic sketch of the petrous ICA and its branches. The inconstant caroticotympanic branch **(1)** arises from the superior aspect of the genu. Small periosteal branches **(2)** are also present. A vidian artery **(3)** is shown arising from the inferior aspect of the petrous ICA, as it does in nearly 30% of all cases. It passes through the foramen lacerum. Branches to the oropharynx anastomose with branches of the ascending pharyngeal **(4)** and accessory meningeal **(5)** arteries. These in turn anastomose with branches of the descending **(6)** and ascending **(7)** palatine arteries. The latter is a branch of the facial artery. The vidian artery may terminate in the oropharynx or continue anteriorly as the artery of the pterygoid canal **(outlined arrows).**

NORMAL GROSS AND ANGIOGRAPHIC ANATOMY OF THE CERVICAL AND PETROUS INTERNAL CAROTID ARTERY

Gross Anatomy

The internal carotid artery normally originates from the common carotid artery at the C3–C4 or C4–C5 level. The left common carotid bifurcation is higher than the right in 50% while the right bifurcation is higher in 22% of all cases.[27] The ICA runs cephalad deep to the sternomastoid muscle in a neurovascular bundle together with the internal jugular vein and vagus nerve. The internal jugular vein lies lateral to the ICA while the vagus nerve courses between these two vessels.

The ICA initially lies posterolateral to the external carotid artery (ECA) (Figs. 3-1, 4-1). As the cervical ICA ascends, it usually courses medial to the main trunk of the ECA. The extracranial or cervical component terminates as the ICA enters the carotid canal of the petrous temporal bone just anterior to the jugular foramen.

There are two segments to the petrous portion of the ICA: a vertical or ascending segment and a horizontal segment. Initially the ICA ascends anterior to the jugular fossa and lies just behind the Eustachian tube. The horizontal segment begins where the ICA turns anteromedially in front of the tympanic cavity and cochlea (Fig. 4-1). Here, dura or a thin plate of bone separates the carotid artery from the middle ear structures as well as the Gasserian ganglion.[21] Then, the ICA sometimes courses slightly inferiorly, emerging from the carotid canal near the apex of the petrous temporal bone by crossing over the cranial part of the foramen lacerum and passing into the cavernous sinus.

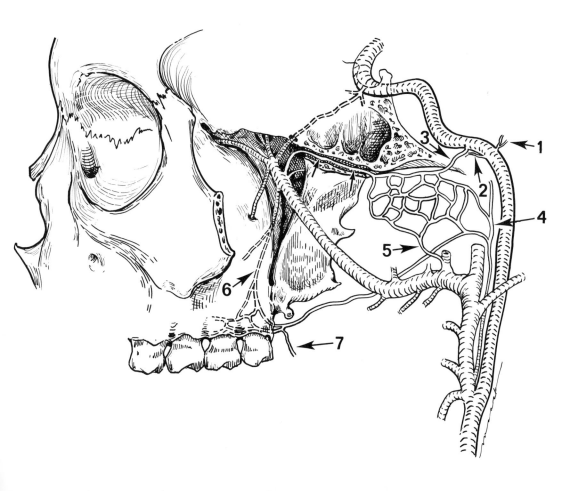

Cervical Branches. No named branches arise from the cervical portion of a normal ICA although numerous authors have reported anomalous origins of a variety of other vessels from the extracranial ICA (see below).

Intrapetrous Carotid Artery Branches have recently been identified in 23% of normal carotid angiograms and 38% of neurosurgical dissections.[22] The most frequently identified branch arising from the petrous segment of the ICA is the **vidian artery**, also termed the artery of the pterygoid canal.[22] This vessel usually arises from the maxillary artery (an ECA branch) within the pterygopalatine fossa and courses above the nasopharynx at the base of the pterygoid plates.[15] However, the vidian artery originates from the petrous ICA in one-quarter to one-third of all cases and contributes to vascular anastomoses within the mucosa of the posterosuperior nasopharynx. The vidian artery may also continue anteriorly as the artery of the pterygoid canal to anastomose with small branches of the maxillary artery within the pterygomaxillary fissure and pterygopalatine fossa (Fig. 4-2).[20A, 21A] The **caroticotympanic artery** is a small branch that arises from the ICA near its genu and passes superiorly to supply the tympanic cavity (Fig. 4-2). The caroticotympanic artery is not usually identified unless it supplies a glomus tympanicum tumor or is seen as part of a persistent stapedial artery, a rare anomaly.[10, 16] Small **periosteal branches** arise from the anteroinferior portion of the horizontal ICA and may occasionally be visualized on normal angiographic studies.

Radiographic Anatomy

Although the cervical ICA is relatively constant in diameter throughout its course (Fig. 4-3), it may normally have a slight bulbous dilatation called the **carotid sinus** at its origin (Fig. 4-4). Usually the proximal portion of the ICA initially lies posterolateral to the ECA, then ascends, running medial to the ECA (Fig. 4-4A). Normally the cervical ICA has no angiographically identifiable branches.

As it enters the carotid canal the ICA ascends for approximately 1 cm, then angles

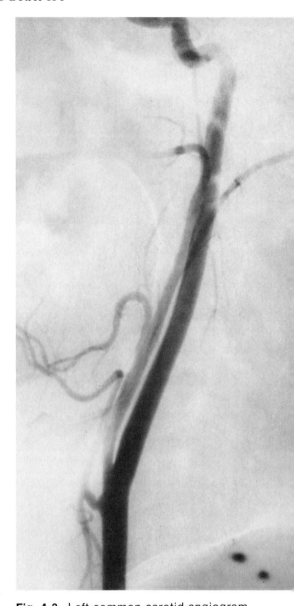

Fig. 4-3. Left common carotid angiogram (mid-arterial phase, lateral view). The course as well as caliber of the internal carotid artery is normal. A low bifurcation is present (adjacent to C5).

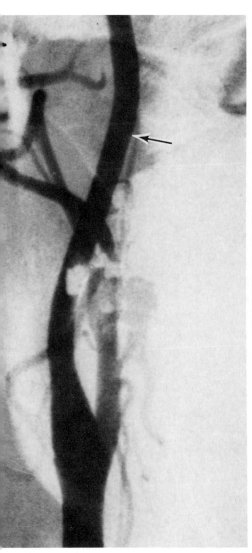 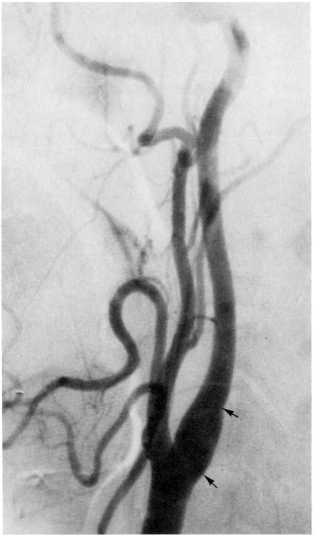

A B

Fig. 4-4. Normal common carotid angiogram, AP **(A)** and lateral **(B)** views. A slight dilatation at the origin of the internal carotid artery represents the carotid bulb **(B, black arrows).** Note that as the ICA ascends, it initially lies lateral to the external carotid artery but then crosses medially **(A, outlined arrows).**

sharply forward as it courses anteromedially toward the apex of the petrous temporal bone (Fig. 4-4B). The petrous ICA branches are small and are seen only in a minority of magnification-subtraction angiograms.[20A, 21A]

Normal Variants and Anomalies of the Cervical and Petrous Internal Carotid Artery

Rarely, the ECA and ICA arise from the aortic arch as separate branches.[3] Although the normal common carotid artery bifurcation is usually near the level of the upper border of the thyroid cartilage (about the C4 level), it can be as high as the arch of C1 or as low as the body of T2 (Fig. 4-3). Initially, the proximal ICA may course medial to the ECA instead of following its usual posterolateral course (Fig. 4-5), a configuration found in six percent of left common carotid angiograms and 18% of right-sided studies.[1]

Tortuousity or Kinking of the Cervical ICA is common in both young children and older adults. While a tortuous ICA is usually without clinical significance it may cause cranial nerve impairment on occasion.[5, 25, 31] Coiling of the cervical ICA occurs in 5 to 15% of patients in unselected angiographic series and is thought to be at least partially developmental, unrelated to either age or hypertension (Fig. 4-6).[31]

Congenital Absence of the ICA is a very rare anomaly.[6] Only 29 cases of total unilateral and seven cases of complete bilateral absence of the ICA have been reported.[26] An abnormally high percentage of these cases has been associated with intracranial aneurysms. In cases of ICA atresia, a portion of the vessel often remains; the terminal (intracranial) segment may fail to develop or the ICA may be aplastic up to its cavernous portion. In the latter instance, the siphon is the only part that develops.[17]

Hypoplasia of the ICA has been reported both as an isolated anomaly and in conjunction with anencephaly, neurofibromatosis, and basal telangiectasia. Diffuse narrowing of the ICA associated with arteritis, dissecting aneurysm, tubular fibromuscular dysplasia, or segmental stenosis with reduced flow should not be confused with hypoplasia (see below).[11] In developmental hypoplasia or aplasia tomograms of the petrous temporal bone will demonstrate a small or absent carotid canal.

Anomalous Branches occasionally arise from the cervical ICA. **Inferior** and **ascending pharyngeal, vidian** and **occipital arteries** have been described as originating from the cervical ICA.[17, 30] Other anomalous branches that may arise from the ICA are the various persistent

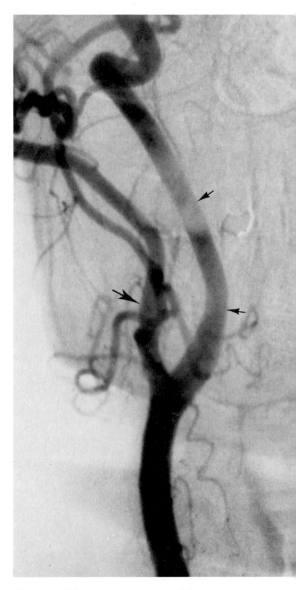

Fig. 4-5. Right common carotid angiogram (arterial phase, AP view). The ICA **(small black arrows)** arises medial to the ECA **(large black arrow).**

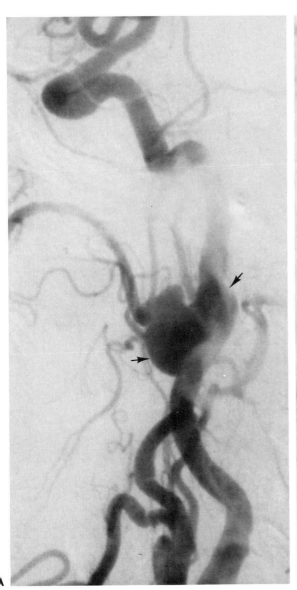

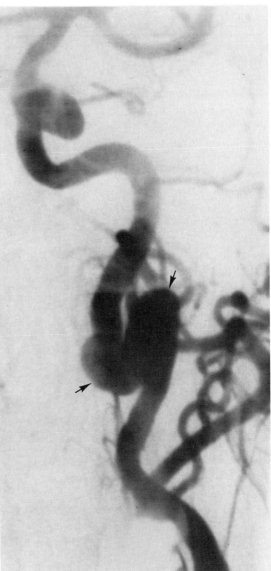

Fig. 4-6. Left common carotid angiogram (arterial phase). Lateral **(A)** and AP **(B)** views demonstrate a very tortuous, redundant ICA. The ICA forms almost a complete loop **(arrows).** On a single view, this could be mistaken for a cervical aneurysm.

embryonic carotid-basilar anastomoses. A **persistent proatlantal intersegmental artery** originates from the cervical ICA (rarely from the ECA) and courses posterosuperiorly to rest on the transverse process of the atlas (Fig. 4-7). It then pursues a characteristic horizontal suboccipital course to enter the foramen magnum and anastomose with the ipsilateral vertebral artery.[1, 29] A **persistent hypoglossal artery,** another type of residual embryonic anastomosis, connects the cervical ICA to the basilar artery (see Fig. 6-13).

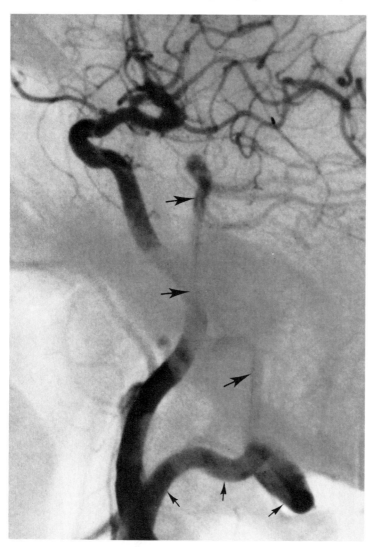

Fig. 4-7. Left common carotid angiogram (arterial phase, lateral view). A proatlantal intersegmental artery **(small arrows)** arises from the cervical ICA. Note filling of the basilar artery system **(large arrows).** *(Anderson RE, Sondheimer FK: Neuroradiology 11:113–118, 1976)*

The **persistent stapedial artery** is a rare variant that represents a continuation of the primitive hyoid branch of the ICA and presents as a branch of the petrous ICA. The stapedial artery runs superiorly where it courses through the obturator foramen of the stapes.[2] It passes anteriorly for a short distance within the facial canal and enters the middle cranial fossa through a bony foramen along the anterior aspect of the petrous bone. It terminates as the middle meningeal artery.[10]

A rare but clinically important anomaly is the **aberrant petrous ICA.** Here, the ICA traverses the middle ear cavity and presents as a retro-tympanic pulsatile mass. As an ancillary finding all the external carotid branches arise from a single vessel that passes superiorly from the aortic arch to the petrous canal. No carotid bifurcation is present. The ICA then enters the temporal bone posterior to the external auditory meatus, ascending between the facial canal and the jugular bulb. Entering the middle ear fossa, the ICA is sharply angulated anteriorly (Figs. 4-8A, B). Tomography in these cases discloses an absent vertical portion of the carotid canal. The soft tissue outline of the aberrant ICA may be identified within the middle ear cavity. Clinically, an

(Text continues on p. 96)

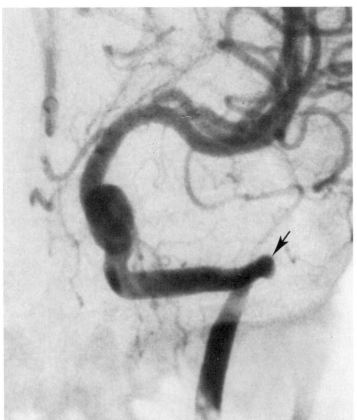

Fig. 4-8. Left internal carotid angiogram (arterial phase). AP **(A)** and lateral **(B)** views demonstrate an aberrant ICA. Note the more lateral course of the ICA and its sharp anterior angulation **(arrow)** in the middle ear cavity. Its petrous portion appears elongated.

A
B

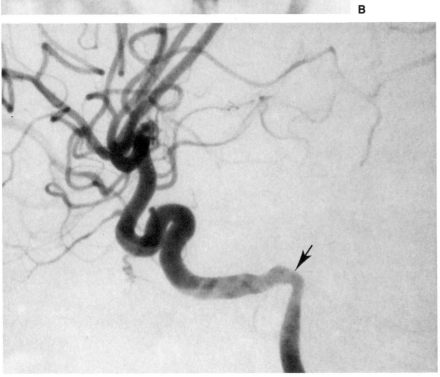

aberrant carotid artery can simulate a glomus tympanicum tumor (paraganglioma). Such cases have resulted in sudden, fatal hemorrhage if surgery is performed without preoperative angiography.[8, 14, 28]

ABNORMALITIES OF THE CERVICAL AND PETROUS INTERNAL CAROTID ARTERY

Atherosclerosis

The common carotid artery bifurcation and the proximal portion of the ICA are the most common sites of significant atherosclerotic disease involving the aortic arch and its branches. As with atherosclerotic disease elsewhere, the affected carotid artery may appear elongated, narrowed, or ulcerated (Figs. 4-9, 4-10, 4-11). While irregular contours are frequently associated with mural thrombus or intimal ulceration, they may also represent smooth cul de sacs within fibrotic plaques or intramural hemorrhage and subintimal hematoma. Some frank ulcers also occur in smooth, benign-appearing plaques and are too small to be detected by angiography.[6A, 7]

Recent evidence indicates that carotid plaques usually begin as areas of fibrointimal thickening and evolve to their symptomatic stages when they are altered by supervening events such as intraplaque hemorrhage.[12] Severe involvement may progress to complete occlusion of the proximal ICA (see Fig. 3-6). The differentiation between a completely occluded ICA and a very tightly stenotic one is an important clinical distinction since, with some exceptions,[4, 13] total carotid occlusion is generally considered a contraindication to surgery. If even a slight trickle of antegrade flow is present and the vessel patent, endarterectomy remains a consideration.

The patterns of extracranial to intracranial collateral blood flow occurring with hemodynamically significant ICA stenosis are described in Chapter 3. Intracranial sources of collateral flow are discussed in Chapters 6 and 9.

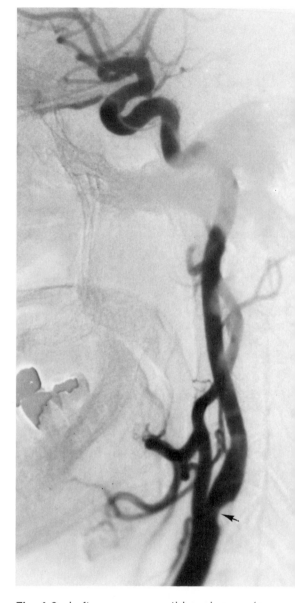

Fig. 4-9. Left common carotid angiogram (arterial phase, lateral view). A smooth, non-hemodynamically significant plaque **(arrow)** is present on the posterior wall of the ICA at its origin.

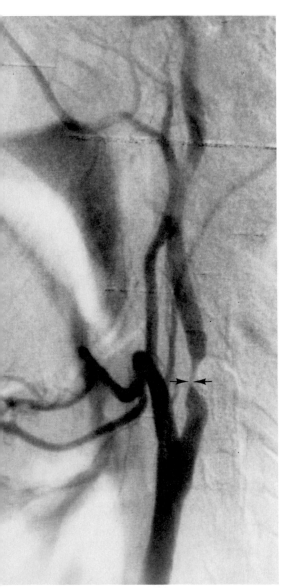

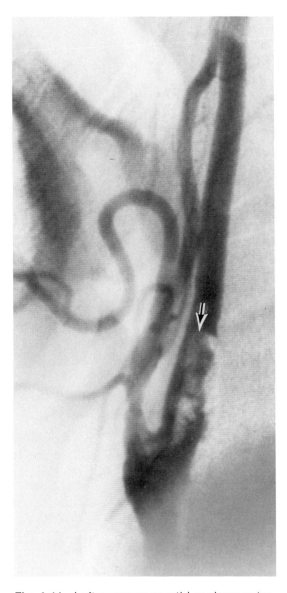

Fig. 4-10. Left common carotid angiogram (arterial phase, lateral view). The ICA is almost occluded by atheromatous plaque. The lumen is reduced to a threadlike opening **(arrows),** but some antegrade blood flow is present and the vessel remains patent.

Fig. 4-11. Left common carotid angiogram (arterial phase, lateral view). An irregular, ulcerated plaque involves both the ECA and ICA. An intraluminal thrombus **(arrow)** is present at the site of ICA stenosis. At surgery, fresh hemorrhage was present in the plaque and presence of an intraluminal thrombus documented.

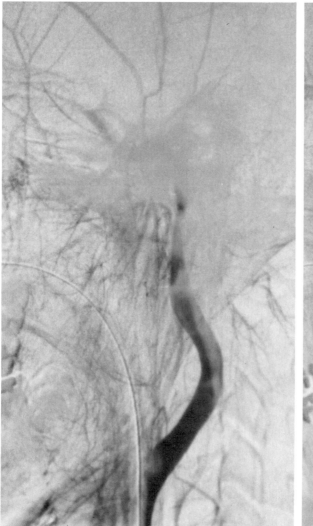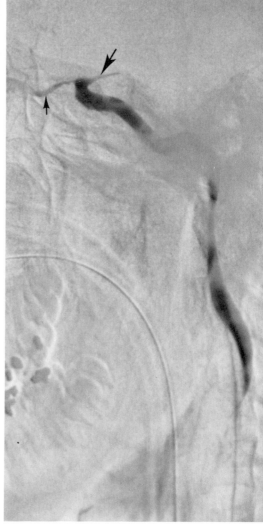

A B

Fig. 4-12. Left common carotid angiogram (lateral view) depicting clinical and angiographic evidence of brain death. Films obtained at 6 seconds **(A)** and 24 seconds **(B)** following contrast injection show contrast stasis in the ICA with no filling of the intracranial vessels **(large arrow)**. Some flow through the ophthalmic artery **(small arrow)** is present.

Non-atheromatous Stenosis

Occlusion of the cervical ICA has been reported in association with a variety of non-atheromatous disease processes.[19] Cerebral circulatory arrest from increased intracranial pressure, fibromuscular dysplasia, arteritis, blunt trauma, arterial thrombosis, and invasive neoplasms of the neck may cause stenosis or occlusion of the proximal ICA.

Narrowing or occlusion of the cervical ICA may occur when the cerebral perfusion pressure falls to zero secondary to markedly increased intracranial pressure.

Cerebral Circulatory Arrest ("brain death") is documented angiographically either by selective common carotid and vertebral studies or by using the aortocervical technique (aortic arch injection with simultaneous filming over the head). Non-filling of the cerebral vessels with prolonged stasis of contrast in the carotid artery is present (Fig. 4-12). On occasion, the contrast may disappear from the ICA through the ophthalmic artery. It should be noted that selective pressure injection into the ICA itself in such cases may produce some artifactual filling of the intracranial arteries.[23]

Fibromuscular Dysplasia (FMD) is a non-atheromatous angiopathy of unknown etiology that has been identified in a number of small and medium-sized arteries. Originally thought to affect the cephalic vessels only rarely, FMD is now recognized as one of the most common non-atheromatous conditions producing irregularities and dilatation of the cervical ICA.[11] Cervical FMD is bilateral in approximately 65% of all cases. Nearly a third of all cases are associated with intracranial aneurysm. Formerly regarded as primarily an incidental angiographic finding, current studies indicate that many patients with FMD present with significant clinical symptomatology.[20] The symptoms are usually those of transient ischemic attacks, actual cerebral infarction, or subarachnoid hemorrhage from a co-existing aneurysm.

The lesions of cervical FMD are located in the mid-portion of the internal carotid or vertebral artery adjacent to the first and second cervical vertebrae. Characteristically, changes of FMD extend from the C1 or C2 level to the entrance of the ICA into the petrous carotid canal. Rarely does FMD involve the petrous or cavernous ICA. The common carotid bifurcation and proximal ICA are spared in nearly all cases.

The most common angiographic appearance of FMD is the so-called "string of beads" pattern created by multiple arterial dilatations separated by irregularly spaced concentric stenosis (Fig. 4-13). A less common appearance is unifocal or multiple smooth concentric tubular stenoses (Fig. 4-14). Rarely the arterial dilatations associated with FMD progress to actual pseudoaneurysm formation (Fig. 4-15).

While the "string of beads" appearance is quite characteristic of FMD and is usually associated with medial fibroplasia, the angiographic differential diagnosis includes circular spastic contractions of the extracranial carotid and vertebral arteries (Fig. 4-16). In this latter entity, the constrictions are more regular, evenly spaced, and occur without the dilatation of intervening segments so typical of FMD. They are probably related to vascular irritation produced by the catheterization and subsequent injection of contrast or may occur when contrast is injected into a vessel with reduced distal run-off.

The angiographic findings with tubular FMD are less specific. The differential diagnosis includes arterial hypoplasia, arteritis (see below), diminished vessel caliber secondary to decreased distal blood flow (Fig. 4-12), and vascular spasm from the catheterization itself. Rarely atherosclerosis and dissecting or traumatic aneurysm mimic FMD.

Arteritis of various types may produce stenosis or progressive obliteration of the cervical ICA. While Takayasu's and other arteritides involving the aortic arch and its major branches usually affect the origins and proximal segments of these vessels (see Fig. 2-18), the angiographic appearance of arteritis may, on occasion, be indistinguishable from tubular FMD or arterial hypoplasia.

Trauma to the cervical ICA may result in thrombosis, stenosis or occlusion, or aneurysm formation. The ICA is relatively unprotected in its cervical course and is therefore vulnerable to traumatic injury from a variety of causes. Blunt, intraoral, or penetrating trauma to the ICA may result in thrombosis (Fig. 4-17), intimal tears, dissection, stenosis or occlusion, arteriovenous fistula (Fig. 4-18), or false aneurysm.[28A] Sudden deceleration or hyperextension injury produces strong shearing forces at the point where the

(Text continues on p. 106)

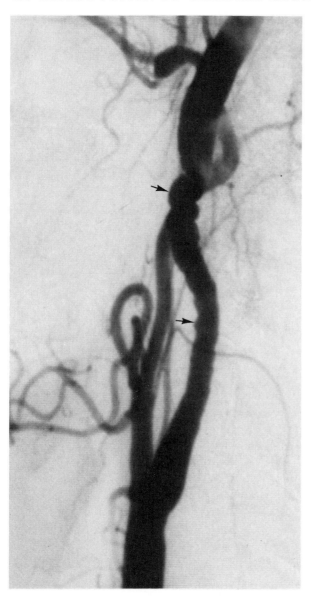

Fig. 4-13. Left common carotid angiogram (arterial phase, lateral view) of fibromuscular dysplasia (FMD). The ICA has alternating areas of dilatation and stenosis that produce a "string of beads" appearance **(arrows),** the classical angiographic appearance of FMD. Note sparing of the carotid bifurcation, a characteristic finding. *(Osborn AG, Anderson RE: Angiographic spectrum of cephalocervical fibromuscular dysplasia. Stroke 8:617–626, 1977. By permission of the American Heart Association, Inc.)*

Fig. 4-14. Left common carotid angiogram (arterial phase, lateral view) of surgically documented FMD. The entire cervical ICA shows diffuse, tubular narrowing **(arrows)** extending from just beyond the carotid bulb to the petrous canal. This angiographic appearance is indistinguishable from other arteridites. *(Osborn AG, Anderson RE: Angiographic spectrum of cephalocervical fibromuscular dysplasia. Stroke 8:617–626, 1977. By permission of the American Heart Association, Inc.)*

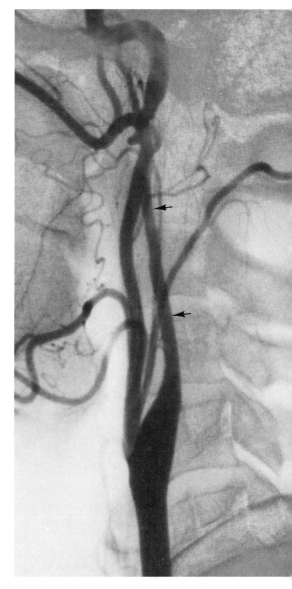

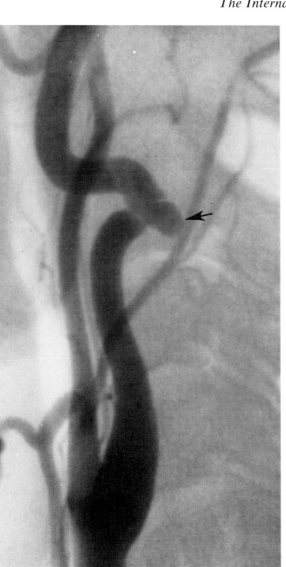

Fig. 4-15. Common carotid angiogram (arterial phase, lateral view) of documented FMD. A pseudoaneurysm is present **(arrows)** and was removed surgically. Again, the location adjacent to C2 is characteristic. *(Osborn AG, Anderson RE: Angiographic spectrum of cephalocervical fibromuscular dysplasia. Stroke 8:617–626, 1977. By permission of the American Heart Association, Inc.)*

Fig. 4-16. Left common carotid angiogram (arterial phase, lateral view). The multiple smooth, symmetrical, regularly spaced constrictions **(arrows)** represent arterial circular spastic contractions. *(Osborn AG, Anderson RE: Angiographic spectrum of cephalocervical fibromuscular dysplasia. Stroke 8:617–626, 1977. By permission of the American Heart Association, Inc.)*

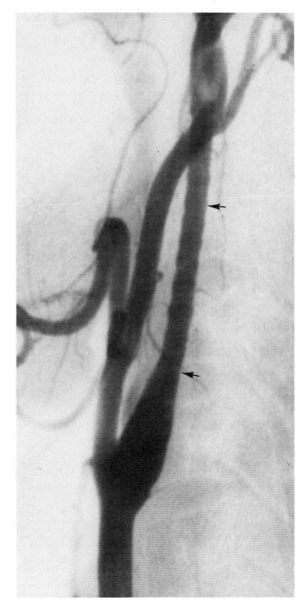

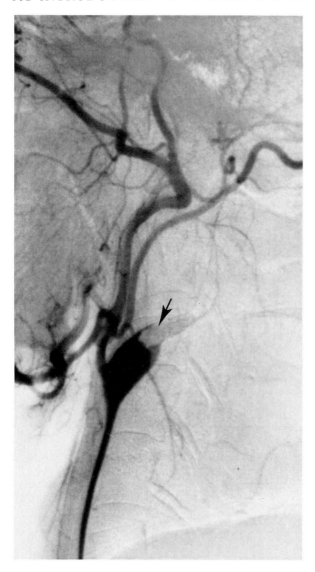

Fig. 4-17. Left common carotid angiogram (late arterial phase, lateral view) of blunt trauma to the neck. A thrombus is present in the ICA **(arrows).**

Fig. 4-18. Left internal carotid angiogram (early arterial phase) of deceleration injury and a traumatic arteriovenous fistula. The ICA has been occluded at its entrance into the petrous carotid canal **(large arrow)** where it communicates with a markedly dilated inferior petrosal sinus **(small arrows).** Retrograde filling of the basilar venous plexus and cavernous sinus is present.

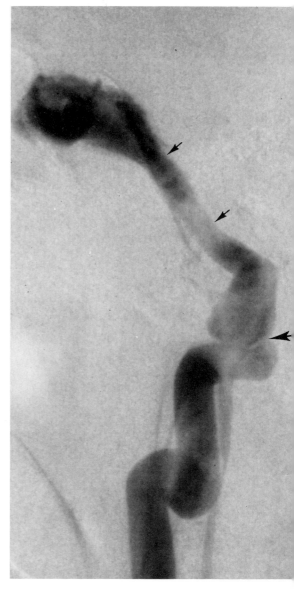

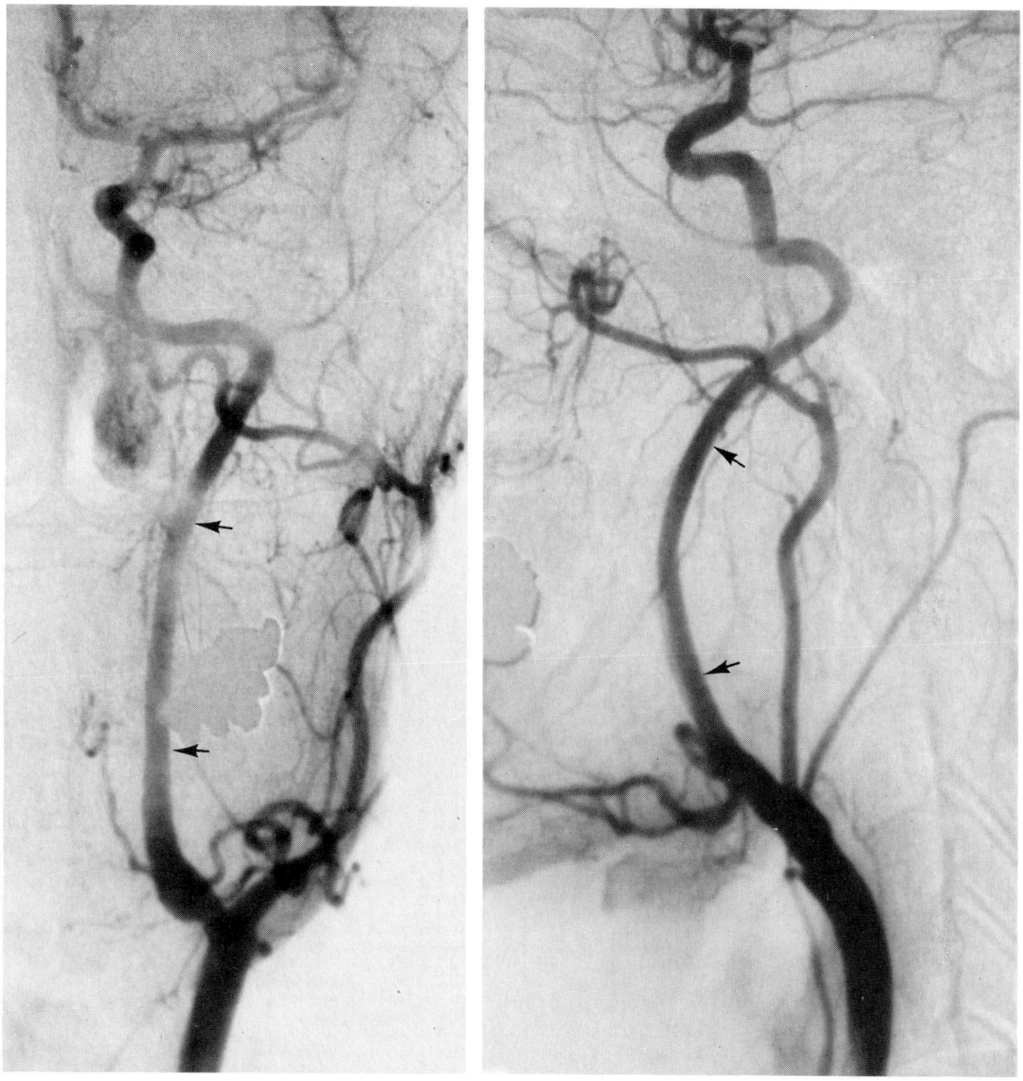

A B

Fig. 4-19. Left common carotid angiogram (arterial phase) of a huge chondrosarcoma arising from the skull base. AP **(A)** and lateral **(B)** views. The ICA is stretched and bowed **(arrows)** around a large avascular cervical mass.

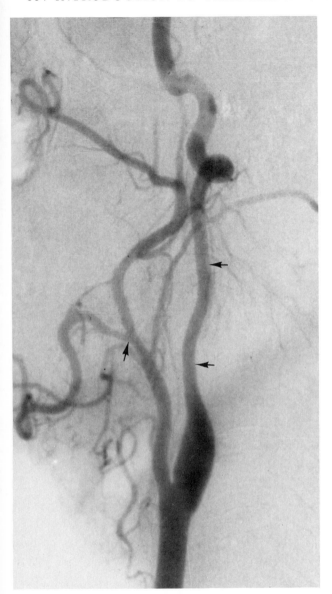

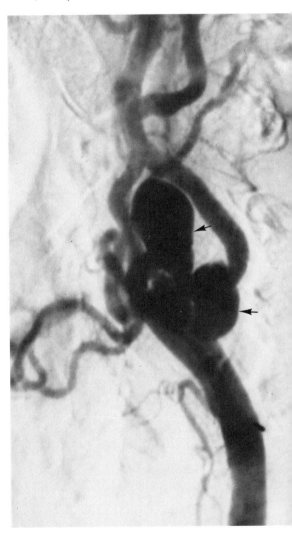

Fig. 4-21. Left common carotid angiogram (arterial phase, oblique view) in a hypertensive patient with a cloverleaf-shaped pseudoaneurysm **(arrows)** of the ICA. *(Courtesy of B. McIff, M.D.)*

Fig. 4-20. Left common carotid angiogram (arterial phase, lateral view) of a squamous cell carcinoma. The cervical ICA is encased and narrowed as are segments of the ECA **(arrows).**

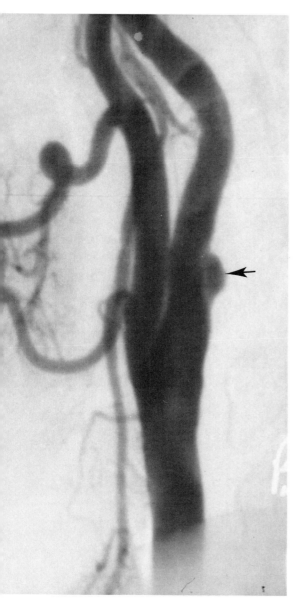

Fig. 4-22. Left common carotid angiogram (arterial phase, lateral view) in a patient who had had a previous arteriogram performed by direct puncture. A small aneurysm **(arrow)** is present at the previous puncture site.

Fig. 4-23. Right common carotid angiogram (arterial phase, AP view) of an anterior communicating artery aneurysm **(small black arrow).** During a previous angiogram, the guidewire produced subintimal dissection of the ICA. The subintimal flap is no longer apparent but a post-traumatic pseudoaneurysm **(large arrow)** has been formed.

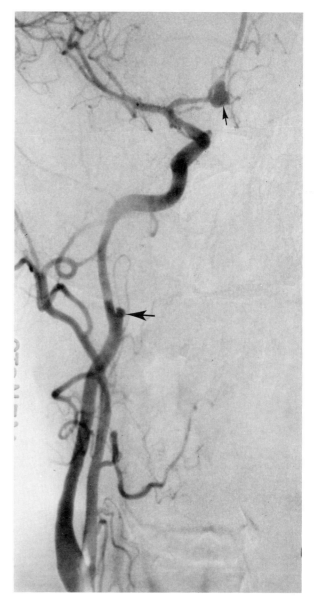

relatively flexible, unprotected cervical ICA enters the rigid petrous carotid canal. Most traumatic occlusions of the ICA result in rapid thrombosis of the entire vessel between the carotid bulb and ophthalmic artery regardless of the site at which the occlusion originated.[9]

Mass Lesions

Mass lesions of sufficient size may displace the ICA. The precise type of displacement depends on the relationship of the mass to the ICA. Lesions commonly displacing the cervical ICA include paraganglioma (Fig. 3-24), neurofibroma, enlarged cervical lymph nodes (Fig. 3-38), and thyroid masses (Fig. 3-36). Infiltrating malignant neoplasms can displace and compress the cervical ICA (Figs. 4-19A, B). Vascular encasement and narrowing are occasionally present (Fig. 4-20). These neoplasms rarely produce occlusion of the ICA.

Aneurysms

Extracranial aneurysms of the ICA are relatively uncommon but not as unusual as once believed.[18, 24] They are most often post-traumatic or atherosclerotic, although congenital and mycotic aneurysms do occur. Aneurysms of the cervical ICA are also occasionally associated with cystic medial necrosis, some connective tissue disorders, and fibromuscular dysplasia. False aneurysms of the cervical ICA have been reported following endarterectomy.[3A]

Atherosclerotic or hypertensive aneurysms of the extracranial ICA are usually identified in elderly hypertensive patients and are found distal to the common carotid artery bifurcation (Fig. 4-21). They are often located in an area of severe atherosclerotic involvement.

Penetrating injury may result in a false saccular ICA aneurysm. Blunt trauma may cause either a dissecting or a saccular aneurysm. A less common cause of traumatic extracranial ICA aneurysm is direct percutaneous needle puncture (Fig. 4-22) or subintimal wedging of the catheter or guidewire during selective angiography (Fig. 4-23).

Some authors have pointed out that the diagnosis of congenital or developmental aneurysm is usually one of exclusion when no previous history of trauma or infection or sign of atherosclerosis is present.[18] Defects or abnormalities of the arterial media may be a contributory factor. An extracranial saccular aneurysm that arose from an area of surgically documented fibromuscular dysplasia is illustrated in Fig. 4-15.

REFERENCES

1. **Anderson RA, Sondheimer FK:** Rare carotid vertebrobasilar anastomoses with notes on the differentiation between proatlantal and hypoglossal arteries. Neuroradiology 11:113–118, 1976

2. **Ascherl GF Jr, Dilenge D:** Anatomic variations of the ophthalmic and middle meningeal arteries and their relationship to the embryonic stapedial artery. Am J Neuroradiol 1:45–53, 1980

3. **Bryan RN, Drewyer RG, Gee W:** Separate origins of the left internal and external carotid arteries from the aorta. Am J Roentgenol 130:362–365, 1978

3A. **Chaudhary MY, Puljics, Clauss RH:** Bilateral false aneurysms after carotid endarterectomy. Neuroradiology 18:215–216, 1979

4. **Countee RW, Vijayanathan T:** Reconstitution of "totally" occluded internal carotid arteries. J Neurosurg 50:747–757, 1979

5. **Desai B, Tooke JF:** Kinks, coils and carotids: a review. Stroke 6:649–653, 1975

6. **Dilenge D, Heon M:** The internal carotid artery. In Newton TH, Potts DG (eds): Radiology of the Skull and Brain, Vol 2, pp 1202–1245. St Louis, CV Mosby, 1974

6A. **Edwards JH, Kricheff II, Gorstein F, et al:** Atherosclerotic subintimal hematoma of the carotid artery. Radiology 133:123–129, 1979

7. **Edwards JH, Kricheff II, Riles T et al:** Angiographically undetected ulceration of the carotid bifurcation as a cause of embolic stroke. Radiology 132:369–373, 1979

8. **Glasgold AI, Harrigan WD:** The internal carotid artery presenting as middle ear tumor. Laryngoscope 82:2217–2221, 1972

9. **Glickman MG:** Angiography in head trauma. In Newton TH, Potts DG (eds): Radiology of the Skull and Brain, Vol 2, pp 2639–2649. St. Louis, CV Mosby, 1974

10. **Guinto FC Jr, Garrabrant EC, Radcliffe WB:** Radiology of the persistent stapedial artery. Radiology 105:365–369, 1972

11. **Houser OW, Baker, HL:** Fibromuscular dysplasia and other uncommon diseases of the cervical carotid artery: angiographic aspects. Am J. Roentgenol 104:201–212, 1968

12. **Imparato AM, Riles TS, Gorstein F:** The carotid bifurcation plaque: pathological findings associated with cerebral ischemia. Stroke 10: 238–245, 1979

13. **Kusunoki T, Rowed DW, Tator CH et al:** Thromboendarterectomy for total occlusion of the internal carotid artery: a reappraisal of risks, success rate and potential benefits. Stroke 9:34–38, 1978

14. **Lapayowker MS, Liebman EP, Ronis ML et al:** Presentation of the internal carotid artery as a tumor of the middle ear. Radiology 98:293–297, 1971

15. **Lasjaunias P, Moret J:** Hyperselective angiography in the study of the nasopharynx. J Neuroradiol 5:103–112, 1978

16. **Lasjaunias P, Moret J:** Normal and non-pathological variation in the angiographic aspects of the arteries of the middle ear. Neuroradiology 15:213–219, 1978

17. **Lie TA:** Congenital anomalies of the carotid artery. Amsterdam, Excerpta Medica, 1968

18. **Margolis MT, Stein, RL, Newton TH:** Extracranial aneurysms of the internal carotid artery. Neuroradiology 4:378–389, 1972

19. **Momose KJ, New PF:** Non-atheromatous stenosis and occlusion of the internal carotid artery and its main branches. Am J Roentgenol 118:550–566, 1973

20. **Osborn AG, Anderson RE:** Angiographic spectrum of cephalocervical fibromuscular dysplasia. Stroke 8:617–626, 1977

20A. **Osborn AG:** The vidian artery: Normal and pathologic anatomy. Radiology, 1980 (in press)

21. **Paullus WS, Pait TG, Rhoton AL Jr:** Microsurgical exposure of the petrous portion of the carotid artery. J Neurosurg 47:713–726, 1977

21A. **Quisling RG:** Intrapetrous carotid artery branches: Pathological application. Radiology 134:109–113, 1980

22. **Quisling RG, Rhoton AL Jr:** Intrapetrous carotid artery branches: radioanatomic analysis. Radiology 131:133–136, 1979

23. **Rosenklint A, Jorgensen PB:** Evaluation of angiographic methods in the diagnosis of brain death. Correlation with local and systemic arterial pressure and intercranial pressure. Neuroradiology 7:215–219, 1974

24. **Ruffato C, Valenta R, Liessi G et al:** Bilateral aneurysms of the cervical internal carotid arteries. Neuroradiology 14:271–273, 1978

25. **Scotti G, Melancon D, Olivier A:** Hypoglossal paralysis due to compression by a tortuous internal carotid artery in the neck. Neuroradiology 14:263–265, 1978

26. **Servo A:** Agenesis of the left internal carotid artery associated with an aneurysm on the right carotid siphon. J Neurosurg 46:677–680, 1977

27. **Smith D, Larsen JL:** On the symmetry and asymmetry of the bifurcation of the common carotid artery. Neuroradiology 17:245–247, 1979

28. **Steffen TN:** Vascular anomalies of the middle ear. Laryngoscope 78:171–197, 1968

28A. **Stringer WL, Kelly DL Jr:** Traumatic dissection of the extracranial internal carotid artery. Neurosurg 6:123–130, 1980

29. **Suzuki S, Nobechi T, Itoh I et al:** Persistent proatlantal intersegmental artery and occipital artery originating from internal carotid artery. Neuroradiology 17:105–109, 1979

30. **Teal JS, Rumbaugh CL, Segall HE et al:** Anomalous branches of the internal carotid artery. Radiology 106:567–573, 1973

31. **Vannix RS, Joergenson EJ, Carter R:** Kinking of the internal carotid artery. Clinical significance and surgical management. Am J Surg 134:82–89, 1977

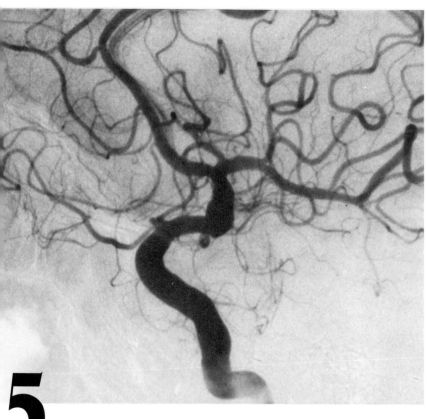

5 The Internal Carotid Artery: Cavernous and Supraclinoid Segments

NORMAL GROSS ANATOMY OF THE CAVERNOUS AND SUPRACLINOID INTERNAL CAROTID ARTERY

The precise point where the internal carotid artery (ICA) enters the cavernous sinus is difficult to determine. For this reason, it is subdivided into presellar and juxtasellar segments instead of precavernous and intracavernous portions.[5]

Presellar Segment

After the ICA emerges from the carotid canal near the petrous tip it lies just above the intracranial aspect of the foramen lacerum. Initially, the ICA ascends within the cavernous sinus and courses slightly medial toward the posterior clinoid process.

Juxtaseller Segment

Lateral to the posteroinferior corner of the sella turcica, the ICA angles sharply forward

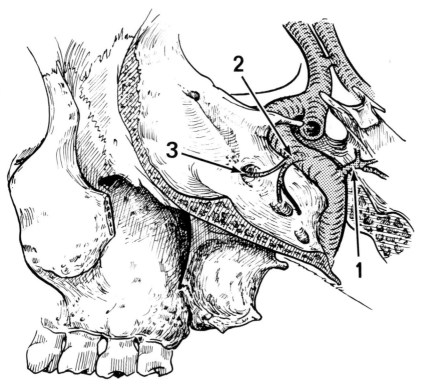

Fig. 5-1. Anatomic diagram of the cavernous ICA. The cavernous sinus has been removed. Note the double curvature of the carotid siphon. The meningo-hypophyseal trunk **(arrow 1),** the lateral main stem artery **(arrow 2),** and the artery of the foramen rotundum **(arrow 3)** are shown.

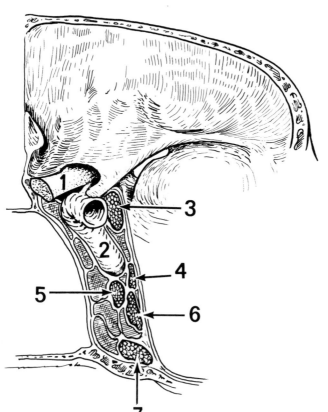

Fig. 5-2. Cross-sectional anatomic diagram of the cavernous sinus, ICA and the related cranial nerves as viewed from above and behind. **1.** Optic nerve (CN II). **2.** Internal carotid artery. **3.** Oculomotor nerve (CN III). **4.** Trochlear nerve (CN IV). **5.** Abducent nerve (CN VI). **6.** Ophthalmic nerve (CN V_1). **7.** Maxillary nerve (CN V_2).

(and often slightly downward) along the sphenoid sinus, then again curves upward on the medial side of the anterior clinoid process (Fig. 5-1). This double curvature, which resembles the letter "S", is termed the *carotid siphon.* The juxtasellar course of the ICA is often marked by a groove in the body of the sphenoid bone which is called the *carotid sulcus.* In most instances, the ICA bulges slightly into the sphenoid sinus itself. In some cases, underlying bone is absent and the ICA and sphenoid sinus are separated only by dura matter and sinus mucosa.[6, 22B]

The carotid artery is the most medial neurovascular structure within the cavernous sinus. The oculomotor, trochlear, and the first and second divisions of the fifth cranial nerve (CN V) lie between the two dural leaves of the lateral sinus wall and are therefore lateral to the ICA. The abducent nerve (CN VI) courses within the sinus itself and is usually directly adjacent to the lateral wall of the ICA (Fig. 5-2).

Within the cavernous sinus, the ICA gives rise to three small but important branches: the meningohypophyseal trunk, the artery of the inferior cavernous sinus (lateral main stem artery), and the capsular arteries (of McConnell).

The Meningohypophyseal Trunk is the largest and most proximal intracavernous branch. This vessel is found in virtually 100% of all anatomic specimens and arises near the apex of the initial curve of the juxtasellar ICA (Fig. 5-3).[7, 19] Adjacent to the cavernous sinus roof,

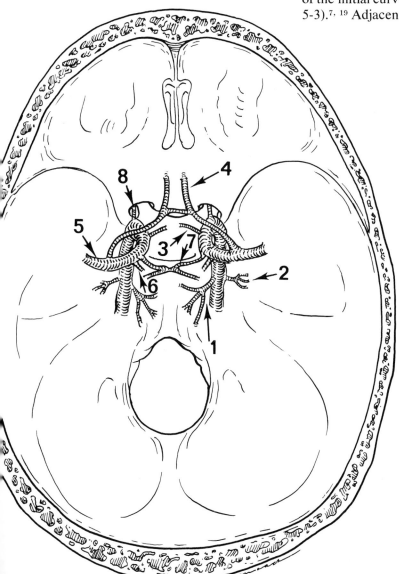

Fig. 5-3. Anatomic sketch of the cavernous and supraclinoid ICA branches. **1.** Meningohypophyseal trunk. **2.** Lateral main stem artery. **3.** Superior hypophyseal artery. **4.** Anterior cerebral artery. **5.** Middle cerebral artery. **6.** Anterior choroidal artery. **7.** Posterior communicating artery. **8.** Ophthalmic artery.

the meningohypophyseal trunk typically gives rise to three branches: the tentorial artery (also called the artery of Bernasconi and Cassinari), the dorsal meningeal artery, and the inferior hypophyseal artery. Less frequently the artery of the inferior cavernous sinus may arise as a branch of the meningohypophyseal trunk.

The **tentorial artery** is the most constant branch of the meningohypophyseal trunk. It passes posterolaterally along the free margin of the tentorium to the incisural apex where it anastomoses with its counterpart from the opposite side and with meningeal branches of the ophthalmic artery (Fig. 5-4).[7]

The second major branch of the meningohypophyseal trunk is the **dorsal meningeal artery** (clival branch). It is present in 90% of anatomic specimens. This vessel runs posteriorly and medially through the cavernous sinus, passing over the dorsum sellae and rostral clivus to anastomose with the opposite dorsal meningeal artery (Fig. 5-4).[22, 29]

The third and least frequently identified branch of the meningohypophyseal trunk is the **inferior hypophyseal artery.** This vessel courses anteromedially to the pituitary sulcus. Branches from the inferior hypophyseal artery encircle the hypophysis, primarily supplying the posterior lobe and the dura of the sella turcica and cavernous sinus. This vessel also anastomoses with its mate from the contralateral ICA.

The Artery of the Inferior Cavernous Sinus is also termed the inferolateral trunk or lateral main stem artery (Figs. 5-1, 5-4). This vessel has been identified in 80 to 85% of all anatomic specimens. It corresponds to the proximal remnant of the embryonic dorsal ophthalmic artery and originates from the inferolateral aspect of the juxtaseller ICA.[14] After curving over the sixth cranial nerve, the lateral main stem artery gives rise to branches that supply the dura of the cavernous sinus and the cranial nerves within the cavernous sinus. Its most important branch is the **artery of the foramen rotundum.** This vessel passes through the foramen rotundum and anas-

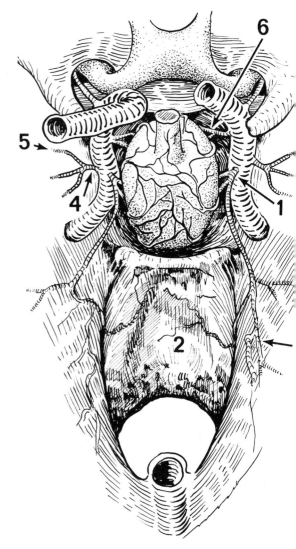

Fig. 5-4. Anatomic diagram of the cavernous ICA and its relationship to adjacent structures. The optic tracts and chiasm have been retracted anteriorly. **1.** Meningohypophyseal trunk. **2.** Dorsal meningeal branches of the meningohypophyseal trunk. **3.** Marginal tentorial artery (artery of Bernasconi and Cassinari). **4.** Lateral main stem artery. **5.** Artery of the foramen rotundum. **6.** McConnell's capsular arteries.

tomoses with its counterpart from the ipsilateral ECA.[14]

Numerous anastomoses are present between rami of the lateral main stem artery and branches of the ophthalmic, maxillary, accessory meningeal, and middle meningeal arteries. These may assist in supplying a variety of vascular lesions at the skull base as well as provide an important source of collateral blood flow in ICA occlusion (see Chapter 3).[8, 25]

McConnell's Capsular Arteries are the most distal and least constant set of branches arising from the intracavernous ICA (Fig. 5-4). They are found in slightly less than 30% of all ana-

tomic specimens.[7] The **inferior capsular artery** courses inferomedially to supply the floor of the sella turcica. It anastomoses with its counterpart from the opposite side as well as with branches from the inferior hypophyseal artery. The **anterior capsular artery** courses medially along the roof of the sella.

Intracranial ICA Segment

After passing anteriorly in the cavernous sinus, the ICA ascends to pierce the dura mater on the medial aspect of the anterior clinoid process (Fig. 5-1). Once it emerges from the dura, the ICA courses superiorly and slightly laterally between the optic and oculomotor nerves. Just below the anterior perforated substance, it divides into its two terminal branches, the anterior and middle cerebral arteries.

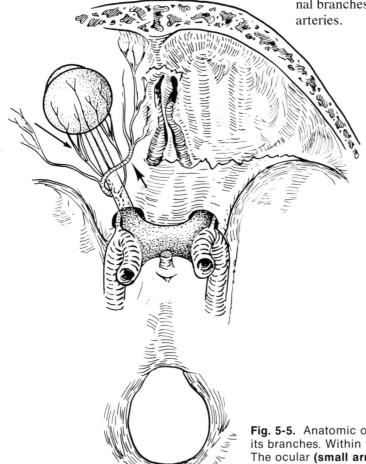

Fig. 5-5. Anatomic of the ophthalmic artery (OA) and its branches. Within the orbit it crosses the optic nerve. The ocular **(small arrow)** and orbital **(large arrow)** branches are indicated. The extraorbital branches are not shown in this intracranial view.

Branches of the Extracavernous Intracranial ICA. Prior to its terminal bifurcation into the anterior and middle cerebral arteries, the intracranial ICA gives rise to the superior hypophyseal, ophthalmic, posterior communicating, and anterior choroidal arteries. The intracranial ICA also sends small branches to the hypothalamus and optic nerve and chiasm.

The **superior hypophyseal artery** and its mate from the opposite side form an arterial collar or plexus around the base of the hypophyseal stalk. Branches from this plexus also supply the optic chiasm and anterior lobe of the hypophysis. This artery is usually not identified on routine normal angiographic studies.

The **ophthalmic artery** (OA) arises from the antero- or superomedial surface of the infra-clinoid ICA as it emerges from the cavernous sinus (Fig. 5-3, 5-5). The OA origin is intradural in 89% of anatomic dissections.[22A] Occasionally the OA may arise from the middle meningeal artery, other branches of the ECA, or the proximal cavernous ICA (Fig. 5-11).[3]

The OA courses anteriorly through the optic canal along the undersurface of the optic nerve. Within the orbit it crosses either under or over the optic nerve, then runs forward on the medial orbital wall below the trochlea. The OA supplies the globe and orbital contents. It forms extensive anastomoses with branches of the ECA which may become an important source of intracranial collateral blood flow in ICA occlusive disease (see Chapter 3).[8, 28]

The OA has three major groups of branches: ocular branches (the central retinal and ciliary arteries), orbital branches (lacrimal and muscular arteries), and extraorbital branches. The latter group includes the supraorbital, anterior and posterior ethmoidal, dorsal nasal, palpebral, medial frontal, and supratrochlear arteries.[8] The ethmoidal arteries pass superiorly through their respective foramina to supply the dura of the cribriform plate and planum sphenoidale. They also have small branches that anastomose with ethmoidal branches of the sphenopalatine artery to supply part of the nasal fossa. The anterior falx artery arises from the anterior ethmoidal branch of the OA and supplies part of the falx cerebri. Occasionally the middle meningeal artery may arise from the OA (Fig. 5-12) or vice versa.

The last two major branches of the extracavernous ICA prior to its terminal bifurcation are the **posterior communicating** and **anterior choroidal arteries** (Fig. 5-3). (See chapters 6 and 7.) Two or three small perforating arteries also arise from the supraclinoid ICA distal to the posterior communicating artery (Fig. 6-3A). These small vessels supply part of the optic tract and chiasm, anterior hypothalamus, tuber cinereum, and medial temporal lobe.[23]

NORMAL RADIOGRAPHIC ANATOMY OF THE CAVERNOUS AND SUPRACLINOID INTERNAL CAROTID ARTERY

Cavernous Branches of the ICA

The roentgen anatomy of the cavernous ICA is relatively simple. The presellar segment extends superiorly and slightly medially from the petrous apex to the sella turcica. Once it enters the cavernous sinus, the juxtasellar ICA first turns anteroinferiorly before it ascends to pierce the dura at the anterior clinoid process. On lateral carotid angiograms this course results in a somewhat S shaped curve and forms the carotid siphon (Fig. 5-6).

On AP projections, the anterior and posterior portions of the juxtasellar segments are partially superimposed. The most medial loop of the ICA represents the posterior part of the juxtasellar segment (Fig. 5-7A). On submentovertex views, the intracranial ICA is clearly seen (Fig. 5-7B). Here again the most medial part of the vessel represents the posterior part of the juxtasellar segment.

The cavernous branches of the ICA can sometimes be visualized on subtracted films of selective internal carotid angiograms, particularly the lateral view. The cavernous branches are also well seen in many types of vascular lesions (see below). The meningohypophyseal trunk arises from the posterosuperior curve of the juxtasellar segment (Fig. 5-6). The tentorial and dorsal meningeal arteries can also be identified occasionally. A not infrequent normal angiographic finding is a distinct localized blush in the posterior pituitary lobe (Fig. 5-8), seen in approximately 20% of cases.[22C]

The Ophthalmic Artery

Selective internal carotid angiography with magnification-subtraction radiography permits identification of the ophthalmic artery and many of its branches. On lateral projections, the OA appears to originate from the anterior convexity of the ICA just below the anterior clinoid process (Fig. 5-9). Base, AP, or modified Water's views may be required to delineate its exact site of origin.

(Text continues on p. 118)

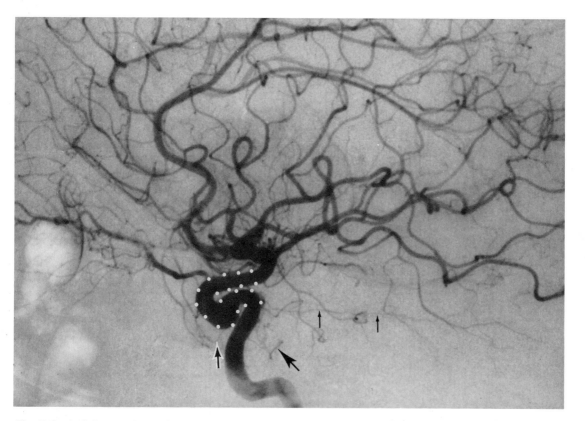

Fig. 5-6. Left internal carotid angiogram (arterial phase, lateral view). The tentorial branch of the meningohypophyseal trunk **(small arrows),** the dorsal meningeal artery **(large arrow),** and the small branches of the lateral main stem artery **(outlined arrow)** are shown. The carotid siphon is indicated by the white dots.

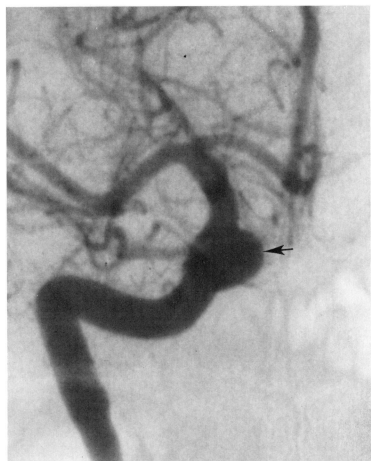

Fig. 5-7. A. Right internal carotid angiogram (mid-arterial phase, AP view). The loops of the juxtasellar ICA are overlapped in this projection. The most medial part of the vessel **(arrow)** is the posterior aspect of the juxtasellar segment. **B.** Right common carotid angiogram (submentovertex view) of a right middle cerebral artery aneurysm **(small arrow).** Note the most posterior segment of the cavernous ICA **(large arrow)** is also the most medial. Contrast this normal juxtasellar ICA with the displaced cavernous segment seen in Figure 5-26.

A
B

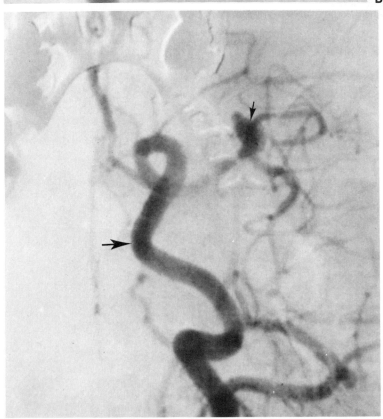

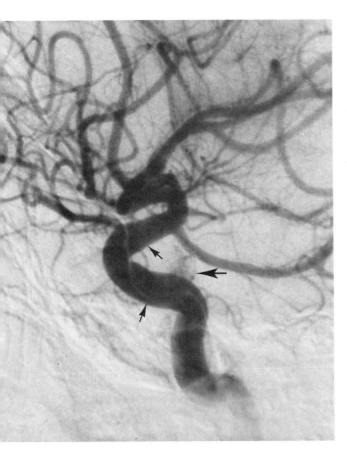

Fig. 5-8. Left common carotid angiogram (arterial phase, lateral view). The loops of the juxtasellar ICA **(small arrows)** form the carotid siphon. Note the distinct posterior pituitary blush **(large arrow).**

Fig. 5-9. Normal internal carotid angiogram (arterial phase, lateral view). The OA and its branches are well shown. Note the definite angulation where the artery passes over the optic nerve **(large arrow).** Note the ocular choroidal crescent **(small arrows).** **1.** Ocular branches (ciliary arteries). **2.** Orbital (muscular) branches. Extraorbital branches: **3.** Medial frontal branch. **4.** Supraorbital artery. **5.** Palpebral branch. **6.** Nasal branch. **7.** Lacrimal artery.

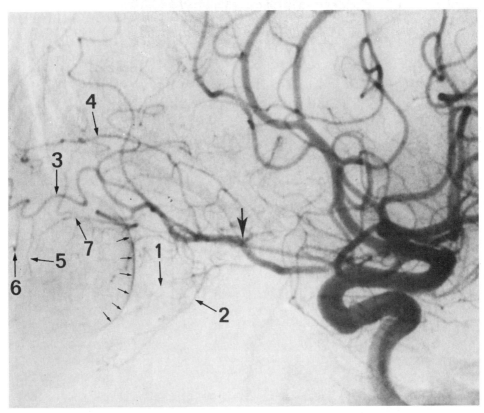

The OA courses anterolaterally and slightly downward through the optic canal to enter the orbit. A distinct superomedial angulation of the OA is present where it crosses either over or under the optic nerve (Fig. 5-9). The OA then runs forward and medial along the medial orbital wall.

The OA gives rise to numerous branches that supply the globe, orbit, and adjacent structures. The central retinal artery is rarely identified angiographically. The only ocular branches routinely seen are the ciliary arteries. The short ciliary arteries form a portion of the choroidal blush (see below). The long posterior ciliary arteries follow a sinusoidal course anteriorly. These vessels also contribute to the choroidal crescent.

In contrast to the ocular branches, the orbital and extraorbital branches of the OA are seen more often (Fig. 5-9). The supraorbital, muscular, palpebral, frontal, nasal, and ethmoidal arteries can frequently be identified.

The choroidal plexus of the eye is a dense vascular network comprised of capillaries as well as small arteries and veins. On lateral carotid angiograms, the ocular choroidal crescent appears as a distinct semicircular blush projected slightly in front of the zygomaticofrontal border of the orbit (Figs. 5-9, 5-10). The choroidal blush can be identified on the late arterial or capillary phase in virtually all normal internal or common carotid angiograms and is hence a constant, reliable finding.[17]

Fig. 5-10. Left internal carotid angiogram (late arterial phase, lateral view). The ocular choroidal crescent (**arrows**) is well delineated.

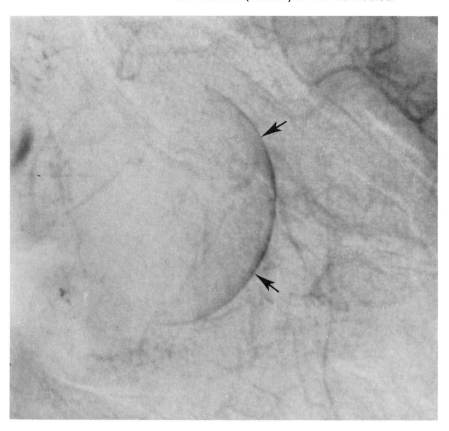

Intracranial Branches of the ICA

The normal radiographic appearance of the posterior communicating, anterior choroidal, anterior cerebral, and middle cerebral arteries is discussed in Chapters 6 through 9.

ANOMALIES OF THE INTERNAL CAROTID ARTERY AND ITS CAVERNOUS AND SUPRACLINOID BRANCHES

A persistent trigeminal artery (see Chapter 6), one of the fetal carotid-basilar anastomotic channels, arises from the ICA proximal to the origin of the meningohypophyseal trunk (Fig. 6-12). Rarely, anastomotic channels between the cavernous ICA and either the superior or posterior inferior cerebellar artery are present.[13] Anomalous transsellar collateral vessels that connect the intracavernous portions of the carotid arteries have also been reported.[26]

In eight percent of anatomic dissections, the ophthalmic artery (which usually arises just as the ICA pierces the dura) arises more proximally within the cavernous sinus (Fig. 5-11).[7, 9] Another relatively common anomaly is the origin of the middle meningeal artery from the OA (Fig. 5-12). This variant is identified in 0.5% of all cases.[3]

Fig. 5-11. Left common carotid angiogram (arterial phase, lateral view). The OA originates from the proximal intracavernous ICA **(arrow)**.

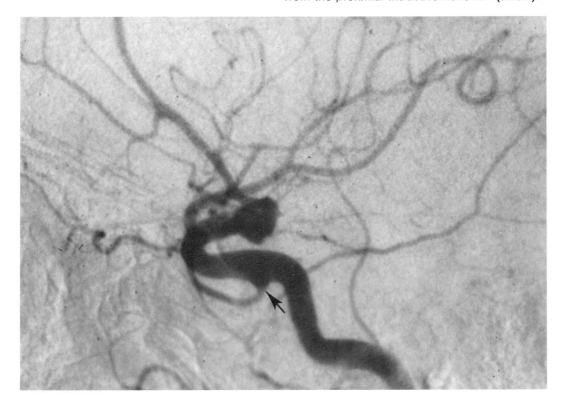

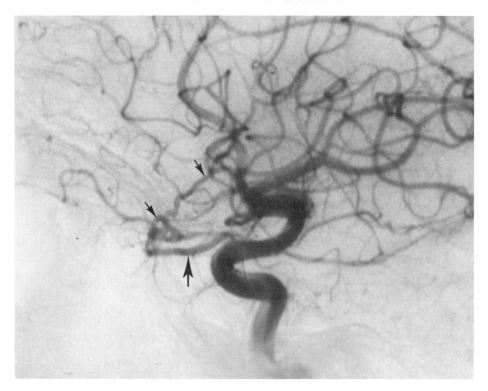

Fig. 5-12. Left internal carotid angiogram (arterial phase, lateral view). The middle meningeal artery **(small arrows)** originates from the OA **(large arrow).**

Fig. 5-13. Left internal carotid angiogram (arterial phase, lateral view) of an asymptomatic cavernous ICA aneurysm **(arrow).**

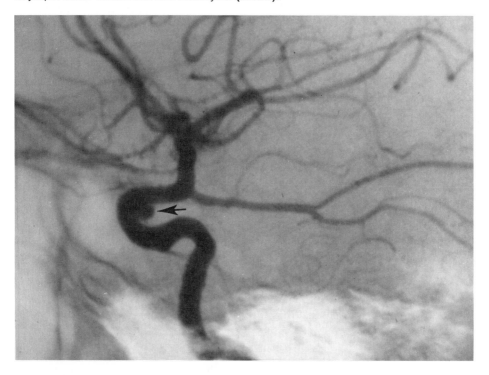

ABNORMALITIES OF THE CAVERNOUS AND SUPRACLINOID INTERNAL CAROTID ARTERY

Aneurysms

Most aneurysms involving the ICA arise from the circle of Willis (see Chapter 6), usually at the origin of the posterior communicating artery. Aneurysms arising below the posterior communicating artery origin represent approximately 5% of all intracranial aneurysms.[2] Two percent are completely extradural.[22A] Intracavernous aneurysms are often asymptomatic (Fig. 5-13). However, juxtasellar saccular aneurysms of sufficient size may compress the nerves that lie within the wall of the cavernous sinus (Fig. 5-14). Palsy of the third cranial nerve is the most common clinical finding. If the aneurysm involves the inferior aspect of the optic chiasm homonymous hemianopsia may be present. Rupture of an intracavernous aneurysm can produce a carotid-cavernous sinus fistula with resultant pulsating exophthalmos, conjunctival injection, and orbital bruit. Fusiform or saccular aneurysms of the extracavernous-intracranial ICA may produce unilateral optic nerve compression (Fig. 5-15). Occasionally these lesions may become so large that they mimic an intracranial neoplasm (Fig. 5-16).

(Text continues on p. 125)

Fig. 5-14. Left internal carotid angiogram (arterial phase, lateral view) of a large intracavernous ICA aneurysm **(arrows).** *(Courtesy of W. H. Marshall, M.D.)*

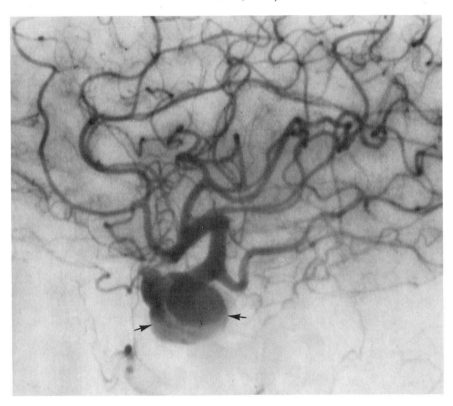

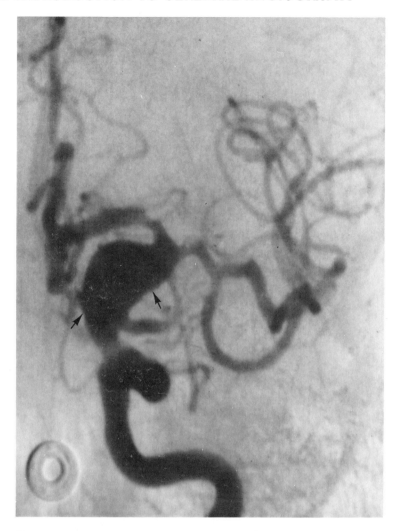

Fig. 5-15. Left internal carotid angiogram (arterial phase, AP view) of a fusiform aneurysm **(arrows)** of the supraclinoid ICA.

Fig. 5-16. Right internal carotid angiogram (arterial phase) of a giant saccular ▶ aneurysm **(arrows)** of the supraclinoid ICA. **A.** AP view. **B.** Lateral view.

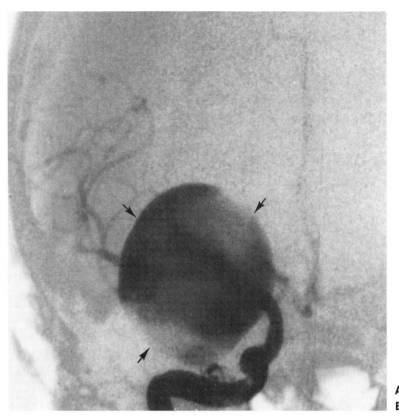

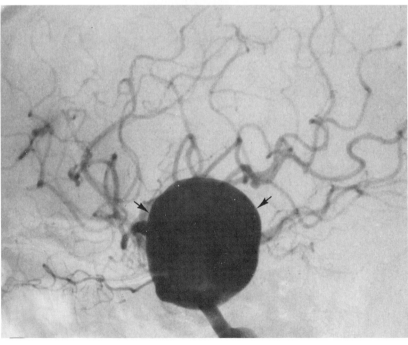

A
B

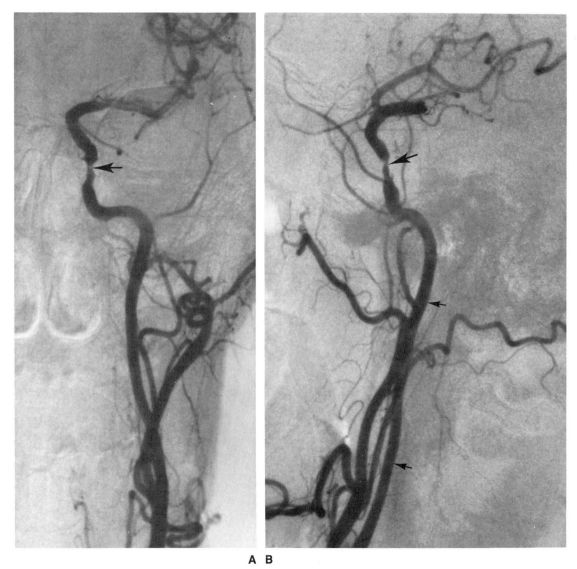

A B

Fig. 5-17. Left common carotid angiogram (arterial phase) of severe atherosclerotic stenosis of the juxtasellar ICA **(large arrow). A.** AP view. **B.** Lateral view.
Note the slightly decreased caliber of the cervical ICA **(small arrows)** secondary to
diminished blood flow.

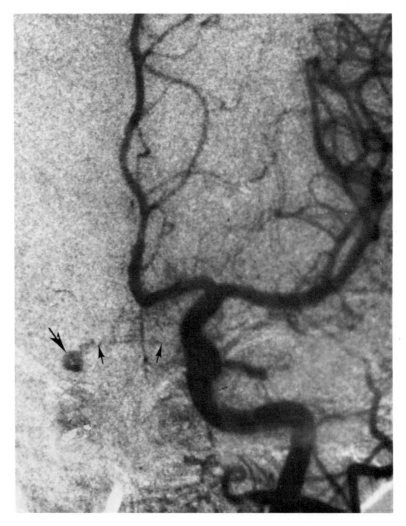

Fig. 5-18. Left internal carotid angiogram (arterial phase, AP view) of complete occlusion of the right ICA. Cavernous collaterals **(small arrows)**, probably around the superior hypophysis or diaphragm sellae, supply the right supraclinoid ICA **(large arrow).**

Atherosclerosis

Atherosclerotic disease often affects the juxtasellar segment of the ICA. Involvement of the carotid siphon may also become severe (Fig. 5-17). Tortuousity and ectasia of the supraclinoid ICA can also be associated with diffuse atheromatous disease.

In the case of ICA occlusion below the level of the cavernous sinus, significant collateral flow may occur via the numerous dural ECA branches that anastomose with cavernous branches of the ICA (see Fig. 3-42) or orbital and ethmoidal branches of the ophthalmic artery (see Figs. 3-39, 3-40, 3-41). Rarely, intracavernous branches of the contralateral ICA provide angiographically detectable collateral flow (Fig. 5-18).

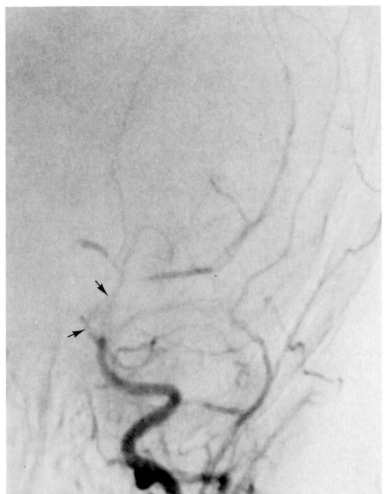

Fig. 5-19. Left common carotid angiogram, (arterial phase) of a child with severe basilar meningitis. The supraclinoid and juxtasellar segments of the ICA are markedly narrowed **(arrows). A.** AP view. **B.** Lateral view.

A
B

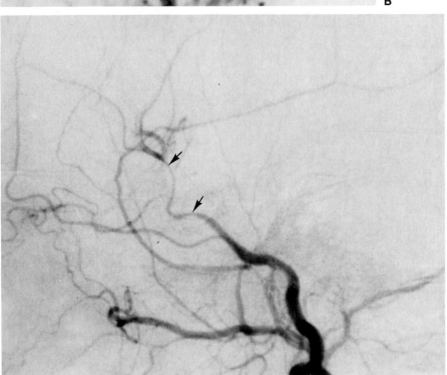

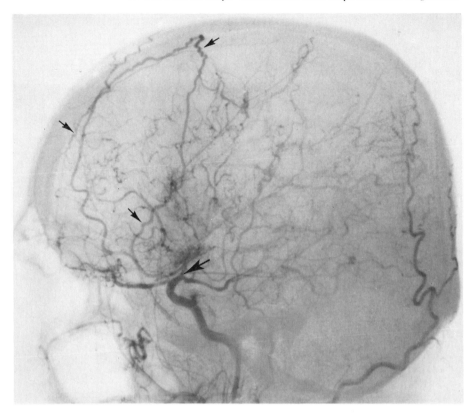

Fig. 5-20. Left carotid angiogram (late arterial phase, lateral view) of idiopathic occlusive vascular disease. The ICA is occluded **(large arrow)** just above the posterior cerebral artery origin. Numerous meningeal branches **(small arrows)** of the ECA and basilar branches of the ICA provide collateral flow. The tortuous, pseudoangiomatous network of collateral vessels resembles a puff of smoke and is the basis for the Japanese term for this condition— moyamoya disease.

Nonatheromatous Stenosis

Nonatheromatous stenosis of the juxtasellar or supraclinoid ICA is relatively uncommon and can be caused by tumors such as meningioma, craniopharyngioma, or other neoplasms involving the skull base. Inflammatory disease in the sphenoid sinus or basilar meninges may cause severe ICA narrowing (Fig. 5-19).[9, 24, 30] Arteritis, fibromuscular dysplasia, radiation therapy, vascular spasm from subarachnoid hemorrhage, trauma, and increased intracranial pressure are additional causes.[3A] Systemic vascular involvement with Menkes' kinky hair syndrome and the neurocutaneous disorders such as neurofibromatosis have also

been reported as nonatheromatous causes of ICA stenosis.[1, 10, 26A, 27]

Rarely, progressive stenosis of the carotid siphon is seen in children and young adults.[10] The development of a network of small collateral vessels at the base of the brain may become striking in these cases (Fig. 5-20).[26B]

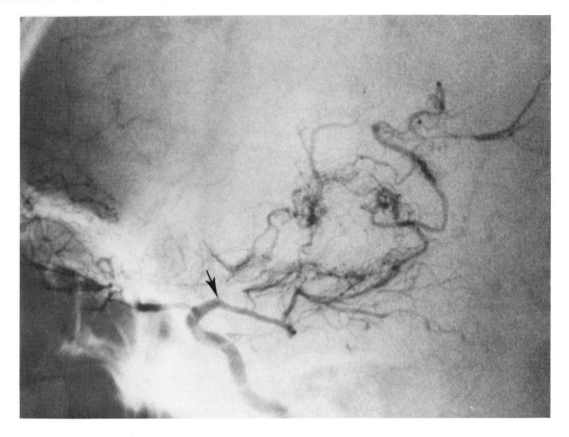

Because this pseudoangiomatous network bears a superficial resemblance to a cloud or puff of smoke, the Japanese termed this radiographic entity "moyamoya." Initially thought to represent a form of basilar telangiectasia, this unusual angiographic pattern is now generally recognized as a nonspecific radiological syndrome resulting from the extensive development of multiple parenchymal, leptomeningeal, and transdural collateral pathways. It is not usually a primary angiomatous process. "Moyamoya" may be seen in progressive arterial occlusive disease resulting from many causes, ranging from atherosclerotic disease (Fig. 5-21) or radiation arteritis to the idiopathic variety.[4, 11]

A related abnormality is the "carotid rete." The small branches of the cavernous ICA have extensive anastomoses with each other, their counterparts from the opposite side, and with meningeal branches from the external ca-

rotid, ophthalmic, and vertebral arteries. This vascular plexus has been misnamed the carotid rete or carotid rete mirabile because of its similarity to the basilar network of freely anastomosing arteries seen in certain animals and lower vertebrates. In those species, branches of the ECA form a network at the base of the brain that reforms within the cavernous sinus into one or two short branches. These become the major source of vascular supply to the circle of Willis. This vascular plexus also provides direct communication between peripheral perforating branches of the ECA and the intracranial circulation. While true carotid rete mirabile in man is rare, a few cases associated with a hypoplastic ICA have been reported. More often, the "rete" is simply an acquired source of extra- to intracranial collateral blood flow in patients with progressive intracranial vascular occlusive disease (Fig. 5-20).[15, 16]

Fig. 5-21. Left internal carotid angiogram (arterial phase, lateral view) of severe atherosclerotic disease. The ICA is occluded **(arrow)** above the posterior communicating artery. Numerous choroidal, thalamoperforating, and ophthalmic branches provide tortuous collateral supply to distal rami of the occluded vessel.

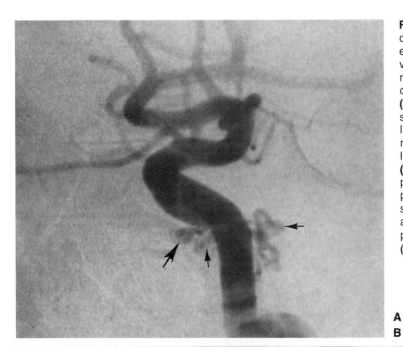

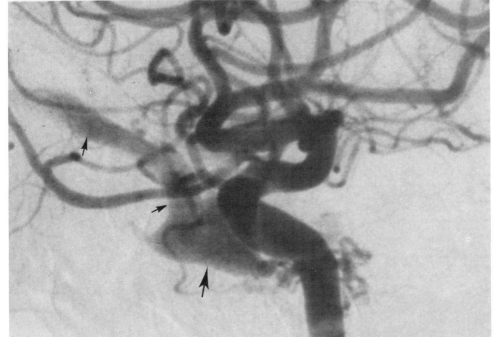

Fig. 5-22. A. Left internal carotid angiogram (very early arterial phase, lateral view) of a carotid-cavernous fistula. The site of communication is identified **(large arrow)** and the lesion is supplied by enlarged branches of the meningohypophyseal and lateral main stem arteries **(small arrows). B.** Same patient as **A** (mid-arterial phase). The cavernous sinus **(large arrow)** drains anteriorly into a dilated superior ophthalmic vein **(small arrows).**

A
B

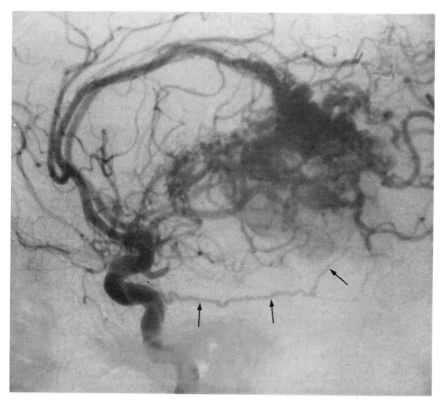

Fig. 5-23. Left internal carotid angiogram (arterial phase, lateral view) of a massive pial-dural arteriovenous malformation. A markedly enlarged tentorial branch **(arrows)** of the meningohypophyseal trunk supplies the lesion. (Same patient as Figure 3-12.)

Vascular Malformations

Carotid-cavernous fistulae (Fig. 5-22) or arteriovenous malformations (Fig. 5-23) may derive some contribution from enlarged cavernous branches.[18]

Carotid Cavernous Fistulae may be congenital, spontaneous (often secondary to atherosclerotic involvement of the siphon), or traumatic. Dural cavernous sinus fistulas occur between meningeal branches of the ICA and cavernous sinus. The ICA itself may also communicate directly with the cavernous sinus (the so-called direct type of fistula). Most internal carotid-cavernous sinus fistulae seem to be acquired and are often a complication of severe head trauma. However, external carotid-cavernous fistulae are usually based on the pre-existence of abnormal arteriovenous communications that open spontaneously or become functional secondary to other factors (such as hypertension).[21]

Initial symptoms of cavernous sinus fistulae often include orbital bruit, chemosis, and pulsating exophthalmos secondary to the transmission of arterial pressure into the dural cavernous sinus. Angiographic features of carotid-cavernous fistulae include rapid, dense opacification of the cavernous sinus (which is usually enlarged) with drainage into a dilated superior ophthalmic vein (Fig. 5-22). Collateral venous drainage into the contralateral cavernous sinus, pterygoid and petrosal veins, and inferior ophthalmic veins may also be present. Spontaneous cavernous sinus thrombosis with closure of the fistula is not uncommon, particularly with dural carotid-cavernous shunts. Filling defects within the cavernous sinus and its tributaries, atypical venous drainage patterns, venous stasis, and an abnormally shaped cavernous sinus are angiographic findings that should suggest venous thrombosis.[23A]

While the angiographic diagnosis of carotid-cavernous fistulae is usually easy, its exact localization is often difficult to determine since the actual site of communication is frequently obscured by rapid opacification of the cavernous sinus. Very fast multiplanar serial angiographic studies are required in these cases. In addition, selective vertebral angiography during temporary compression of the ipsilateral cervical carotid artery may be helpful in localizing the site or sites of communication.[12]

While the major vascular supply in carotid cavernous fistulae is usually from the ICA, small branches from the ECA may also participate (see Chapter 3).

Arteriovenous Malformations may derive significant vascular supply from enlarged cavernous branches of the ICA (Figs. 5-23, 5-24) and usually represent the mixed pial-dural type of malformation. Occasionally they participate in supplying pure dural AVMs in the posterior fossa.

Mass Lesions

Sellar and juxtasellar neoplasms of sufficient size may displace the cavernous ICA. The degree and direction of displacement depend on the exact size and location of the mass. For example, large pituitary adenomas may displace the posterior juxtasellar segment later-

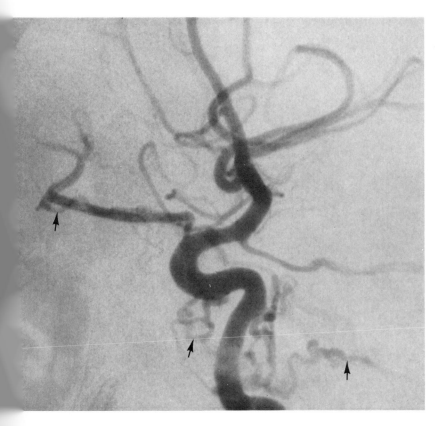

Fig. 5-24. Left internal carotid angiogram (early arterial phase, lateral view) of a massive occipital dural arteriovenous malformation (not shown). Several hypertrophied cavernous branches of the ICA and the recurrent meningeal branch of the ophthalmic artery **(arrows)** assist in supplying the vascular malformation.

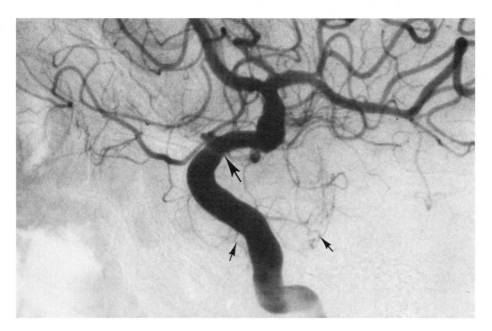

Fig. 5-25. Left internal carotid angiogram (arterial phase, lateral view) of a large chromophobe adenoma. The carotid siphon is opened **(large arrow),** giving this structure a "C" shape instead of its usual "U" or "S" configuration. Enlarged, stretched branches of the meningohypophyseal trunk and lateral main stem artery **(small arrows)** supply the somewhat vascular mass.

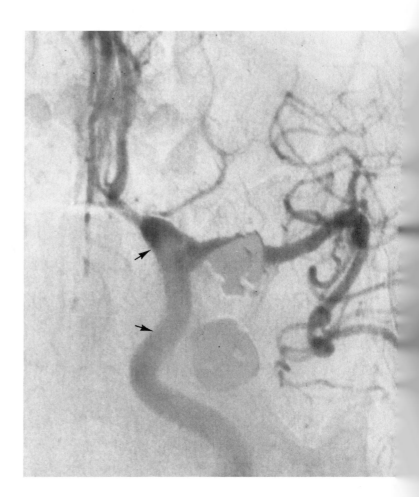

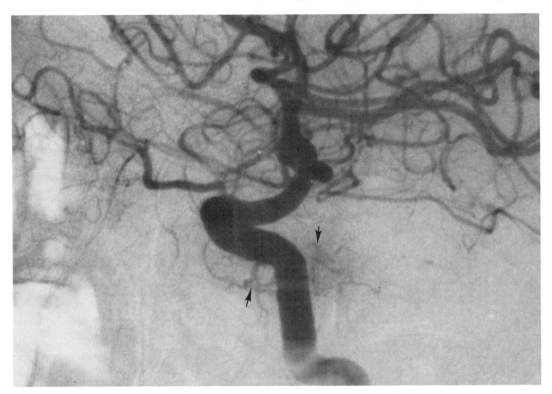

Fig. 5-27. Left internal carotid angiogram (mid-arterial phase, lateral view) of a large sphenoid wing meningioma. The tumor has extended medially to involve the dura of the sella turcica. Enlarged dural branches of the meningohypophyseal and lateral stem arteries supply the lesion **(arrows).**

ally and posteroinferiorly, as well as elevate the supraclinoid portion (Fig. 5-25). Craniopharyngiomas and other large suprasellar masses can also displace the supraclinoid ICA.[20] Sufficiently large sellar masses can distort the carotid siphon, transforming its normal S-shaped configuration into a "C" shape. Angiograms obtained in a submentovertex position may demonstrate lateral displacement of the juxtasellar ICA segments in some cases (Fig. 5-26). However, lateral displacement of the carotid siphon in this view is not a reliable indicator of lateral tumor extension since it usually occurs beneath the cavernous sinus.[22C]

Intracranial neoplasms such as pituitary adenoma (Fig. 5-25) or meningioma (Fig. 5-27) may derive some blood supply from branches of the meningohypophyseal trunk and lateral main stem artery. Extracranial vascular tumors such as paraganglioma or juvenile nasopharyngeal angiofibroma usually derive most of their blood supply from the ECA. However, cavernous branches of the ICA can also contribute to such lesions (Figs. 5-28, 5-29).

◄ Fig. 5-26. Right internal carotid angiogram (arterial phase, submentovertex view) of a large pituitary adenoma. The juxtasellar ICA is displaced laterally **(arrows).**

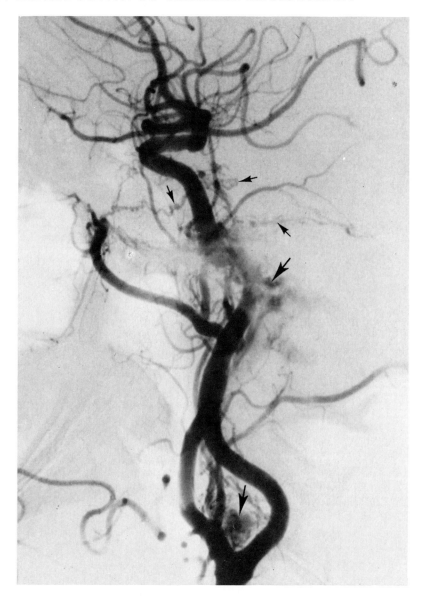

Fig. 5-28. Left common carotid angiogram (arterial phase, lateral view) of multiple paragangliomas **(large arrows).** Numerous hypertrophied cavernous ICA branches **(small arrows)** supply the lesion.

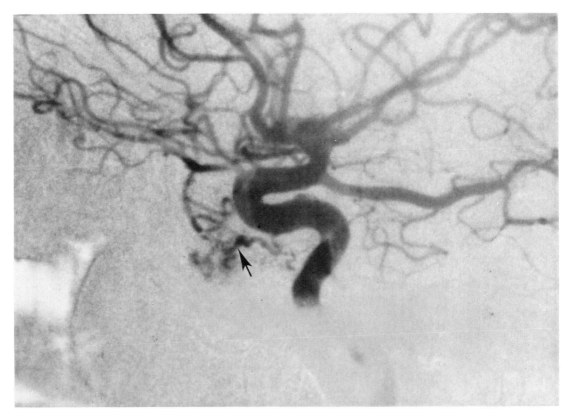

Fig. 5-29. Left internal carotid angiogram (arterial phase, lateral view) of a recurrent nasopharyngeal angiofibroma that has involved the sphenoid sinus. A markedly enlarged artery of the inferior cavernous sinus **(arrows)** supplies the tumor *(Courtesy of Dr. T. S. Roberts.)*

THE ABNORMAL OPHTHALMIC ARTERY

Mass Lesions

Retrobulbar mass lesions often cause posterior flattening or compression of the choroid blush. Lesions of significant size may also cause proptosis (Figs. 5-30, 5-34). Nonneoplastic intraorbital mass effects such as Graves' ophthalmopathy can also produce angiographically detectable exophthalmos. Flattening of the ocular choroidal crescent in patients with increased intracranial pressure and varying degrees of papilledema has also been reported (Fig. 5-31).[17, 28]

In addition to displacing or deforming the choroidal crescent, vascular intraorbital lesions may derive significant blood supply from the OA and its branches. The most common benign orbital neoplasm is hemangioma. These tumors usually occur in infants and children (Fig. 5-32), but may occasionally be found in adults (Fig. 5-33). Other primary orbital tumors include meningiomas (Fig. 5-34), sarcomas, neurofibromata, lacrimal gland neoplasms, and optic nerve gliomas. Non-neoplastic mass-producing lesions, such as fibrous dysplasia and mucocele, may also distort the orbital vessels.

Vascular Lesions

Branches of the OA may be involved in supplying extraorbital vascular lesions such as meningioma or dural arteriovenous malformations (Fig. 5-24).

Occasionally, aneurysms may originate at or adjacent to the OA origin. The OA may be involved with atherosclerotic disease. While stenosis can sometimes be identified, angiography in patients with embolic symptoms and transient monocular blindness usually shows a normal OA although the primary source (such as an ulcerated plaque in the proximal ICA) may be demonstrated.

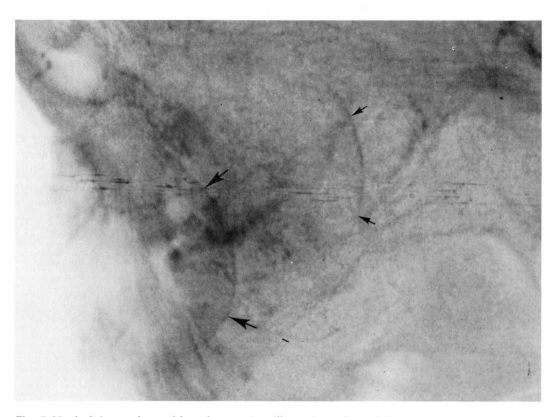

Fig. 5-30. Left internal carotid angiogram (capillary phase, lateral view) in a child with a huge left orbital rhabdomyosarcoma (same patient as Figure 3-35). The right ocular choroidal crescent **(small arrows)** is in normal position. Note the marked left orbital proptosis **(large arrows).** *(Osborn AG, Thurman DJ, Van Dyk HJL: Neuroradiology 15:13–19, 1978)*

Fig. 5-32. Left internal carotid angiogram (arterial phase, lateral view) of a huge orbital hemangioma **(large arrows).** Note the marked enlargement of the OA **(small arrow).**

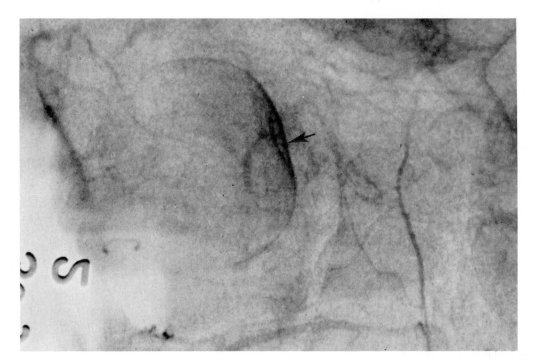

Fig. 5-31. Left internal carotid angiogram (early venous phase, lateral view) of a posterior fossa tumor and a markedly ocular choroidal crescent flattened posteriorly **(arrows)**, presumably due to pressure transmitted along the optic nerve sheath. *(Osborn AG, Thurman DJ, Van Dyk HJL: Neuroradiology 15:13–19, 1978)*

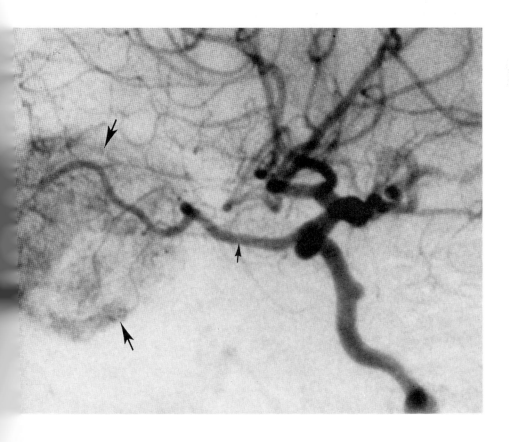

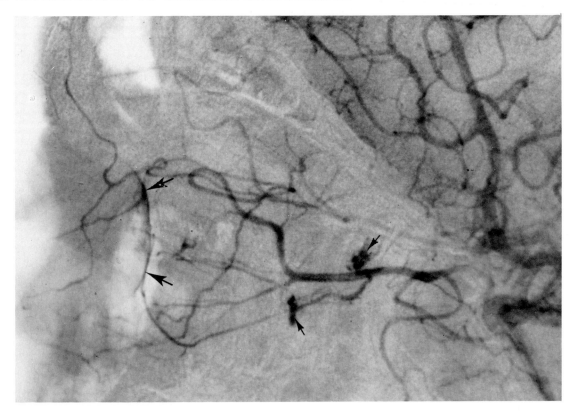

Fig. 5-33. Left internal carotid angiogram (arterial phase, lateral view) in a middle-aged patient with an orbital hemangioma. The mass is mostly avascular, although a few foci of abnormal contrast accumulation are seen **(small arrows).** Note the marked proptosis **(large arrow)** as well as stretching and draping of the ocular and orbital ophthalmic artery branches around the mass.

Fig. 5-34. Left common carotid angiogram (lateral view) of a huge retrobulbar meningioma. Early arterial films **(A)** show buckling and posterior displacement of the distal OA **(large arrow).** Enlarged small orbital branches are present that supply the tumor **(small arrows).** Early venous phase films **(B)** show a distinct retrobulbar vascular blush **(small arrows)** displacing the ocular choroidal crescent anteriorly **(large arrows).**

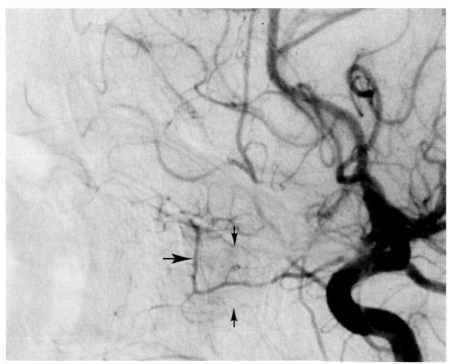

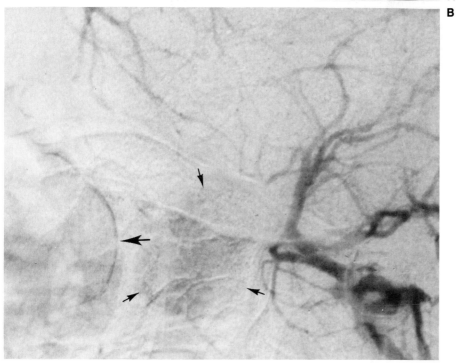

A

B

REFERENCES

1. **Adams PC, Strand RD, Bresnan MJ et al:** Kinky hair syndrome: serial study of radiological findings with emphasis on similarity to the battered child syndrome. Radiology 112:401–407, 1974
2. **Allcock JM:** Aneurysms. In Newton TH, Potts DG (eds): Radiology of the Skull and Brain, Vol 2, pp 2451–2454. St. Louis, CV Mosby, 1974
3. **Ascherl GF Jr, Dilenge D:** Anatomic variations of the ophthalmic and middle meningeal arteries and their relationship to the embryonic stapedial artery. Am J Neuroradiol 1:45–53, 1980
3A. **Brant-Zawadzki M, Anderson M, DeArmond SJ et al:** Radiation-induced large intracranial vessel occlusive vasculopathy. Am J Roentgenol 134:51–55, 1980
4. **Debrun G, Sauvegrain J, Aicardi J et al:** Moyamoya, a nonspecific radiological syndrome. Neuroradiology 2:241–244, 1975
5. **Dilenge D, Heon M:** The internal carotid artery. In Newton TH, Potts DG (eds): Radiology of the Skull and Brain, Vol 2, pp 1204–1245. St. Louis, CV Mosby, 1974
6. **Fujii K, Chambers SM, Rhoton AL Jr:** Neurovascular relationships of the sphenoid sinus. J Neurosurg 50:31–39, 1979
7. **Harris FS, Rhoton AL Jr:** Anatomy of the cavernous sinus. A microsurgical study. J Neurosurg 45:169–180, 1976
8. **Hayreh SS:** The ophthalmic artery. In Newton TH, Potts DG (eds): Radiology of the Skull and Brain, Vol 2, pp 1333–1350. St. Louis, CV Mosby, 1974
9. **Hilal SK, Solomon GE, Gold AP et al:** Primary cerebral arterial occlusive disease in children. I. Acute acquired hemiplegia. Radiology 99:71–86, 1971
10. **Hilal SK, Solomon GE, Gold AP et al:** Primary cerebral arterial occlusive disease in children. II. Neurocutaneous syndromes. Radiology 99:87–93, 1971
11. **Hinshaw DB, Thompson JR, Hasso AN:** Adult arteriosclerotic moyamoya. Radiology 110:633–636, 1976
12. **Huber P:** A technical contribution to the exact angiographic localization of carotid cavernous fistulas. Neuroradiology 10:239–241, 1976
13. **Khodad G:** Persistent trigeminal artery in the fetus. Radiology 121:653–656, 1976
14. **Lasjaunias P, Moret J, Mink J:** The anatomy of the inferolateral trunk (ILT) of the internal carotid artery. Am J Roentgenol 101:34–46, 1977
15. **Margolis MT, Newton TH:** Collateral pathways between the cavernous portion of the internal carotid and external carotid arteries. Radiology 93:834–836, 1969
16. **Newton TH:** The abnormal external carotid artery. In Newton TH, Potts DG (eds): Radiology of the Skull and Brain, Vol 2, pp. 1325–1327. St. Louis, CV Mosby, 1974
17. **Osborn AG, Thurman DJ, Van Dyk HJL:** The angiographic ocular choroidal crescent: distortion with intraorbital and remote intracranial pathology. Neuroradiology 15:13–19, 1978
18. **Palacios E, Azar-Kia Behrooz, Williams V:** The significance of the dural supply from the carotid siphon. Am J Roentgenol 125:815–822, 1975
19. **Parkinson D:** Collateral circulation of cavernous carotid artery: anatomy. Can J Surg 7:251–268, 1964
20. **Miller JH, Peña AM, Segall HD:** Radiological investigation of sellar masses in children. Radiology 134:81–87, 1980
21. **Peeters FLM, Kroger R:** Dural and direct cavernous sinus fistulas. Am J Roentgenol 132:599–606, 1979
22. **Pribram HFW, Boulter TR, McCormick WF:** The roentgenology of the meningohypophyseal trunk. Am J Roentgenol 98:583–594, 1966
22A. **Punt J:** Some observations on aneurysms of the proximal internal carotid artery. J Neurosurg 51:151–154, 1979
22B. **Rhoton AL Jr, Hardy DG, Chambers SM:** Microsurgical anatomy and dissection of the sphenoid bone, cavernous sinus and sellar region. Surg Neurol 12:63–104, 1979
22C. **Richmond IL, Newton TH, Wilson CB:** Indications for angiography in the preoperative evaluation of patients with prolactin-secreting pituitary adenomas. J Neurosurg 52:378–380, 1980
23. **Saeki N, Rhoton AL Jr:** Microsurgical anatomy of the upper basilar artery and the posterior circle of Willis. J Neurosurg 46:563–578, 1977
23A. **Seeger JF, Gabrielsen TO, Giannotta SL et al:** Carotid-cavernous sinus fistulas and venous thrombosis. Am J Neuroradiol 1:141–148, 1980
24. **Sekhar LN, Dujovny M, Rao GR:** Carotid-cavernous sinus thrombosis caused by *Aspergillus fumigatus.* J Neurosurg 52:120–125, 1980
25. **Shields CB, Rice JF:** The superficial recurrent ophthalmic artery: meningeal supply to petrous ridge meningiomas. Neuroradiology 17:173–176, 1979

26. **Staples GS:** Transsellar intracavernous intercarotid collateral artery associated with agenesis of the internal carotid artery. J Neurosurg 50:393–394, 1979

26A. **Taboada D, Alonso A, Moreno J et al:** Occlusion of the cerebral arteries in Recklinghausen's disease. Neuroradiology 18:281–284, 1979

26B. **Takahashi M, Miyauchi T, Kowada M:** Computed tomography of moyamoya disease: Demonstration of occluded arteries and collateral vessels as important diagnositic signs. Radiology 134:671–676, 1980

27. **Tomsick TA, Lukin RR, Chambers AA et al:** Neurofibromatosis and intracranial arterial occlusive disease. Neuroradiology 11:229–234, 1976

28. **Vignaud J, Hasso AN, Lasjaunias P et al:** Orbital vascular anatomy and embryology. Radiology 111:617–626, 1974

29. **Wallace S, Goldberg HI, Leeds NE et al:** The cavernous branches of the internal carotid artery. Am J Roentgenol 101:34–46, 1967

30. **Wollschlaeger G, Wollschlaeger PB, Lopez VF et al:** A rare cause of occlusion of the internal carotid artery. Neuroradiology 1:32–38, 1970

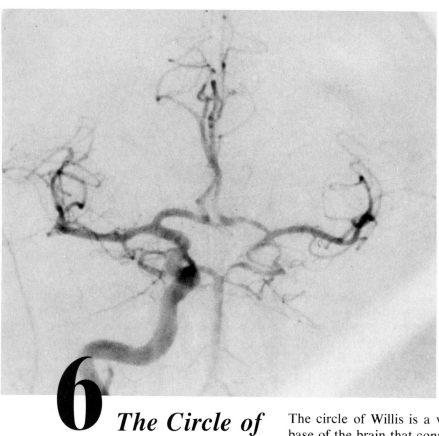

6 *The Circle of Willis*

The circle of Willis is a vascular ring at the base of the brain that connects the two internal carotid systems with each other and with the vertebral-basilar circulation. The anastomoses thus provided by this vascular ring are of great significance when one of the major arteries supplying the brain becomes occluded. The neurologic deficit suffered as well as the ability of a patient to withstand occlusion of one or more of these major vessels depends on the presence of collateral circulation to the affected area. The circle of Willis is the most important potential source of this collateral circulation. Hence, thorough knowledge of the normal anatomy of the circulus arteriosus, its anomalies, and the clinical significance of these variations is important to clinician and neuroradiologist alike.

EMBRYOLOGIC DEVELOPMENT OF THE CIRCULUS ARTERIOSUS

A brief review of the normal embryologic development of the human brain vascular system, its fetal configuration, and subsequent differentiation is helpful in understanding patterns of intracranial circulation in the adult.

In the human embryo, the primitive internal carotid arteries are initially divided into a cranial and a caudal division. The caudal division terminates in the mesencephalon. The trigeminal, otic, and primitive hypoglossal arteries (Fig. 6-1) are transitory anastomoses which develop between the primitive internal carotid arteries and the more dorsally located paired longitudinal neural arteries (precursors of the basilar artery).

At the 4 mm stage, the hindbrain structures are supplied by the anterior (carotid) circulation via the primitive trigeminal artery. During the 5 to 6 mm stage, the caudal division of the internal carotid artery (ICA) anastomoses with its ipsilateral longitudinal neural artery at the mesencephalon. This cranial communication becomes the definitive posterior communicating artery which subsequently replaces the transitory trigeminal artery. The more caudal primitive trigeminal, otic, and hypoglossal arteries usually regress during later development.[1, 8, 9, 11, 20, 25] As the vertebral-basilar circulation develops, the posterior communicating arteries also diminish in size. The proatlantal intersegmental artery is a suboccipital anastomosis between the ICA or external carotid artery (ECA) and the caudal aspect of the longitudinal neural artery (Fig. 6-1). As the vertebral arteries develop this primitive connection regresses.[2, 21]

NORMAL GROSS AND RADIOGRAPHIC ANATOMY OF THE CIRCLE OF WILLIS

Normal Gross Anatomy

The circle of Willis is an arterial polygon that surrounds the ventral surface of the diencephalon adjacent to the optic nerves and optic tracts. The *classical* circle of Willis is

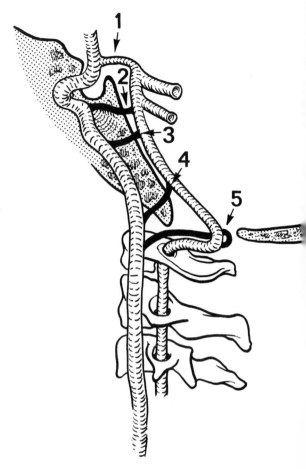

Fig. 6-1. Anatomic diagram of the embryologic carotid-basilar and carotid-vertebral anastomoses. **1.** Posterior communicating artery. **2.** Trigeminal artery. **3.** Otic artery. **4.** Hypoglossal artery. **5.** Proatlantal intersegmental artery.

illustrated in Fig. 6-2A. The anterior portion of the circle consists of the two internal carotid arteries, the horizontal (A1) segments of both anterior cerebral arteries, and the anterior communicating artery. The posterior part of the circle consists of the proximal (P1) segments of both posterior cerebral arteries (these portions are from their origin at the terminal basilar artery bifurcation to their junction with the posterior communicating arteries), and the two posterior communicating arteries themselves. The posterior communicating arteries arise from the posteromedial surface of the ICA and sweep backward

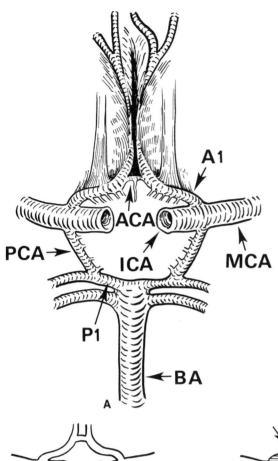

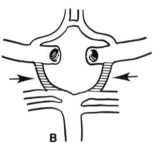

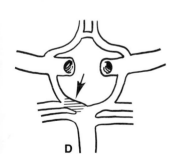

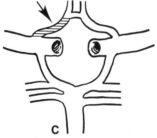

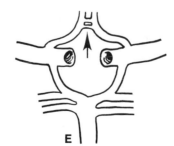

above the third cranial nerve to join the posterior cerebral arteries. Thus, they connect the anterior (carotid) circulation with the posterior (vertebral-basilar) system.

Numerous small branches arise from the circle of Willis to supply important structures at the base of the brain such as the optic nerves, chiasm, optic tracts, infundibulum, internal capsule, and portions of the basal ganglia and thalamus (Fig. 6-3).[16B, 19]

Fig. 6-2. Anatomic diagram of the circle of Willis and its common variations. **(A)** "Classic" circle of Willis. No component is hypoplastic or absent. This balanced configuration is present in only 18 percent of all cases. **(B)** Hypoplasia of one or both posterior communicating arteries; 22 percent. **(C)** Absent or hypoplastic A1 segment of the anterior cerebral artery; 25 percent. **(D)** "Fetal" origin of the posterior cerebral artery with hypoplasia of the P1 segment; 15 percent. **(E)** Multichanneled or duplicated anterior communicating artery; 9 percent. In **B–E,** the absent or hypoplastic segments are shaded **(arrows).**

Normal Variants

The *classic* circle of Willis has well-developed, symmetrical components. No segment is hypoplastic. Such a configuration as this is the exception rather than the rule. While relative bilateral symmetry of the circle of Willis is present during the second trimester, true anomalies of the circulus arteriosus are present in the majority of adults. Careful anatomic studies have demonstrated that only 18 to 20% of all specimens have a classical or balanced configuration.[1, 11, 17]

Most of the variants involving the circle of Willis are due to hypoplasia of one or more of its components. A common normal variant is hypoplasia of one or both posterior communicating arteries. This pattern is seen in 22 to 32% of all cases.[19] Other frequent variations are hypoplasia or absence of the proximal (A1) segment of the anterior cerebral artery (25% of all cases) and direct origin of the posterior cerebral artery from the ICA. In this latter instance, the posterior communicating artery is large and the P1 segment of the posterior cerebral artery is small or hypoplastic. This configuration is seen in 15 to 22% of all cases and is termed the *fetal* origin of the posterior cerebral artery.[1, 19] The posterior cerebral artery rarely arises as the only branch of the ICA.[18] The anterior communicating artery may be hypoplastic, duplicated, or multichanneled (9% of all cases).[15] Common anatomical variants of the circle of Willis are illustrated in Figures 6-2 (B-E).

Normal Radiographic Anatomy

The entire circle of Willis is rarely seen on a single cerebral angiogram. However, on occasion, a patient with a favorable anatomic configuration or occlusion of three of the four major arteries supplying the brain will fill the complete circle from the sole remaining patent vessel. An example of such a case is illustrated in Figure 6-4.

The anterior communicating artery is seldom seen on routine AP and lateral views.

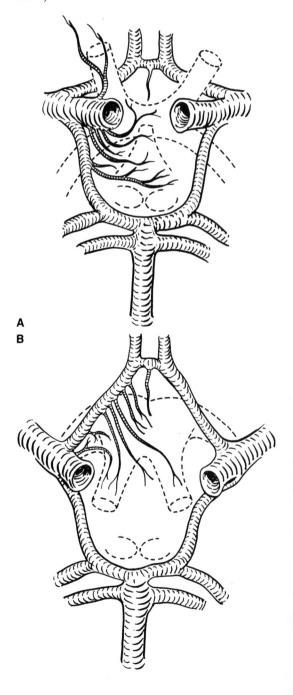

Fig. 6-3. Anatomic diagram of the ventral **(A)** and dorsal **(B)** surfaces of the chiasm, infundibulum, and optic tracts. The circle of Willis sends numerous branches to the chiasm, infundibulum, and other important structures at the base of the brain. *(Adapted from Wollschlaeger G and Wollschlaeger PB, The Circle of Willis. In Newton TH and Potts DG, (eds) Radiology of the Skull and Brain, vol. II, Angiography, p. 1189. St. Louis, C.V. Mosby Co., 1974.)*

A
B

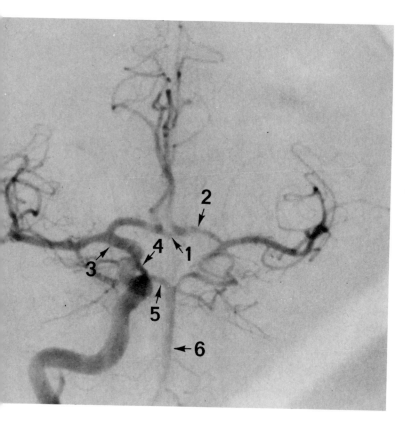

Fig. 6-4. Right common carotid angiogram (mid-arterial phase, AP view) in complete occlusion of both vertebral and left ICAs. The entire circle of Willis is filled via the right carotid artery. **1.** Anterior communicating artery. **2.** A1 segment. **3.** Right internal carotid artery. **4.** Posterior communicating artery. **5.** P1 segment, posterior cerebral artery. **6.** Basilar artery.

Oblique (Fig. 6-5A), Water's (Fig. 6-5B), or an axial (base) view may be necessary to demonstrate clearly the anterior communicating artery. Occasionally temporary cross-compress of the contralateral common carotid artery during contrast injection may be also required.

All or part of the posterior communicating arteries are often demonstrated when the ICA or vertebral artery is injected. Temporary reflux of contrast into the posterior communicating arteries may render them transiently visible (Fig. 6-6).

Most of the small vessels arising from the circle of Willis are too small to be seen on routine angiographic studies. However, a few of the larger branches can sometimes be identified. One of these is the recurrent artery of Heubner, a small vessel that originates from the A1 portion of the anterior cerebral artery (Fig. 6-7). It doubles back on its parent vessel,

accompanying both the anterior and middle cerebral arteries for a variable distance before entering the brain. The recurrent artery then passes posteriorly and laterally following the course of the lenticulostriate arteries to supply part of the basal ganglia, internal capsule, and hypothalamus.[15]

Anterior thalamoperforating arteries arise from the posterior communicating arteries and pass superiorly to supply the tuber cinereum, ventral and paraventricular thalamic nuclei, mammillary bodies, posterior hypothalamus and subthalamic nucleus, posterior chiasm, part of the cerebral peduncles, and the posterior limb of the internal capsule.[19] These thalamoperforating vessels surround the third ventricle and are best demonstrated by magnification vertebral angiography when the posterior communicating arteries are refluxed (Fig. 6-6).

(Text continued on p. 151)

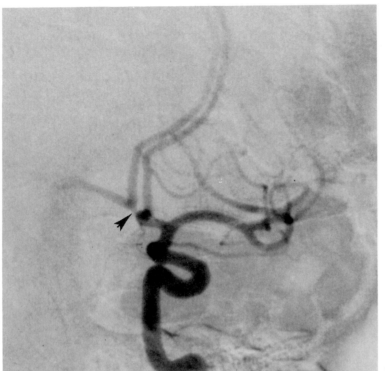

A

B

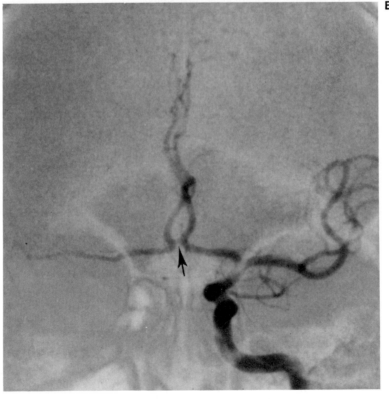

Fig. 6-5. Left internal carotid angiograms (mid-arterial view. Oblique **(A)** and Water's **(B)** views were obtained during temporary cross compression of the contralateral carotid artery. The anterior communicating artery **(arrows)** is well visualized on both these special projections.

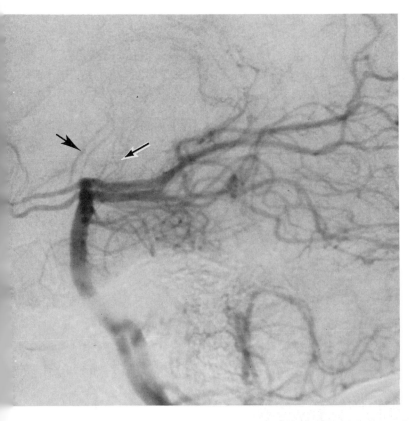

Fig. 6-6. Left vertebral angiogram (arterial phase, lateral view). The posterior communicating arteries have both been refluxed. Anterior thalamoperforating arteries arise from the posterior communicating arteries **(black arrow).** Posterior thalamoperforating arteries **(outlined arrow)** originate from the proximal posterior cerebral artery.

Fig. 6-7. Left carotid angiogram (arterial phase, AP view). The recurrent artery of Heubner **(arrows)** is indicated.

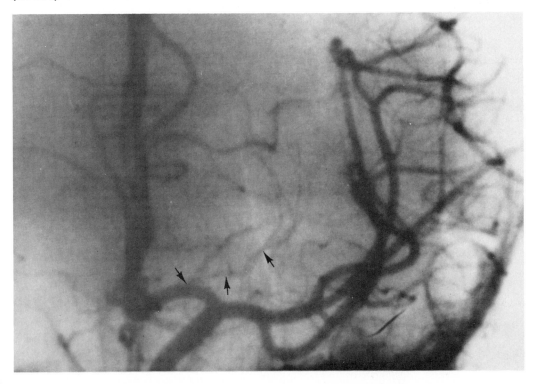

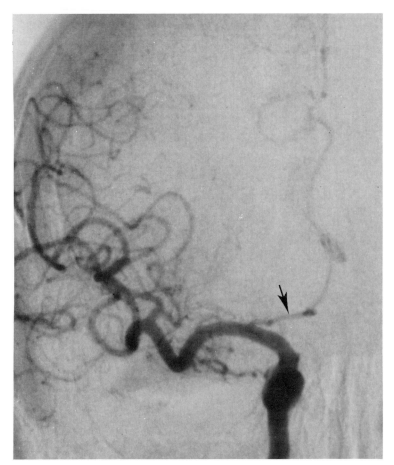

Fig. 6-8. Right carotid angiogram (mid-arterial phase, AP view) in hypoplasia of the right A1 anterior cerebral artery segment **(arrow).**

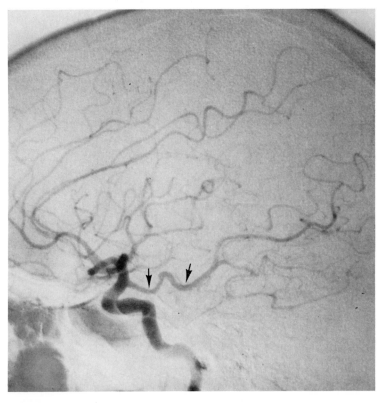

Fig. 6-9. Left carotid angiogram (mid-arterial phase, lateral view) in fetal origin of the left posterior cerebral artery **(arrows).**

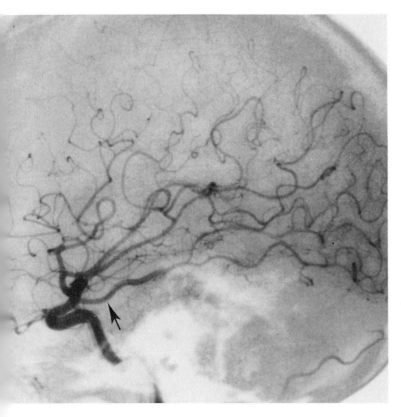

Fig. 6-10. Left internal carotid angiogram (mid-arterial phase, lateral view) Fetal origin of the posterior cerebral artery is present **(arrow)**. The middle cerebral artery and its cortical branches are well visualized. The left A1 segment was absent, hence the anterior cerebral artery territory is not filled. Both anterior cerebral arteries were supplied by the right ICA.

Some variants of the circle of Willis can be identified angiographically. Hypoplasia of the horizontal or A1 segment of the anterior cerebral artery (Fig. 6-8) and fetal origin of the posterior cerebral artery (Fig. 6-9) are easily recognized.

Variations in the Circle of Willis

The circle of Willis is the most important source of potential collateral blood flow to the cerebral cortex. Since its components are notoriously subject to frequent variations, hypoplasia of one or more segments of the circle may preclude the development of adequate collateral blood flow. In Figure 6-10, a rather striking example of such a case is illustrated. Note that in this left carotid angiogram the middle cerebral artery is well filled. However, the posterior cerebral artery has a fetal type of configuration (*i.e.*, a carotid origin) and the an-

terior cerebral circulation is not visualized. Hence, both the ipsilateral A1 anterior cerebral artery segment and the P1 portion of the posterior cerebral artery are probably hypoplastic. In this individual, sudden occlusion of the left ICA—the sole vessel capable of supplying the middle and posterior cerebral circulations in the dominant hemisphere—would probably result in death or profound neurologic impairment.

The opposite example is illustrated in Figure 6-11. A left vertebral angiogram was performed in a 54-year-old truck driver who had occluded both internal carotid arteries. The right vertebral artery was hypoplastic. The entire intracranial circulation was supplied by the patent left vertebral artery via a balanced circle of Willis. This patient's only complaint was that he occasionally fainted when he turned his head to peer out the side window of his rig!

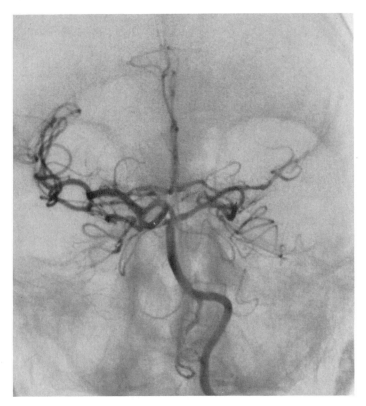

Fig. 6-11. Left vertebral angiogram (mid-arterial phase, AP view) in occlusion of both ICAs. Note that the entire intracranial circulation is now supplied by the left vertebral artery via a balanced circle of Willis.

Fig. 6-12. Left internal carotid angiogram (mid-arterial phase, lateral view) in large persistent trigeminal artery **(arrow).**

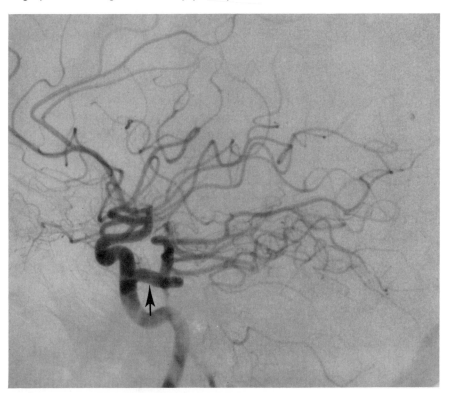

THE RADIOLOGY OF PERSISTENT CAROTID-VERTEBROBASILAR ANASTOMOSES

As was discussed previously, the primitive trigeminal, otic, and hypoglossal arteries are transient embryologic anastomoses between the internal carotid arteries and precursors of the basilar artery system (Fig. 6-1). If these vessels fail to regress normally during subsequent development, a persistent carotid-basilar anastomosis results. These anomalous connections may be demonstrated by cerebral angiography.

The most common carotid-basilar anastomosis is a persistent trigeminal artery (Fig. 6-12). This anomaly is found in about 0.1 to 0.2% of all cases.[24] A persistent trigeminal artery arises from the ICA below the abducens nerve as the ICA enters the cavernous sinus.[13] The anomalous vessel then passes posteriorly and slightly inferiorly to join the upper basilar artery. A persistent trigeminal artery is usually associated with small posterior communicating and vertebral arteries and a hypoplastic basilar artery caudal to the anastomosis.

Carotid-basilar anastomoses are usually identified as incidental angiographic findings. However, aneurysms of the circle of Willis, arteriovenous malformations, other persistent primitive anastomoses, and anomalous origins of the superior and inferior cerebellar arteries have occurred in conjunction with trigeminal artery.[12, 13, 24] Microembolization from an ulcerated carotid artery to both occipital lobes via a persistent trigeminal artery has also been reported.[16A]

The rare, persistent otic artery is an anastomosis between the anterior inferior cerebellar artery and the intrapetrous portion of the ICA. Only a few cases have been demonstrated and most of these have been found at postmortem examination.[18, 24]

A persistent hypoglossal artery is an uncommon form of carotid-basilar anastomosis that passes through the anterior condyloid foramen and joins the cervical ICA to the basilar artery (Fig. 6-13).[2, 4]

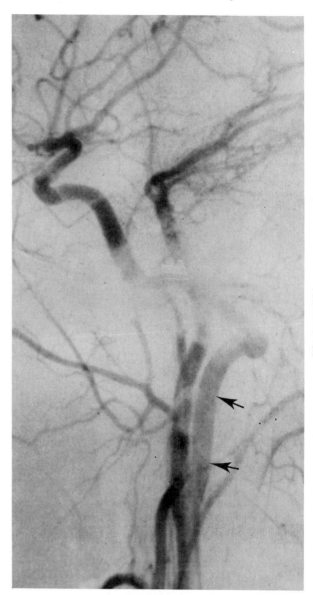

Fig. 6-13. Left common carotid angiogram (arterial phase, lateral view). A persistent hypoglossal artery **(arrows)** is present.

A suboccipital or proatlantal intersegmental artery is a rare anomaly. Unlike the primitive hypoglossal artery (which joins the basilar artery), a proatlantal artery originates from the ECA or cervical ICA and has a suboccipital anastomosis with the horizontal portion of the vertebral artery (see Figs. 4-7, 5-1). Its distal intracranial course is identical to that of the vertebral artery.[2] Some authors feel a persistent proatlantal segmental artery is embryologically identical to the distal ascending portion of the occipital artery.[10]

ANEURYSMS OF THE CIRCLE OF WILLIS

Aneurysms are saccular or fusiform arterial dilatations that may be developmental, arteriosclerotic, traumatic, or mycotic in origin. Congenital saccular or berry aneurysms commonly affect the circle of Willis and arise predominantly at the bifurcation between two arterial branches. Gaps in the media at the bifurcations of cerebral arteries are important for aneurysm formation but are not the sole factor involved.[22]

Age, impact of blood flow, and arterial hypertension may also be important factors in the development, growth, and rupture of these lesions.[2A] Intracranial aneurysms are rare in children since the incidence of aneurysms increases with age. Women between the ages of 40 and 60 are usually affected. The most common clinical presentation is rupture with subarachnoid hemorrhage. Rarely, aneurysms may be a cause of cerebral emboli or ischeia.[6, 20A]

The reported frequency of occurrence at each location in the circle of Willis varies. At the University of Utah Medical Center, approximately 20% of all intracranial aneurysms arise from the middle cerebral artery bifurcation (see Chapter 9). About 30% arise from the anterior communicating artery (Fig. 6-14) and 20 to 30% arise from the ICA at the origin of the posterior communicating artery. Fifteen percent are located at the basilar tip or, less commonly, within the posterior fossa circulation. Another five percent were found in miscellaneous locations, such as on peripheral arteries or at the origin of the anterior choroidal artery.

From 15 to 20% of intracranial aneurysms are multiple (Fig. 6-15). When a patient with subarachnoid hemorrhage has more than one aneurysm it may be difficult to determine which one ruptured. Actual extravasation of contrast medium from a ruptured aneurysm is a rare diagnostic sign.[9A] Helpful findings include an adjacent mass effect caused by an associated intracerebral hemotoma; spasm (narrowing) of adjacent vessels; size (the largest aneurysm is statistically the most likely to have ruptured); and irregularity, lobulation, or an apical "tit."

The exact timing of angiographic studies in the patient with an intracranial aneurysm is important. Vascular spasm, a frequent complication of subarachnoid hemorrhage, is often absent for the first 1 to 3 days. Half of these patients will develop vascular spasm later. While there is no constant relationship between clinical grade and the presence of vascular spasm as demonstrated by angiography, significant arterial spasm does increase operative morbidity and mortality. Therefore, some investigators recommend that angiographic studies be performed within 24–72 hours prior to contemplated surgery regardless of the findings on initial arteriography.[22A] Other studies have shown that there is a direct correlation between clinical grade and the extent of subarachnoid blood as demonstrated by CT as well as a relationship between the extent of hemorrhage and severity of vasospasm identified at angiography.[58] CT scans may therefore be helpful in management of these patients.[18A]

It should be noted that aneurysms arising from the circle of Willis may cause localized compression of the cranial nerves. For example, a saccular aneurysm of the intracavernous carotid may compress the nerves as they pass through the wall of the cavernous sinus (see Chapter 5). Most commonly there is pain in the area of the ophthalmic division of CN V

(Text continued on p. 158)

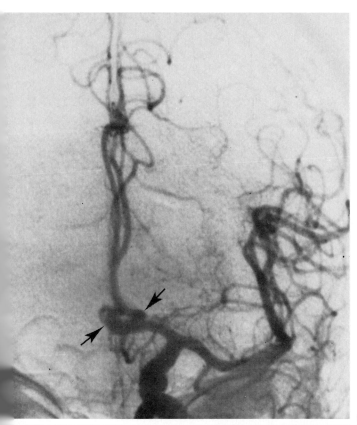

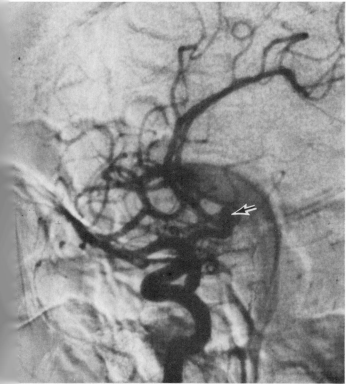

Fig. 6-14. Left internal carotid angiogram (mid-arterial phase). Routine AP projection **(A)** shows several vascular loops **(arrows)** in the area of the anterior communicating artery but no definite aneurysm. An oblique view **(B)** demonstrates a saccular aneurysm of the anterior communicating artery **(arrow).**

A
B

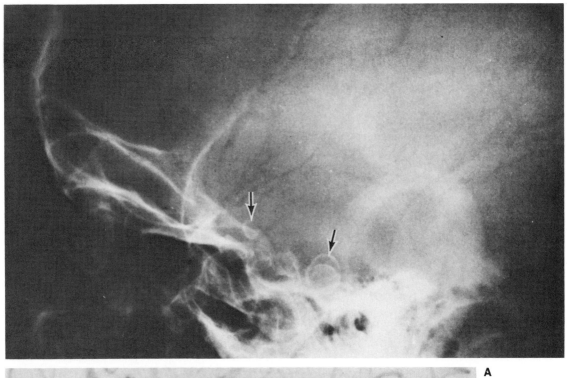

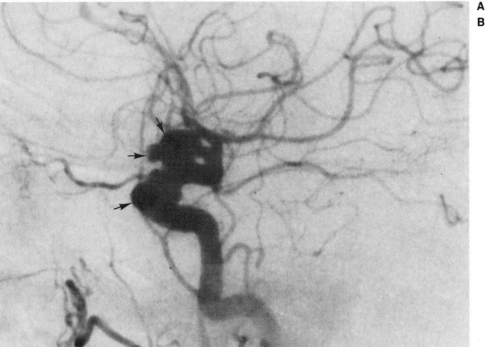

A
B

Fig. 6-15. Plain skull film **(A)** and lateral common carotid angiogram **(B)** in a patient with multiple calcified aneurysms of the circle of Willis **(arrows)**.

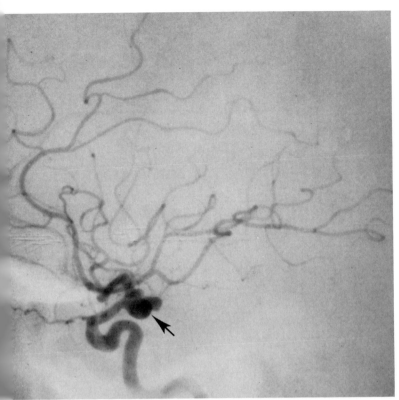

Fig. 6-16. Left internal carotid angiogram (mid-arterial phase). Routine lateral view **(A)** shows a lobulated aneurysm arising from the ICA at the origin of the posterior communicating artery **(arrows).** Angled lateral view **(B,** the patient's head was tilted 15° away from the film changer) clearly shows a somewhat broad-based bilobed aneurysm of the posterior communicating artery **(large arrow).** A smaller, *separate* aneurysm at the origin of the anterior choroidal artery **(small arrow)** is also demonstrated.

A

B

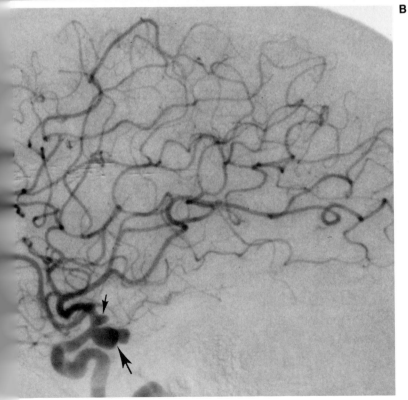

as well as in a CN III palsy. Palsy of cranial nerves IV and V may also be present. Fusiform or saccular aneurysms of the extracavernous intracranial carotid artery may occasionally produce optic nerve compression (Figs. 6-15, 6-16).

Anterior communicating artery aneurysms usually present with subarachnoid hemorrhage but if of sufficient size they may compress the superior chiasm and thus produce bilateral inferior field defects with involvement of macular vision.

Posterior communicating artery aneurysms (Fig. 6-16) frequently produce isolated sudden third nerve palsy with ptosis, pupillary dilatation, and lateral strabismus.

Fusiform, tortuous basilar artery aneurysms may coil in the cerebellopontine angle cistern and produce hemifacial spasm, dizziness, ataxia, nystagmus, or deafness. Trigeminal neuralgia and supranuclear bulbar palsy have also been observed.[5A]

Angiographically, saccular aneurysms usually appear as rounded or lobulated contrast-filled projections arising from the circle of Willis or middle cerebral artery bifurcation (Fig. 6-15). Most of these aneurysms are readily demonstrated on routine angiographic studies. Occasionally, additional special views may be necessary. Oblique or submentovertex (base) projections are helpful in distinguishing between an aneurysm and superimposed vascular loops that may mimic such a lesion. An example of this distinction is illustrated in Figure 6-15. Here, routine AP views show overlapping vascular structures in the area of the anterior communicating artery but no definite aneurysm. However, oblique views demonstrate a definite saccular aneurysm. Oblique, base, or angled lateral views are also helpful in identifying the exact origin of an aneurysm and delineating the size of its neck (Fig. 6-16).

Fusiform aneurysms appear as irregularly dilated and elongated arterial segments. This form of aneurysm most commonly affects the basilar, posterior, and middle cerebral arteries (Fig. 6-17).

Sometimes an aneurysm may be partially or completely thrombosed. These lesions are often incompletely visualized at angiography. They are detected either by visualization of the aneurysm remnant or by identification of an associated mass effect. CT scans are often helpful in delineating partially thrombotic aneurysms.[16, 19A]

A funnel-shaped dilatation of the posterior communicating artery can be seen in approximately five percent of normal angiograms (Fig. 6-18). This triangular outpouching is

Fig. 6-17. Left vertebral angiogram (mid-arterial phase, lateral view). Showing a partially thrombosed fusiform aneurysm of the basilar artery **(arrows).** The basilar artery appears elongated, ectatic and somewhat irregular.

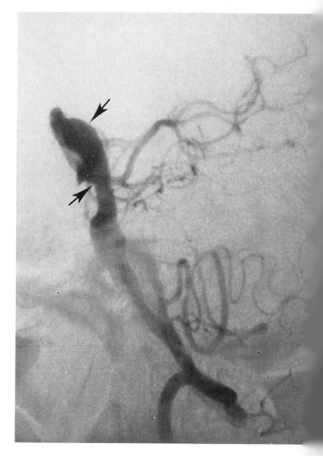

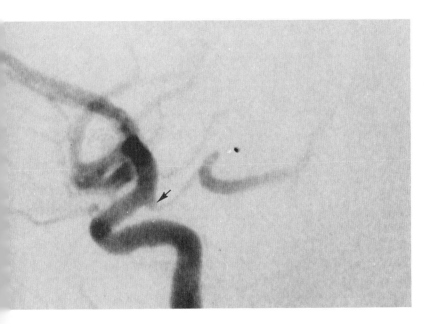

Fig. 6-18. Left internal carotid angiogram (early arterial phase, lateral view). Demonstrating infundibular widening of the posterior communicating artery **(arrow).**

known as an *infundibulum* and is sometimes associated with defects in the arterial media. An infundibulum represents symmetrical enlargement of the anterior aspect of the posterior communicating artery. This dilatation is considered to represent a true aneurysm if: it is larger than 3 mm, if its origin from the ICA is narrower than the localized dilatation itself, or if the posterior communicating artery arises asymmetrically instead of directly from its apex. While many authors have considered an infundibulum to be a benign incidental angiographic finding, some have considered them preaneurysmal. One documented case of a ruptured infundibulum as a cause of subarachnoid hemorrhage has been reported.[3]

OTHER LESIONS AFFECTING THE CIRCLE OF WILLIS

Atherosclerotic Disease

The most frequent and severe atheromatous changes in the cerebral vascular system itself are localized to the circle of Willis and the large arteries at the base of the brain (Fig. 6-19). The upper basilar artery, the ICA bifurca-tion, the proximal aspect of the M1 segment of the middle cerebral artery (see Chapter 9), and the P1 segment of the posterior cerebral artery (see Chapter 10) are most commonly involved.

As with atherosclerotic lesions elsewhere angiographic findings include arterial calcification, ectasia, tortuousity, irregularities of the intima, actual ulcerations, and stenosis (Fig. 6-20).

The clinical sequellae of actual vascular occlusions involving the circle of Willis and its small branches vary depending on the level of the occlusion, the branches implicated, and the available collateral flow. Sudden occlusion of the ICA is often accompanied by severe contralateral hemiplegia and hemianesthesia. If the dominant hemisphere is affected, complete aphasia will be present. If occlusion occurs gradually and collateral blood flow through the circle of Willis is adequate (Fig. 6-7), there may be few or no symptoms.

Isolated infarcts of the anterior cerebral territory are uncommon. Occlusion of the proximal portion of this vessel (including the recurrent artery of Heubner) results in a severe contralateral spastic hemiplegia due to involvement of the anterior part of the internal capsule and the paracentral lobule. Mental changes—memory loss, retardation, confusion, disorientation, emotional lability, and dementia—may occur. If the lesion is on the dominant side, there may be temporary expressive aphasia. Apraxia may be present but masked by the paresis. There is often sensory impairment of the lower extremity.[7, 14, 23]

(Occlusion of the anterior cerebral artery distal to the recurrent artery of Heubner and the anterior communicating artery is discussed in Chapter 8.)

Occlusion of the medial striate artery (Heubner's artery) results in weakness of the contralateral arm and paresis of the lower part of the face and tongue. An extrapyramidal type of rigidity or involuntary movement may be present.[7, 14, 23]

The clinical symptoms resulting from occlusion of the posterior communicating artery and its thalamoperforating branches are inconstant because of the rich and variable blood supply to the structures at the base of the brain.

Early anatomic reports have stated that the anterior communicating artery either has no branches or a single variable branch. However, recent microsurgical studies have demonstrated several small but important branches arising from the anterior communicating artery to supply part of the optic chiasm, lamina terminalis and hypothalamus, parolfactory area of Broca, cingulate gyrus, genu of the corpus callosum, and pillars of the fornix (Fig. 6-3).[5, 15] While these vessels are not often spontaneously occluded, they may

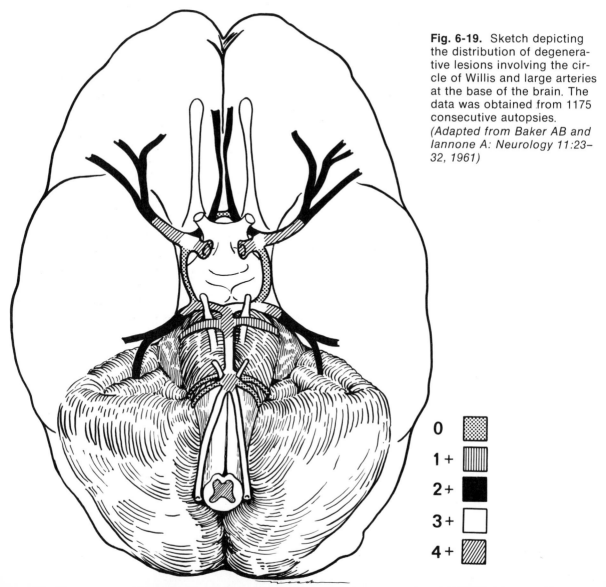

Fig. 6-19. Sketch depicting the distribution of degenerative lesions involving the circle of Willis and large arteries at the base of the brain. The data was obtained from 1175 consecutive autopsies.
(Adapted from Baker AB and Iannone A: Neurology 11:23–32, 1961)

0

1 +

2 +

3 +

4 +

be obliterated during surgery performed for anterior communicating artery aneurysm. The results of disregarding these smaller arteries and their branches may include altered personality, severe recent memory deficits, aphasia, hemiplegia, visual field defects, coma, and even death.[15]

Mass Lesions at the Base of the Brain

Sufficiently large suprasellar mass lesions, such as craniopharyngioma, hypothalamic glioma, and pituitary adenoma may elevate the horizontal portion of the anterior cerebral artery (see Chapter 8). However, on occasion, a suprasellar mass may extend superiorly through the circle of Willis without producing displacement of any major blood vessels. In such instances, the small vessels arising from the circle may show deformities while the components of the circle itself appear relatively normal. (Such a case is illustrated in Figure 6-21.) Here, the AP carotid study appears virtually normal; the A1 segment of the anterior cerebral artery is of normal calibre and position. However, subtle but definite lateral displacement of the anterior choroidal and posterior communicating arteries is present. Study of the vertebrobasilar system disclosed marked posterior displacement of the thalamoperforating arteries by an avascular suprasellar mass. At surgery, a large craniopharyngioma was found. The small perforating vessels arising from the circle of Willis may also enlarge if they supply a vascular lesion at the base of the brain (Fig. 6-22).

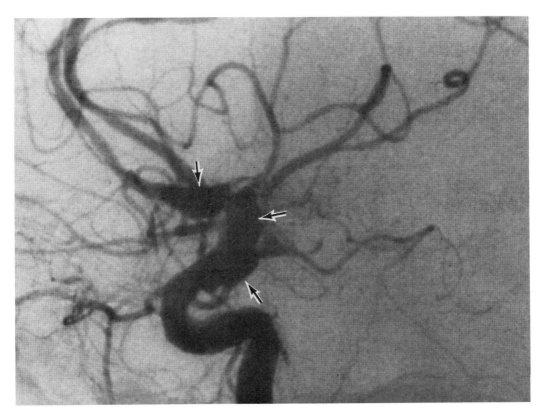

Fig. 6-20. Left common carotid angiogram (mid-arterial phase, lateral view) in diffuse atherosclerotic vascular disease. Note the irregular, ectatic internal carotid and anterior cerebral arteries **(arrows).**

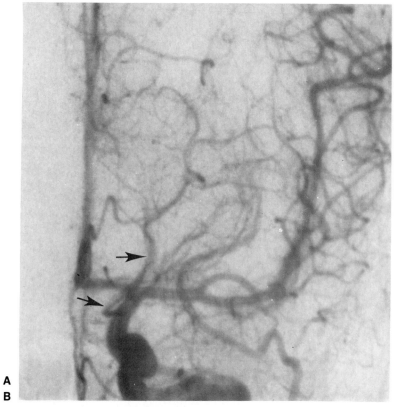

A
B

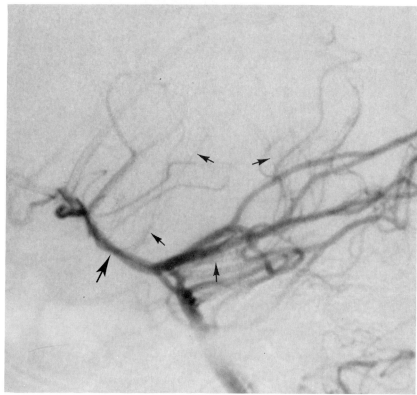

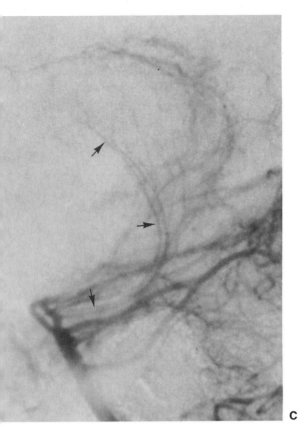

C

Fig. 6-21. Left common carotid angiogram (**A**, arterial phase, AP view) in a large craniopharyngioma. The distal anterior cerebral artery appears straightened (secondary to obstructive hydrocephalus), but the A1 segment is not elevated. Slight lateral displacement of the posterior communicating and anterior choroidal arteries can be seen (**arrows**). (B, C) Left vertebral angiogram (lateral view). (Same case as Fig. 6–21A.) Early arterial phase (**B**). The posterior communicating arteries (**large arrow**) have been refluxed. Stretching of the anterior and bowing of the posterior thalamoperforating arteries around the mass is apparent (**small arrows**). Late arterial phase (**C**). The precise posterior extension of the mass is delineated by the posteriorly displaced thalamoperforating branches (**arrows**).

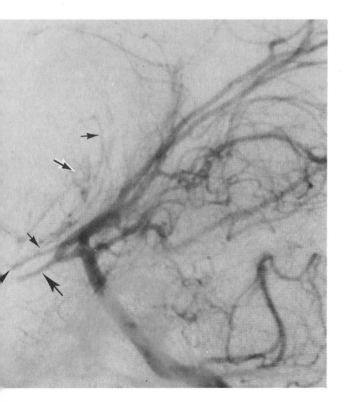

Fig. 6-22. Left vertebral angiogram (mid-arterial phase, lateral view) of a vascular hypothalamic glioma (**outlined arrow**). The posterior communicating arteries have been refluxed (**large black arrows**) and the enlarged anterior thalamoperforating arteries (**small black arrows**) are stretched and bowed posteriorly around the mass.

REFERENCES

1. **Alpers BJ, Beery RG, Paddison RM:** Anatomical studies of the circle of Willis in normal brain. Arch Neurol Psychiatry 81:409–418, 1959

2. **Anderson RA, Sondheimer RK:** Rare carotid-vertebrobasilar anastomoses with notes on the differentiation between proatlantal and hypoglossal arteries. Neuroradiology 11:113–118, 1976

2A. **Andrews RJ, Spiegel PK:** Intracranial aneurysms: Age, sex, blood pressure and multiplicity in an unselected series of patients. J Neurosurg 51:27–32, 1979

3. **Archer CR, Silbert S:** Infundibula may be clinically significant. Neuroradiology 15:247–251, 1978

4. **Brismar J:** Persistent hypoglossal artery, diagnostic criteria. Acta Radiol [Diagn] (Stockh) 17:160–166, 1976

5. **Crowell RM, Morawitz RB:** The anterior communicating artery has significant branches. Stroke 8:272–273, 1977

5A. **Deeb ZL, Jannetta PJ, Rosenbaum AE, Kerber CW, Drayer BP:** Tortuous vertebrobasilar arteries causing cranial nerve syndromes: Screening by computed tomography. J Comp Asst Tomogr 3:774–778, 1979

5B. **Davis JM, Davis KR, Crowell RM:** Subarachnoid hemorrhage secondary to ruptured intracranial aneurysm: Prognostic significance of cranial CP. Am J Neuroradiol 1:17–21, 1980

6. **Duncan AW, Rumbaugh CL, Caplan L:** Cerebral embolic disease: a complication of carotid aneurysms. Radiology 133:379–384, 1979

7. **Haymaker W:** Bing's Local Diagnosis in Neurological Diseases. St. Louis, CV Mosby, 1956

8. **Hodes PJ, Campay F, Riggs HE et al:** Cerebral angiography: fundamentals in anatomy and physiology. Am J Roentgenol 70:61–82 1953

9. **Kier EL:** Development of cerebral vessels, Section I: Fetal cerebral arteries: A phylogenetic and ontogenetic study, in Newton TH and Potts DG (eds), Radiology of the Skull and Brain, vol 2, pp 1089–1130, 1974

9A. **Koenig GH, Marshall WH Jr, Poole GJ et al:** Rupture of intracranial aneurysms during cerebral angiography: Report of ten cases and review of the literature. Neurosurg 5:314–324, 1979

10. **Lasjaunias P, Theron J, Moret J:** The occipital artery. Neuroradiology 15:31–37, 1978

11. **Lie A:** Congenital Anomalies of the Carotid Arteries. Amsterdam, Excerpta Medica Foundation, 1968

12. **Naruse S, Odake G:** Primitive trigeminal artery associated with an ipsilateral intracavernous giant aneurysm – A case report. Neuroradiology 17:259–264, 1979

13. **Parkinson D, Shields CB:** Persistent trigeminal artery: Its relationship to normal branches of the cavernous carotid. J Neurosurg 40:244–248, 1974

14. **Patten W:** Neurological Differential Diagnosis. Springer Verlag, New York, 1977

15. **Perlmutter D, Rhoton AL Jr:** Microsurgical anatomy of the anterior cerebral-anterior communicating recurrent artery complex. J Neurosurg 45:259–272, 1976

16. **Pinto RS, Kricheff II, Butler AR et al:** Correlation of computed tomographic, angiographic, and neuropathological changes in giant cerebral aneurysms. Radiology 132:85–92, 1979

16A. **Quencer RM, Simon J:** Transient bilateral occipital lobe ischemia: Microembolization through a trigeminal artery. Neuroradiology 18:273–275, 1979

16B. **Rhoton AL Jr, Saeki N, Perlmutter D et al:** Microsurgical anatomy of common aneurysm sites. Clin Neurosurg 26:248–306, 1979

17. **Riggs HE, Rupp C:** Variations in form of the circle of Willis. Arch Neurol 8:24–30, 1963

18. **Rothberg M, Mattey WE, Bastidas J:** Anomalous internal carotid-posterior cerebral artery circulation: One form of congenital incomplete circle of Willis. Am J Roentgenol 128:153–155, 1977

18A. **Saito, I, Shigeno T, Aritake K et al:** Vasospasm assessed by angiography and computerized tomography. J Neurosurg 51:466–475, 1979

19. **Saeki N, Rhoton AL Jr:** Microsurgical anatomy of the upper basilar artery and the posterior circle of Willis. J Neurosurg 46:563–578, 1977

19A. **Schubiger O, Valavanis A, Hayek J:** Computed tomography in cerebral aneurysms with special emphasis on giant intracranial aneurysms. J Comp Asst Tomogr 4:24–32, 1980

20. **Stephens RB, Stilwell DL:** Arteries and Veins of the Human Brain. Chas. C Thomas, 1969 Springfield Ill.

20A. **Stewart RM, Samson D, Diehl J et al:** Unruptured cerebral aneurysms presenting as recurrent transient neurologic deficits. Neurology 30:47–51, 1980

21. **Suzuki S, Nobechi T, Itoh I et al:** Persistent proatlantal intersegmental artery and occipital artery originating from internal carotid artery. Neuroradiology 17:105–109, 1979

22. **Suzuki J, Ohara H:** Clinicopathological study of cerebral aneurysms. J Neurosurg 48:505–514, 1978

22A. **Tenner MS, Cooper PR, Hussian SK:** Correlation of preoperative arteriographic spasm and outcome from aneurysm surgery. Presented at the American Society of Neuroradiology, 18th

Annual Meeting, Los Angeles, California. Mar 16–21, 1980

23. **Tichy F:** The syndromes of the cerebral arteries. Arch Pathol 48:475–488, 1949

24. **Tomsick TA, Lukin RR, Chambers AA:** Persistent trigeminal artery: Unusual associated abnormalities. Neuroradiology 17:253–257, 1979

25. **Wollschlaeger G, Wollschlaeger PB:** The circle of Willis, in Newton TH and Potts DG (eds), Radiology of the Skull and Brain, vol 2, pp 1171–1201, 1974

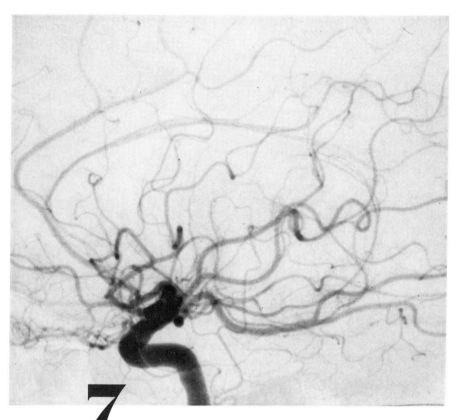

7 *The Anterior Choroidal Artery*

Thorough acquaintance with the normal course and caliber of the anterior choroidal artery (AChA) as well as its relationship to adjacent structures is of great importance to the neuroradiologist. The importance of the AChA is indicated by its extensive area of vascular supply which includes not only the choroid plexus of the temporal horn, but also the optic tract, thalamus, and internal capsule. In addition, the strategic location of the AChA between the uncus (anteromedial tip of the temporal lobe) and cerebral peduncles makes it particularly susceptible to displacement by intracranial mass lesions. The normal gross and angiographic anatomy of the AChA, and appearance of the AChA in vascular lesions, brain herniations, and other abnormalities will be discussed in this chapter.

NORMAL GROSS AND
ANGIOGRAPHIC ANATOMY

Gross Anatomy

The AChA may exist either as a single trunk or, less commonly, a number of small vessels. It normally arises from the posteromedial aspect of the internal carotid artery (ICA) at a variable distance above the posterior communicating artery origin and is the first ICA branch distal to the PCoA in a majority of anatomic specimens.[1A, 7A] Occasionally, the AChA originates either from the middle cerebral or posterior communicating artery or from the terminal ICA bifurcation.[2]

The AChA consists of two main segments. Its proximal aspect (also called the cisternal portion) first courses posteromedially below the optic tract and medial to the uncus of the temporal lobe. Turning laterally, the cisternal AChA continues its course through the crural cistern and around the cerebral peduncle to enter the choroidal fissure of the temporal horn (Fig. 7-1).

The distal or plexal segment of the AChA begins at the choroidal fissure and continues posteriorly in the supracornual cleft of the temporal horn. The AChA may either terminate near the lateral geniculate body or extend around the pulvinar of the thalamus (Fig. 7-2). On occasion it courses with the choroid plexus through the body of the lateral ventricle as far anteriorly as the foramen of Monro.[5]

Branches of the AChA anastomose freely with branches of the lateral posterior choroidal, posterior communicating, and posterior cerebral arteries. A reciprocal relationship is present between the territory supplied by the AChA, posterior cerebral, and lateral posterior choroidal (LPChA) arteries. Because of this reciprocal relationship, branches of the AChA supply an extensive but variable area that includes portions of the temporal lobe (uncus, pyriform cortex, amygdala), the visual system (optic tract, part of the lateral geniculate body, optic radiations), internal capsule (genu and part of the posterior limb of the in-

Fig. 7-1. Anatomic sketch depicting the anterior choroidal artery and its relationship to the choroid plexus of the temporal horn. The left temporal horn has been dissected and is seen as viewed from below. The AChA is indicated **(outlined arrows).** The lateral posterior choroidal artery, a branch of the posterior cerebral artery, is also indicated **(black arrow).**

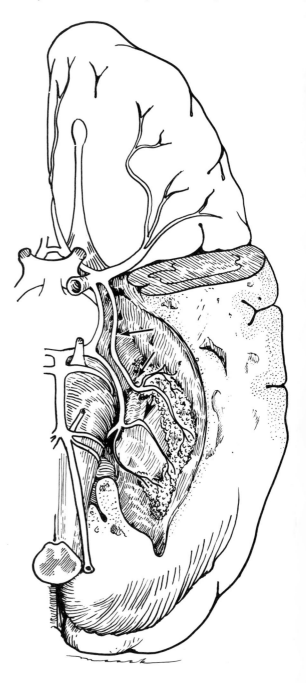

ternal capsule), basal ganglia (medial globus pallidus, tail of caudate nucleus), the diencephalon (part of the lateral thalamus and subthalamus), and the midbrain (middle one-third of the cerebral peduncles and the substantia nigra).[8] The AChA usually supplies the choroid plexus in the inferior portions of temporal horn and atrium. The LPChA (a branch of the posterior cerebral artery) supplies the choroid plexus in the posterior temporal horn, atrium, and body of the lateral ventricle (see Chapter 10). Overlap between these two vessels is common.[1A]

Radiographic Anatomy

The AChA can be identified in approximately 95% of all internal carotid angiograms. The AChA is best delineated on the AP view when caudal angulation of the roentgen beam relative to the orbitomeatal line is at least 15 degrees. As the caudal angulation diminishes, the AChA appears increasingly foreshortened and distorted (Fig. 7-3).

In the anteroposterior projection (Fig. 7-4), the AChA is seen arising from the medial aspect of the ICA. The cisternal AChA first curves medially and posteriorly around the uncus (Fig. 7-4A, arrow 1), then turns laterally around the cerebral peduncle, coursing toward the temporal horn. A definite, abrupt, lateral angulation or "kink" (Fig. 7-4A, arrow 2) is present where the AChA enters the choroidal fissure. The plexal portion of the AChA then follows a gently undulating course through the temporal horn (Fig. 7-4A, arrow 3), first curving laterally, then gradually turning superomedially to reach the atrium and lateral geniculate body.

(Text continued on p. 173)

Fig. 7-2. Anatomic sketch depicting the AChA (lateral view). The "plexal point" (the point where the AChA enters the choroidal fissure) is indicated **(arrow).**

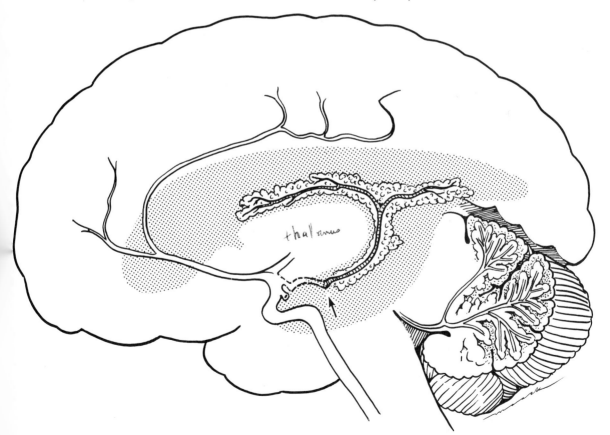

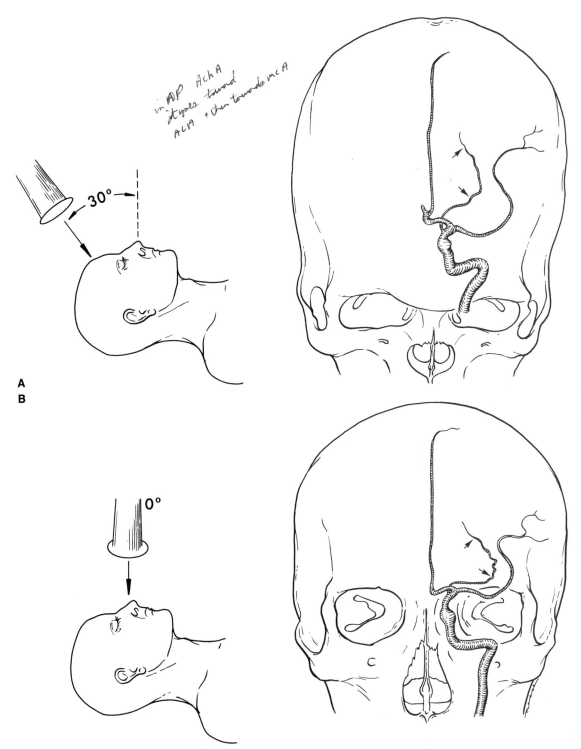

Fig. 7-3. Anatomic sketch depicting the effect of tube angulation on the visualization and appearance of the AChA. **A.** 30° caudal angulation. The AChA **(arrows)** is well delineated. **B.** 0° tube angulation. The AChA **(arrows)** appears foreshortened.

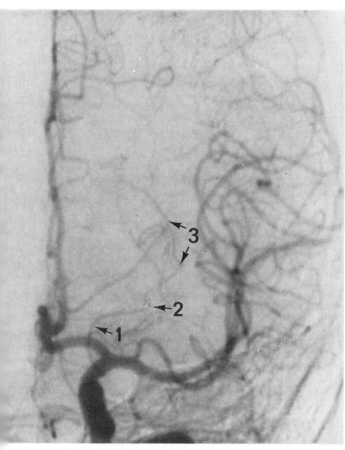

Fig. 7-4. Normal left carotid angiogram (**A,** arterial phase, AP view). The cisternal portion of the AChA as it curves around the uncus **(arrow 1),** the point where the AChA leaves the crural cistern and enters the choroidal fissure of the temporal horn **(arrow 2),** and the plexal portion of the AChA **(arrow 3)** are indicated. Left carotid angiogram (**B,** arterial phase, lateral view). The plexal point of the AChA is indicated **(large arrow).** The course of the AChA as it curves around the pulvinar of the thalamus is also indicated **(small black arrows).**

A
B

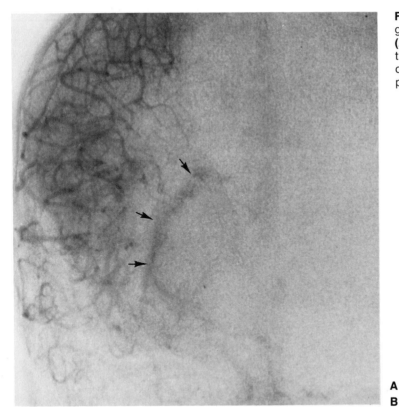

Fig. 7-5. Right carotid angiogram (late arterial phase), AP **(A)** and lateral views **(B)**. Here the dense, rather homogeneous blush of the choroid plexus is indicated **(arrows).**

A
B

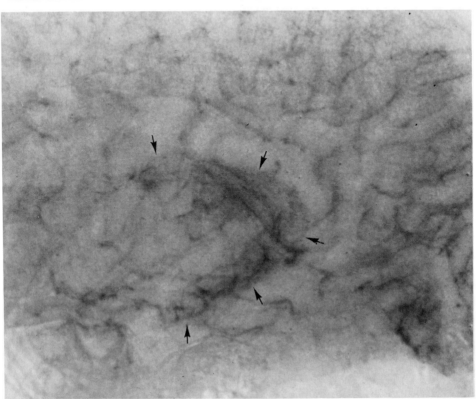

As illustrated in the lateral projection (Fig. 7-4B), the cisternal AChA often runs inferiorly for a short distance before curving upward and posteriorly. The point where the AChA enters the choroid plexus of the temporal horn is termed the *plexal point* (Fig. 7-4B, large arrow) and is usually demarcated by a definite posterosuperior angulation of the AChA. From the plexal point, the AChA follows a broad, concave curve as it extends around the pulvinar of the thalamus (Fig. 7-4B, small arrows).

A dense, homogeneous capillary stain or blush is sometimes seen in the late arterial phase. This blush partially delineates the choroid plexus of the temporal horn and atrium (Fig. 7-5).

A variety of reference lines and measurement methods have been constructed in an attempt to assess minor deviations in the course and caliber of the AChA. However, the exact configuration of the AChA may normally vary within wide limits, particularly in the lateral projection. This wide variability renders most measurements somewhat unreliable.

ABNORMALITIES OF THE ANTERIOR CHOROIDAL ARTERY

Hyperplasia of the Anterior Choroidal Artery

Hyperplasia of the AChA is often difficult to assess. The normal size of the AChA varies widely depending on its terminal area of distribution and its reciprocal relationship with the posterior choroidal and posterior cerebral arteries. Whenever the AChA supplies a portion of the territory ordinarily supplied by the LPChA and posterior cerebral arteries, the AChA will be physiologically enlarged. On the other hand, pathologic hyperplasia of the AChA can occur with vascular neoplasms, arteriovenous malformations, and collateral circulation in occlusive vascular disease.[11]

Some typical abnormalities of the AChA are illustrated in Figures 7-6 through 7-11.

One of the more common lesions producing hyperplasia of the AChA is illustrated in Figure 7-6. Here an enlarged, tortuous AChA (arrows) supplies a vascular glioma involving the thalamus and corpus callosum. In Figure 7-7, an intraventricular meningioma has produced a somewhat similar pattern of AChA enlargement.

Another common cause of hyperplasia of the AChA is shown in Figure 7-8 where subtotal stenosis of the left middle cerebral artery (large arrow) is present in a patient with multiple cerebral vascular occlusions. Enlarged lenticulostriate arteries and an hypertrophied AChA (small arrows) provide extensive collateral circulation to the usual distal middle cerebral artery distribution.

A less common cause of hyperplasia is illustrated in Figure 7-9. Here, a racemose arteriovenous malformation has caused enlargement of both the anterior and posterior choroidal arteries.

Changes in the Anterior Choroidal Artery with Intracranial Mass Lesions

Intracerebral mass lesions of sufficient size may displace one or both segments of the anterior choroidal artery. Lesions immediately adjacent to the AChA may either directly displace the AChA or derive pathologic blood supply from its branches. However, not all displacements of the AChA are caused by lesions adjacent to the artery itself. Remote intracerebral mass lesions of sufficient size can cause characteristic distortions of the AChA as the adjacent uncus or hippocampus is herniated through the tentorial incisura.

Mass effects in certain locations displace the AChA in definite patterns,[4, 5, 10] Anterior temporal lobe masses characteristically stretch and displace the AChA medially. In Figure 7-10A, a large, holotemporal, avascular mass has displaced both the cisternal and plexal portions of the AChA medially. It has also widened the normal initial medial arc of

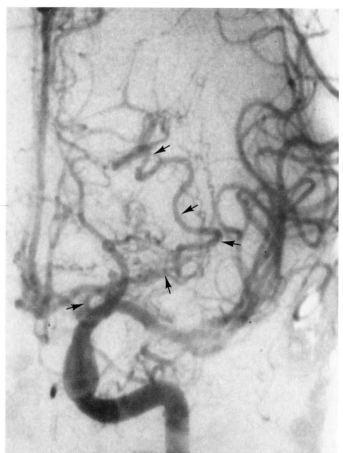

Fig. 7-6. Left carotid angiogram (mid-arterial phase), AP **(A)** and lateral views **(B)** in a moderately vascular thalamic and corpus callosum glioma. The enlarged AChA is indicated **(arrows).**

A
B

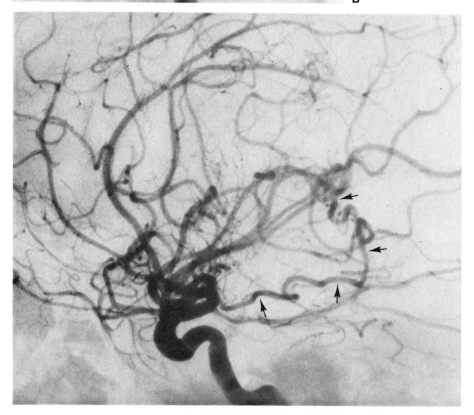

the AChA. If a temporal lobe mass is sufficiently large to produce uncal (*i.e.* anterior descending tentorial herniation) the cisternal AChA will also appear stretched and displaced inferiorly in the lateral projection (Fig. 7-10B, arrows). Note here that the plexal AChA is also displaced inferiorly, indicating the presence of combined uncal and hippocampal transtentorial herniation. Midtemporal and subtemporal extracerebral masses may produce widening and elongation of the cisternal initial medial arc of the AChA. This displacement is usually visible in the AP view (Fig. 7-11A). In the lateral projection, the AChA appears bowed and stretched superiorly (Figs. 7-11B, 7-12).

Inferior temporal masses and lesions in or adjacent to the tentorial incisura also displace the AChA superiorly. In Figure 7-11, a tentorial meningioma has stretched and bowed the cisternal AChA medially and superiorly.

Retrotemporal masses produce anterior displacement of the plexal AChA, causing increased undulation of the cisternal AChA as it is buckled forward by the posteriorly located mass effect. In Figure 7-13 a massive choroid plexus carcinoma (small arrows) has displaced the plexal portion of an enlarged, tortuous AChA (large arrows). Superior retrotemporal lesions will also depress the plexal AChA. Conversely, inferior retrotemporal masses elevate the plexal AChA.

(Text continued on p. 183)

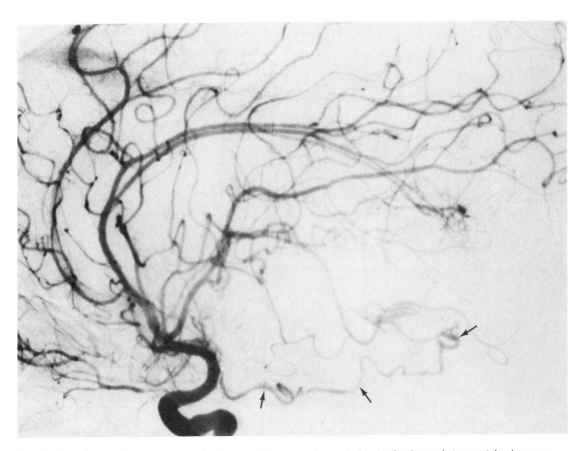

Fig. 7-7. Left carotid angiogram (mid-arterial phase, lateral view) of a large intraventricular meningioma **(small arrows).** The AChA **(large arrows)** is hypertrophied and displaced posteroinferiorly. *(Courtesy of R. Brinton, M.D.)*

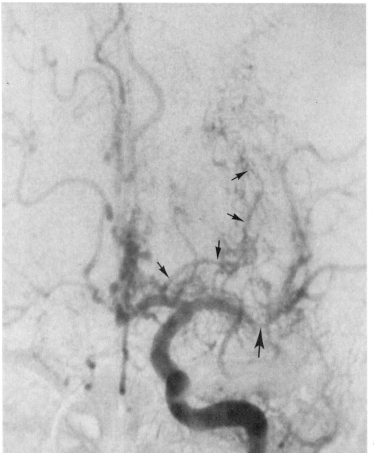

Fig. 7-8. Left common carotid angiogram (mid-arterial phase), AP **(A)** and lateral **(B)** views of multiple intracranial vascular occlusions. The middle cerebral artery is stenotic **(large arrow)** and multiple, tortuous, collateral channels, including a large AChA **(small black arrows)** are present.

A
B

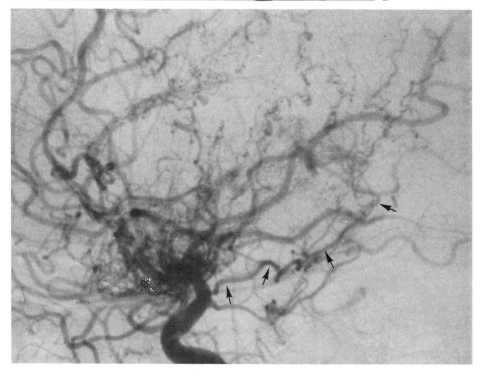

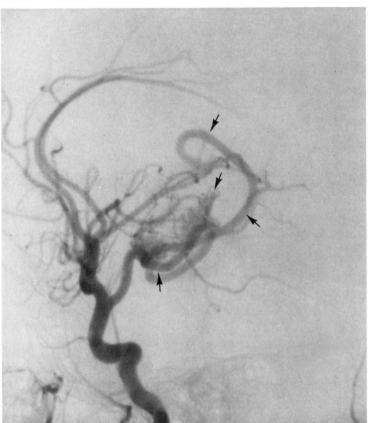

Fig. 7-9. Left common carotid angiogram (lateral view), early arterial **(A)** and mid-arterial phases **(B).** This was seen in a 6-month-old boy. A racemose arteriovenous malformation caused marked enlargement of both the anterior and lateral posterior choroidal arteries **(small arrows).** Aneurysmal dilatation of the vein of Galen and enlargement of the straight sinus are indicated **(large arrows).**

A
B

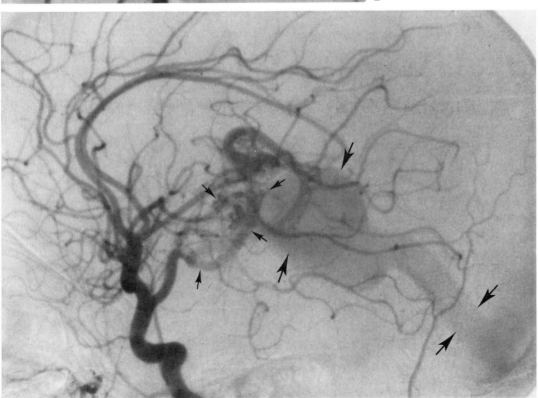

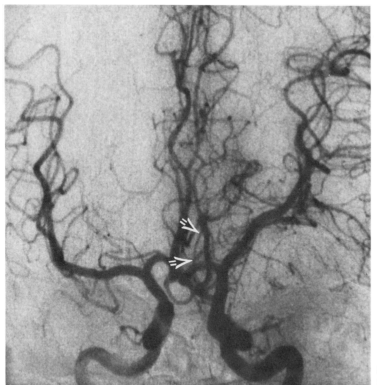

Fig. 7-10. A. Left internal carotid angiogram (arterial phase, AP view) demonstrating an avascular holotemporal mass. The AChA **(arrows)** has been displaced medially almost to the midline. **B.** Same case as 7-10A (lateral view). Descending temporal lobe herniation through the tentorial incisura has produced downward displacement of the AChA **(arrows)**.

A
B

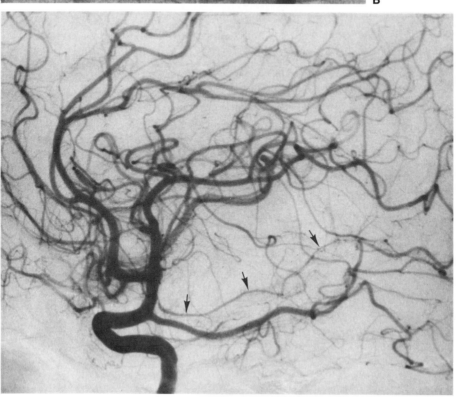

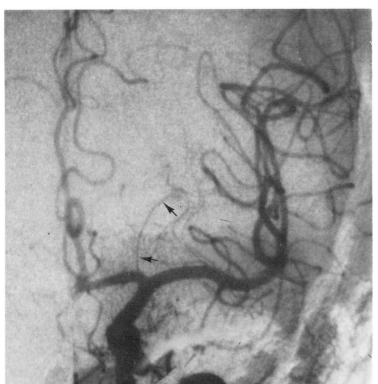

Fig. 7-11. Left common carotid angiogram (arterial phase), AP **(A)** and lateral **(B)** views of a recurrent meningioma at the tentorial incisura. The cisternal AChA is bowed medially and superiorly **(arrows).**

A

B

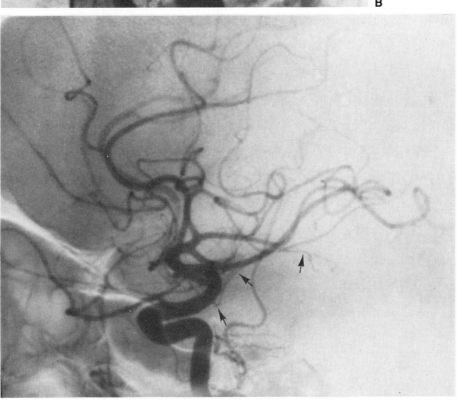

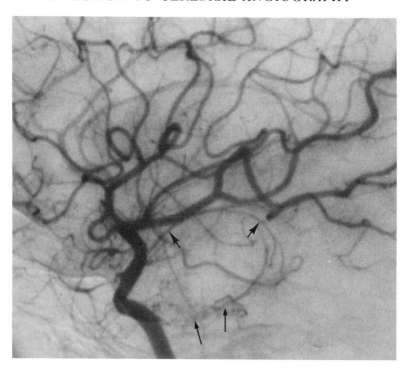

Fig. 7-12. Left internal carotid angiogram (mid-arterial phase, lateral view) outlining a large exophytic vascular mass in the upper midbrain **(small arrows).** The AChA is displaced superiorly **(large arrows).**

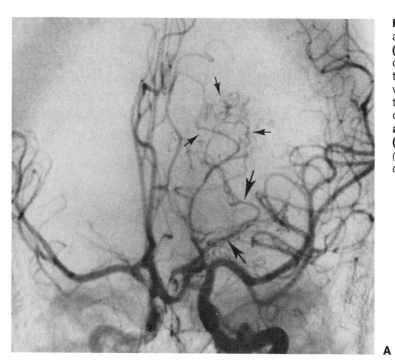

A

Fig. 7-13. Left internal carotid angiogram (arterial phase), AP **(A)** and lateral **(B)** views of a choroid plexus papilloma in the atrium of the left lateral ventricle. The plexal portion of the enlarged AChA has been displaced anteriorly **(large arrows)** by the vascular mass **(small arrows).**
(Fig. 7-13 continued on opposite page, top)

Fig. 7-14. Left internal carotid angiogram AP **(A)** and lateral **(B)** views of large avascular thalamic astrocytoma. The AChA is bowed laterally and posterosuperiorly **(arrows)** around the enlarged thalamus.

(Fig. 7-13
continued)

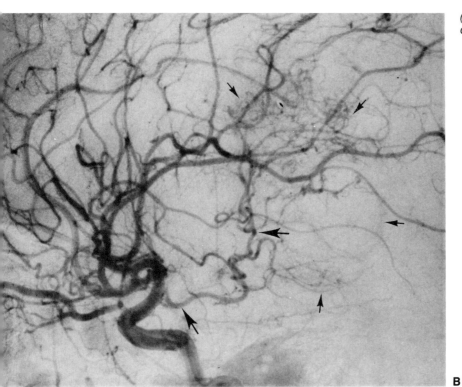

B

A
B

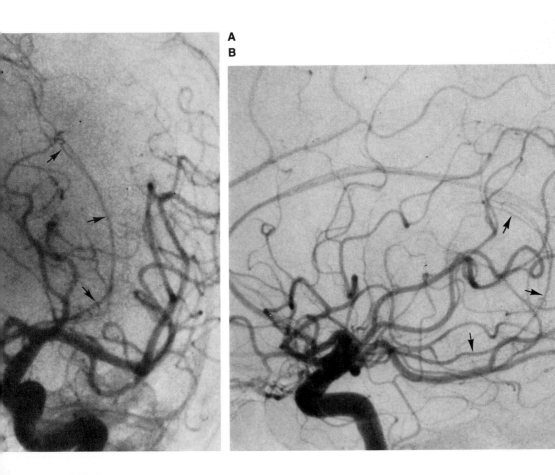

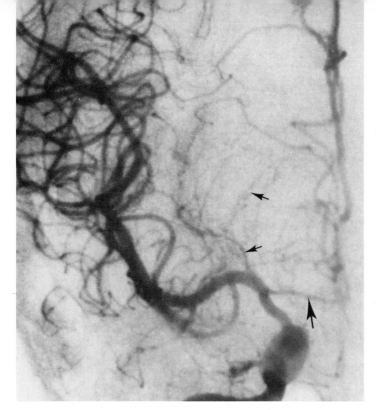

Fig. 7-15. Right internal carotid angiogram (arterial phase, AP view) of a large pituitary adenoma. The anterior cerebral artery **(large arrow)** is normal but the lenticulostriate arteries and AChA **(small arrows)** are displaced laterally.

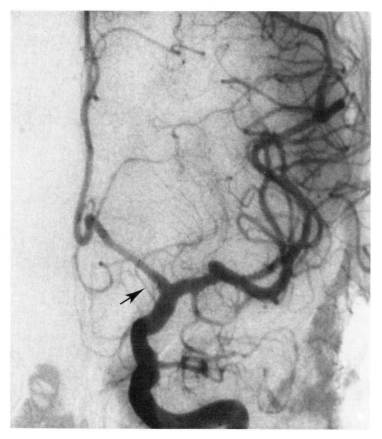

Fig. 7-16. Left internal carotid angiogram (arterial phase, AP view) of a large chromophobe adenoma. The horizontal segment of the anterior cerebral artery is elevated and the initial portion of the cisternal AChA is displaced superolaterally **(arrow)** by the mass.

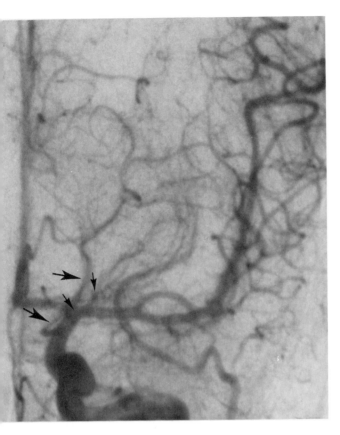

Fig. 7-17. Left carotid angiogram (arterial phase, AP view) of large craniopharyngioma. The horizontal segment of the ACA is normal. The posterior communicating artery **(large arrows)** and the AChA **(small arrows)** are displaced laterally by the mass.

Thalamic masses widen the normal arc of the plexal AChA, bowing it posteriorly, inferiorly, and laterally. An avascular thalamic glioma is illustrated in Figure 7-14. Note the marked accentuation and widening of the AChA arc as it curves around the enlarged pulvinar.

Suprasellar masses may lie almost entirely within the circle of Willis and hence produce little or no displacement of the major cerebral arteries (Fig. 7-15). However, since the cisternal AChA initially courses immediately below the optic tract, slight elevation and lateral displacement of the proximal AChA may be produced if the optic chiasm is displaced superiorly (Figs. 7-15, 7-16). Conversely, lesions directly above the chiasm may compress the proximal cisternal AChA inferiorly. In Figure 7-17, a large avascular suprasellar mass effect is present, caused by a recurrent craniopharyngioma. Note that the horizontal

segment of the anterior cerebral artery is normal. However, both the posterior communicating (large arrows) and proximal anterior choroidal artery (small arrows) have been displaced inferolaterally.

Large temporal lobe masses as well as remote supratentorial mass lesions of sufficient size produce transtentorial herniation of the uncus, hippocampal gyrus, or both. With anterior descending herniation, the uncus is forced over the free edge of the tentorium. The cisternal AChA is consequently displaced medially and inferiorly (Fig. 7-10). Posterior or hippocampal herniation produces medial and inferior displacement of both the cisternal and plexal portions of the AChA. Conversely, large posterior fossa may produce upward herniation of the brainstem or cerebellum through the tentorial notch, displacing the cisternal AChA superiorly (see Chapter 12).

Occlusions of the Anterior Choroidal Artery

Occlusion of the AChA is difficult to determine angiographically. The extensive anastomoses with the LPChA and other branches of the posterior cerebral and posterior communicating arteries are often sufficient to prevent infarction when the AChA is occluded.

In the past, surgical occlusion of the AChA was advocated for the treatment of Parkinson's disease.[1, 7] However, this procedure is no longer used.

The signs and symptoms of AChA occlusion vary depending on the site of occlusion and the variable terminal field of AChA distribution. The classically reported clinical features include contralateral hemiplegia and hemianesthesia (of all sensory modalities but in differing degree). A quadrantic or hemianopic field defect opposite to the side of the lesion is also often present. There is usually sparing of macular vision. Added signs resulting from the involvement of basal ganglia, hippocampus, thalamus, and mesencephalon may be detected.[3, 6, 9] The wide variability in clincal manifestations of AChA occlusion is explained by its anstomoses with branches of the posterior communicating and posterior choroidal arteries.[8]

REFERENCES

1. **Cooper IS:** Surgical occlusion of the anterior choroidal artery in parkinsonism. Surg Gynecol Obstet 99:207–219, 1954
1A. **Fujii K, Lenkey C, Rhoton AL:** Microsurgical anatomy of the choroidal arteries: Lateral and third ventricles. J Neurosurg 52:165–188, 1980
2. **Goldberg HI:** The anterior choroidal artery. In Newton TH, Potts DG (eds): Radiology of the Skull and Brain, Vol 2, pp 1628–1658. St. Louis, CV Mosby, 1974
3. **Haymaker W:** Bing's Local Diagnosis in Neurological Diseases. St. Louis, CV Mosby, 1956
4. **LeMay M, Jackson DM:** Changes in the anterior choroidal artery in intracranial lesions. Am J Roentgenol 92:776–785, 1964
5. **Margolis MT, Hoffman HB, Newton TH:** Choroidal arteries in the diagnosis of thalamic tumors. J Neurosurg 36:287–298, 1972
6. **Patten W:** Neurological Differential Diagnosis. New York, Springer-Verlag, 1977
7. **Rand RW, Brown WJ, Stern WE:** Surgical occlusion of anterior choroidal arteries in parkinsonism. Neurology (Minneap) 6:390–401, 1956
7A. **Rhoton AL Jr, Fugii K, Fradd B:** Microsurgical anatomy of the anterior choroidal artery. Surg Neurol 12:171–187, 1979
8. **Saeki N, Thoton AL Jr:** Microsurgical anatomy of the upper basilar artery and the posterior circle of Willis. J Neurosurg 46:563–578, 1977
9. **Tichy F:** The syndromes of the cerebral arteries. Arch Pathol 48:475–488, 1949
10. **Wackenheim A, Ludwiczak R, Capesius P:** The course of the anterior choroidal artery. Neuroradiology 11:73–75, 1976
11. **Wollschlaeger G, Wollschlaeger PB, Meyer PG, Krautman JJ:** Widening or hyperplasia of the anterior choroidal artery. Radiology 93:1079–1083, 1969

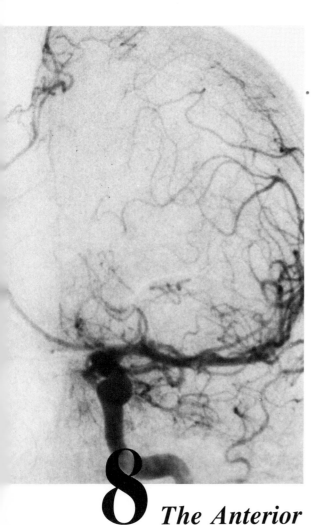

8 *The Anterior Cerebral Artery*

The anterior cerebral artery (ACA) is an important angiographic landmark. Situated between the two cerebral hemispheres, this vessel is an excellent midline marker. Because of its strategic location the ACA is a moderately sensitive indicator of mass lesions in the mid and frontal portions of the brain.

A number of small branches arise from the proximal ACA and course superiorly to supply vital structures at the base of the brain. Distal branches of the ACA irrigate the anterior two-thirds of the medial surfaces of the cerebral hemispheres. Knowledge of the normal anatomy of the anterior cerebral-anterior communicating-recurrent artery complex is also gaining importance as microsurgical techniques in this area become increasingly aggressive. Therefore, a detailed study of both the normal and pathologic ACA is of fundamental importance to the neuroangiographer.

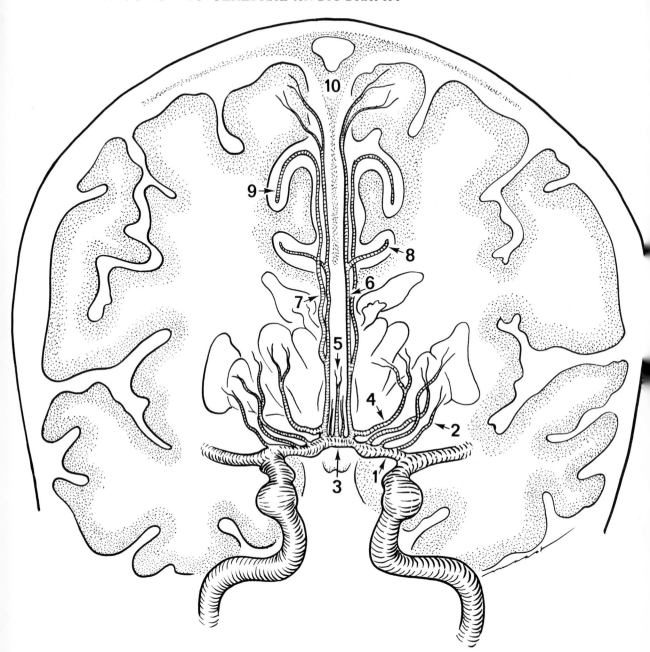

Fig. 8-1. Diagrammatic sketch of the anterior cerebral arteries and their major branches (AP view). **1.** Horizontal (A1) segment. **2.** Medial lenticulostriate arteries. **3.** Anterior communicating artery. **4.** Recurrent artery of Heubner. **5.** Anterior communicating artery branches. **6.** Pericallosal artery. **7.** Callosomarginal artery. **8.** Pericallosal pial plexus. **9.** Callosomarginal artery branches over the cingulate gyrus. **10.** Falx cerebri.

NORMAL GROSS ANATOMY

Horizontal (Precommunicating) Segment

The internal carotid artery (ICA) terminates below the anterior perforated substance by bifurcating into the anterior and middle cerebral arteries. The ACA, the smaller of these two terminal branches, courses medially and somewhat anteriorly over the optic nerve and chiasm to reach the interhemispheric fissure (Fig. 8-1).

The proximal or horizontal portion of the ACA — also termed the A1 segment — extends from the origin of the ACA to its union with the contralateral ACA via the anterior communicating artery. A variable number of small but important penetrating branches (the **medial lenticulostriate arteries**) arise from the horizontal ACA and course posterosuperiorly to supply parts of the anterior perforated substance, subfrontal area, dorsal surface of the optic chiasm and tract, anterior commissure and septum pellucidum, hypothalamus, and paraolfactory structures (see Fig. 6-3B). Some of these small branches have also been described as supplying parts of the anterior pallidum, internal capsule, and Sylvian fissure.[2]

One of the medial striate arteries, the recurrent branch of the ACA (also called the **recurrent artery of Heubner**), originates either from the A1 segment (14%) or the proximal A2 segment (78%) and doubles back on its parent artery at an acute angle, accompanying it a variable distance before penetrating the brain (Fig. 8-1). The parenchymal distribution of the recurrent artery includes the anterior limb of the internal capsule, the anteroinferior portion of the globus pallidus, and the head of the caudate nucleus. Parts of the putamen, hypothalamus, and Sylvian fissure may also be perfused by the recurrent artery.[14]

The **anterior communicating artery** (ACoA) is a short vessel that joins the two ACAs when they reach the interhemispheric fissure (Fig. 8-1). It completes the anterior part of the circle of Willis. The ACoA is a frequent site of congenital berry aneurysms and is a common location for circulus arteriosus anomalies (see Chapter 6). A direct correlation seems to exist between the difference in size of both the A1 segments and the diameter of the ACoA. A small or hypoplastic A1 is usually formed in conjunction with a large ACoA since the contralateral horizontal segment provides most of the vascular supply to both distal ACA territories.

The ACoA has several branches that course superiorly to supply the septal and median paraolfactory nuclei, optic chiasm and nerves, corpus callosum genu, columns of the fornix, septum pellucidum, anterior cingulum, and the anterior hypothalamus (see Figs. 6-3B, 8-1).[1B] This vascular supply to prominent portions of the limbic system is an important consideration in microsurgical manipulation for ACoA aneurysms since inadvertent occlusion may have profound clinical sequelae. Occasionally a large ACoA branch (sometimes termed the median ACA) courses upward and posteriorly over the corpus callosum to supply the paracentral lobules of both hemispheres.[17]

Distal (Postcommunicating) Segment

Distal to the ACoA, the ACA turns superiorly into the interhemispheric fissure. First it courses in front of the lamina terminalis and then passes anterosuperiorly around the genu of the corpus callosum (Figs. 8-2, 8-3). This portion of the ACA is sometimes termed the A2 segment. It extends from the level of the ACoA to the distal ACA bifurcation.

ACA branching is quite variable. The **orbitofrontal artery** is usually the first cortical ACA branch, arising from the A2 segment to supply the gyrus rectus and inferomedial surface of the frontal lobe (Fig. 8-2). In approximately one-third of all cases a branch originates from the ACA near the genu of the corpus callosum and passes anteriorly to supply the ventromedial surface of the frontal lobe. This vessel, the **frontopolar artery,** may arise from a common trunk with the orbitofrontal artery. These arteries perfuse the gyrus rectus and orbital gyri, olfactory bulb

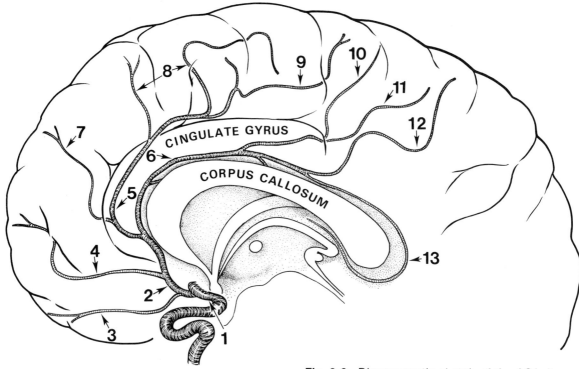

CINGULATE GYRUS

CORPUS CALLOSUM

Fig. 8-2. Diagrammatic sketch of the ACA, its branches, and its relationship to adjacent structures. **1.** Horizontal (A1) segment. **2.** ACA in front of the lamina terminalis. **3.** Orbito-frontal artery. **4.** Frontopolar artery. **5.** Callosomarginal artery. **6.** Pericallosal artery. **7.** Anterior internal frontal artery. **8.** Middle internal frontal arteries. **9.** Posterior internal frontal artery. **10.** Paracentral artery. **11.** Superior internal parietal (precuneal) artery. **12.** Inferior internal parietal artery. **13.** Pericallosal artery extending around the splenium of the corpus callosum.

and tract, and the anterior part of the superior frontal gyrus.

At a variable point near the genu of the corpus callosum, the ACA usually divides into its two terminal branches, a callosomarginal and a pericallosal trunk (Fig. 8-2). The **callosomarginal artery**, usually the smaller of these two branches, passes over the cingulate gyrus and runs posteriorly within the cingulate sulcus. A discrete callosomarginal artery is present in approximately one-half of all cases.[16] When this vessel is small or absent, multiple branches arise directly from the pericallosal artery to supply the usual distribution of the callosomarginal artery. Anterior, middle, and posterior internal frontal arteries arise either from the callosomarginal or pericallosal trunk to supply the medial surface of the hemispheres as far posteriorly as the precental gyrus.[15, 17]

The **pericallosal artery**, the larger of the two terminal ACA branches, is considered the continuation of the ACA. The pericallosal artery runs posteriorly at a variable distance above the corpus callosum. Its major branch, the superior internal parietal or precuneal artery, courses upward to supply the precuneus and superior parietal lobule. Smaller branches supply the paracentral lobule and the inferior aspect of the precuneus. Branches of the pericallosal artery also supply the pial plexus which covers the corpus callosum. Distal or posterior pericallosal branches may also curve around the surface of the splenium and run

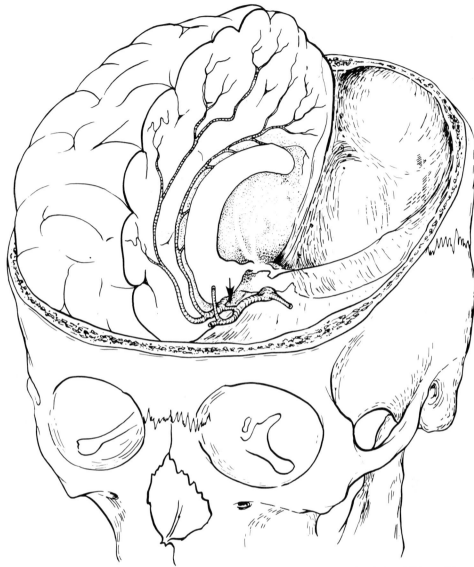

Fig. 8-3. Anatomic sketch of the ACA and its relationship to the corpus callosum. The ACAs initially course anteromedially and are joined in the interhemispheric fissure by the anterior communicating artery **(arrow).** They then course anteriorly around the genu of the corpus callosum curving around it in a postero-superior arc.

forward in the transverse fissure under the belly of the corpus callosum to the foramen of Monro.[17]

Cortical branches of the ACAs extend over the apex of the brain to supply a small strip of cortex along the anterior two-thirds of the superolateral surfaces of both hemispheres where they anastomose with small branches of the middle and posterior cerebral arteries. This so-called "watershed" area is a common site for cerebral infarction.

(Text continued on p. 193)

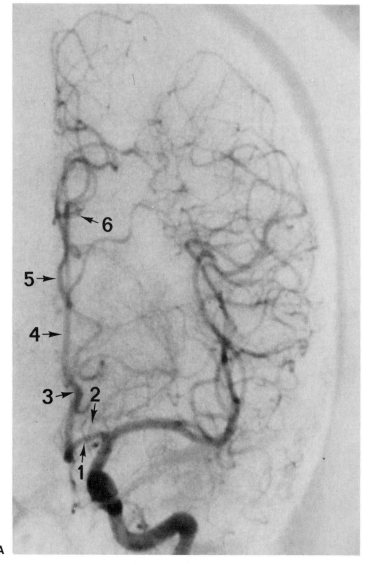

A

Fig. 8-4. Left internal carotid angiogram (**A,** arterial phase, AP view). **1.** Horizontal (A1) segment. **2.** Medial lenticulostriate arteries. **3.** ACA in front of the corpus callosum genu. **4.** Pericallosal artery. **5.** Callosomarginal artery. **6.** Pericallosal artery coursing in the cingulate sulcus above the body of the corpus callosum.

Left internal carotid angiogram (**B,** arterial phase, lateral view) **1.** ACA in the cistern of the lamina terminalis. **2.** Orbitofrontal artery. **3.** Frontopolar artery. **4.** ACA in front of the genu of the corpus callosum. **5.** Callosomarginal artery. **6.** Pericallosal artery in the cingulate sulcus. **7.** Pericallosal artery in the cingulate sulcus just above the corpus callosum.

Left internal carotid angiogram (**C,** arterial phase, lateral view) in an MCA occlusion. The ACA and its branches are therefore seen clearly without overlapping MCA vessels. (The posterior cerebral artery, **[small black arrow]** is opacified on this study.) The callosomarginal artery **(outlined arrow)** territory is supplied by the pericallosal artery which trifurcates **(large black arrow)** into branches supplying the paracentral and internal parietal areas.

(Fig. 8-4 continued on opposite page)

(Fig. 8-4 continued)   *The Anterior Cerebral Artery 191*

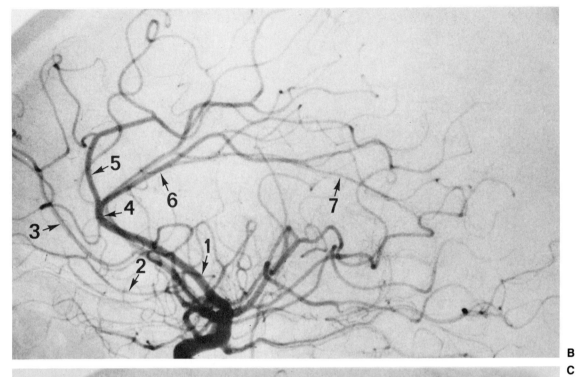

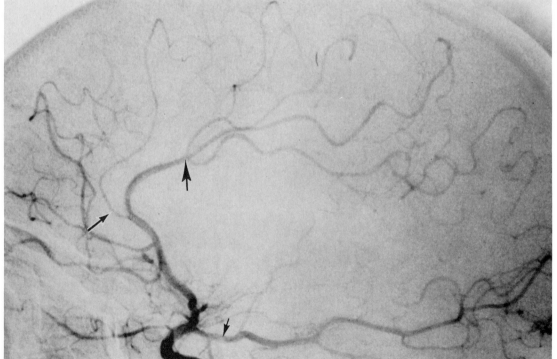

B

C

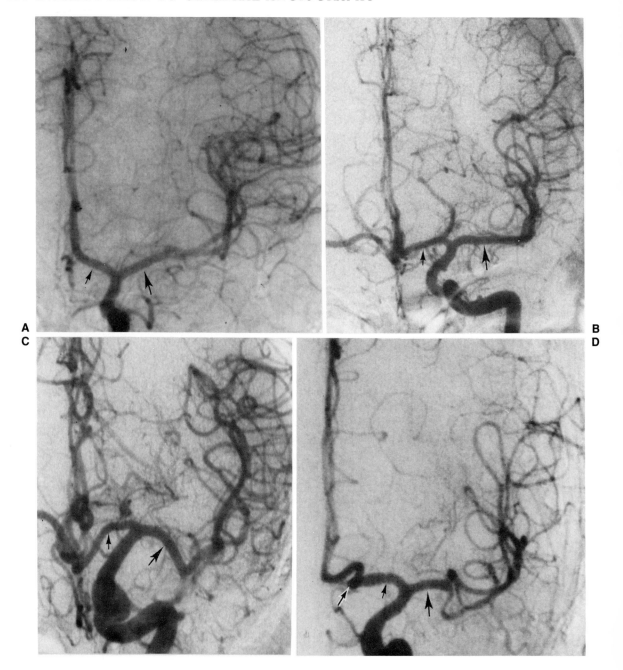

A

C

B

D

◀ **Fig. 8-5.** Series of AP carotid angiograms demonstrating variations in course and configuration of the horizontal ACA **(small arrows).** The M1 segments of the middle cerebral artery (MCA) are indicated **(large arrows). (A)** Six-month-old child, normal study. The horizontal segments of both the ACA and MCA course slightly superiorly. **(B)** 32-year-old female, normal study. The A1 and M1 segments follow a straight, nearly horizontal course. **(C)** 68-year-old male, normal study. The horizontal segments of both and the ACA and MCA have a marked inferior curve. **(D)** 40-year-old male, normal study. The horizontal ACA has a redundant loop **(outlined arrow).**

NORMAL RADIOGRAPHIC ANATOMY

Horizontal (A1) Segment

The distal ICA divides into the anterior and middle cerebral arteries, forming a "T" (Fig. 8-4A). The horizontal or A1 segment of the ACA forms the medial arm of this "T". The contour of the A1 segment varies. As it passes anteriorly and medially toward the interhemispheric fissure and its counterpart from the opposite side the ACA may take a horizontal course, or ascend slightly or descend (Fig. 8-5). This variability makes it difficult to delineate a constant pattern for any particular age group. However, the A1 segment tends to course somewhat more inferiorly with increasing age. Note that an A1 segment that is either perfectly horizontal or slightly convex superiorly should not be misdiagnosed as an indication of displacement by a mass lesion (see below).

The paired A1 segments are joined in the midline by the ACoA. However, the ACoA is often not oriented in a strictly transverse plane since one of the ACAs usually swings somewhat more anterior than its partner. This positional asymmetry together with the close proximity of the ACAs explains why the ACoA is seldom seen on routine AP and lateral views. Angiographic demonstration of the ACoA may require several different radiographic projections. This vessel can often be visualized on oblique, base, or modified AP views. Occasionally special views, *i.e.* an oblique transorbital or reverse oblique half-axial AP projection, may be necessary to delineate the ACoA (see Chapter 6).

Distal Segment

The course of the initial A2 segment in front of the lamina terminalis and corpus callosum genu is quite variable. It may follow a gentle, anteriorly convex curve, a "humped" or inferiorly concave course, or an acutely angled one (Figs. 8-4B, 8-6). Occasionally, it may even appear somewhat blunt or "squared off" at its most anterior extent.

Distal to the ACoA, the ACA passes anterior to the lamina terminalis, then courses around the genu of the corpus callosum. The two major distal ACA branches, the callosomarginal and pericallosal arteries, can usually be identified on routine lateral views where they originate near the corpus callosum genu (Fig. 8-4B). On AP views, however, these two vessels generally appear close together along the midline and may be difficult to differentiate (Fig. 8-4A). Usually the callosomarginal branch can be distinguished from the pericallosal artery by its somewhat more serpentine appearance as it loops into the cingulate sulcus.

Because distal branching of the pericallosal and callosomarginal arteries is quite variable, identification of each individual cortical branch on a particular angiogram may be difficult. A template for identifying these cortical ACA branches on carotid angiograms (lateral view) has been devised (Fig. 8-7). The branches are identified by their terminal areas of distribution instead of by their proximal origin.[11]

In the late arterial or early capillary phases of angiography small distal branches of the pericallosal artery define the superior surface of the corpus callosum. The pericallosal pial

(Text continued on p. 196)

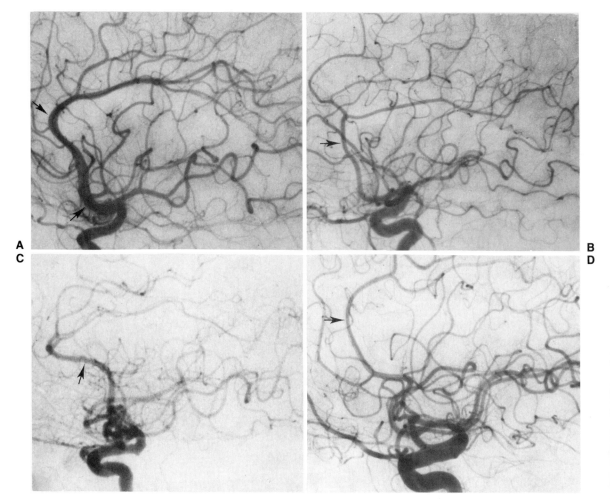

A
B
C
D

Fig. 8-6. Series of normal lateral carotid angiograms demonstrating variations in the course of the distal ACA as it passes around the corpus callosum. **(A)** Anteriorly biconvex configuration **(arrows). (B)** "Squared-off" ACA **(arrow). (C)** Inferiorly concave ACA **(arrow). (D)** Anteriorly convex ACA **(arrow).**

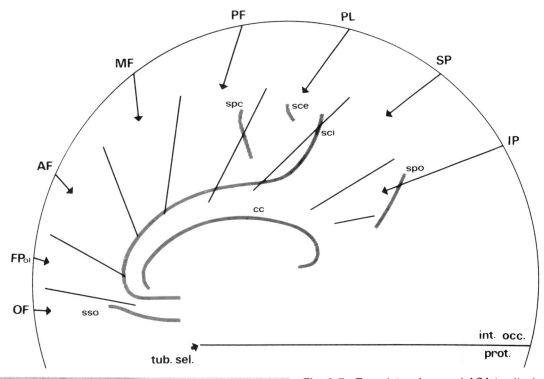

PF   PL

MF   SP

spc   sce

sci

AF   IP

spo

FP_{ol}   cc

OF

sso

int. occ.
prot.

tub. sel.

Fig. 8-7. Template of normal ACA territories that can be superimposed on lateral carotid angiograms. *(Newton TH and Potts DG: Radiology of the Skull and Brain. Vol. 2, p. 1414, St. Louis, CV Mosby Co., 1974)* Orbitofrontal artery **(OF).** Frontopolar artery **(FP).** Anterior internal frontal artery **(AF).** Middle internal frontal artery **(MF).** Posterior internal frontal artery **(PF).** Paracentral lobule artery **(PL).** Superior internal parietal artery **(SP).** Inferior internal parietal artery **(IP).** Tuberculum sellae **(tub. sel.).** Internal occipital protruberance **(int. occ. prot.).**

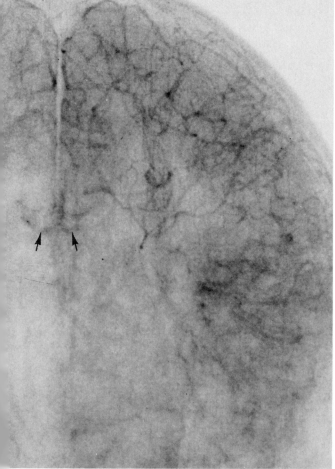

Fig. 8-8. Left internal carotid angiogram (late arterial phase, AP view). The pericallosal pial plexus appears as a faint but definite vascular blush outlining the superior surface of the corpus callosum **(arrows).**

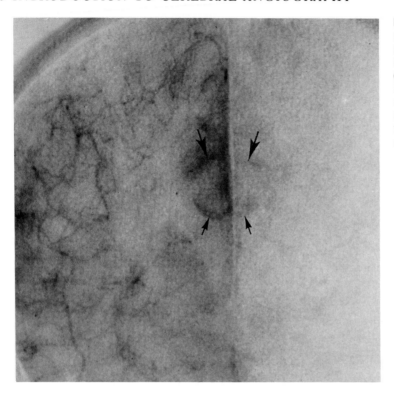

Fig. 8-9. Right internal carotid angiogram (capillary phase, AP view). The pericallosal pial plexus is indicated **(small black arrows).** Branches of the callosomarginal artery have produced a vascular blush that outlines the superior surface of both cingulate gyri **(large arrows).**

plexus often appears as a distinct symmetrical blush (Fig. 8-8). Sometimes the cingulate branches of the callosomarginal artery can also be identified during this phase of angiography (Fig. 8-9).

Midline Measurements

On perfectly straight AP angiograms the ACA should be located at the midpoint between the inner tables of the skull. However, slight rotation of the head will produce the illusory appearance of a deviation in the course of the ACA, distal to the ACoA. If the head is rotated away from the injected side during filming, the ACA will appear slightly convex. If the head is rotated toward the injected side, the ACA will appear somewhat concave (Figs. 8-10, 11). Note that these appearances may give the erroneous impression of a mass lesion.

An approximate correction for head rotation may be made by using the lateral orbital

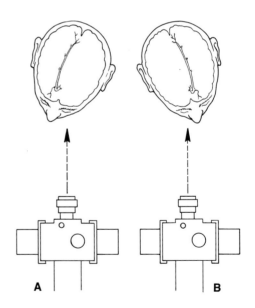

Fig. 8-10. Head rotation during filming of a right carotid angiogram. Rotation towards the side injected **(A)** produces a concave appearing ACA while rotation away from the side injected **(B)** makes the ACA appear convex.

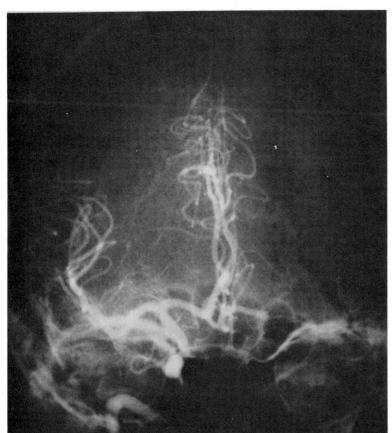

Fig. 8-11. Normal right internal carotid angiogram (**A,** arterial phase, AP view). The patient's head is slightly rotated away from the injected side, producing a somewhat convex appearance of the ACAs. Normal left internal carotid angiogram (**B,** arterial phase, AP view). The patient's head is rotated toward the side injected, producing a concave appearance of the ACA.

A

B

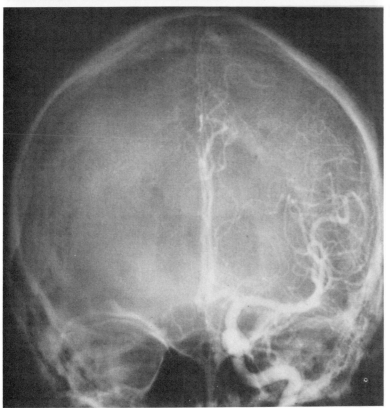

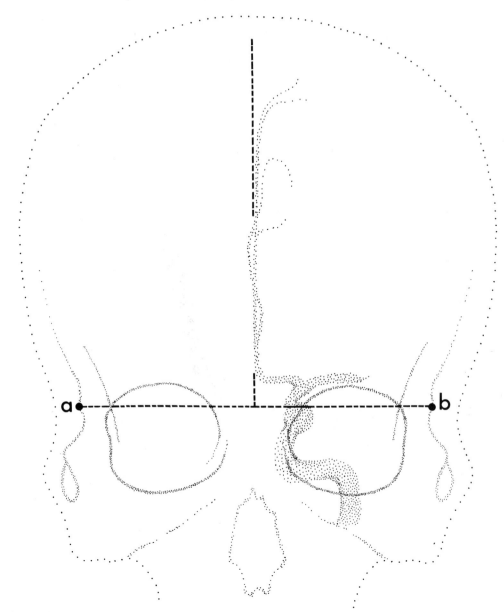

rims as points of reference. Since these bony structures lie in approximately the same plane as the genu of the ACA, they too will be rotated to nearly the same extent. To construct such a midline measurement, the angiographer should:

1. Identify the lateral margins of both orbital rims.
2. Draw a line between these two points.
3. Bisect this line and construct a perpendicular in its midpoint.

Fig. 8-12. Diagrammatic sketch of a left internal carotid angiogram (arterial phase, AP view). Two dots, **a** and **b,** are placed on the lateral margins of the orbital rims. A line is drawn between these two points, bisected, and a perpendicular constructed at its midpoint. The ACA should lie along this line.

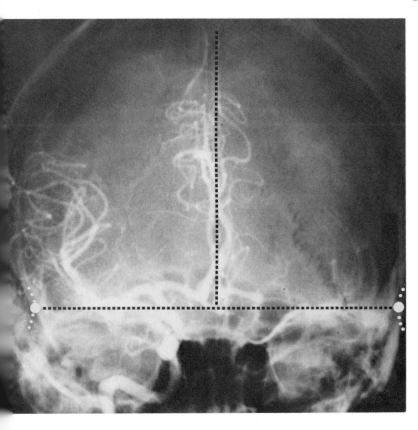

Fig. 8-13. Right internal carotid angiogram (arterial phase, AP view). Same case as 8-11A. The ACA is actually midline, as shown by constructing the measurement depicted in 8-12.

The proximal or lower portion of the ACA should lie along this perpendicular axis (Fig. 8-12). This type of correction for rotation has been applied to Figure 8-13.

NORMAL VARIANTS

Horizontal Segment and ACoA

The anterior portion of the circle of Willis, composed of the paired ACAs and the ACoA, is a common site for congenital anomalies (see Chapter 6). The most common normal variant of the ACA identified on cerebral angiograms is hypoplasia of the horizontal segment (Fig. 8-14). Complete absence of the horizontal ACA (Fig. 8-15) is unusual. In both of these cases, the opposite A1 supplies the ACAs distal to the hypoplastic or absent segment via a large anterior communicating artery. Patients with anomalies of the horizontal ACA also

have a slightly higher incidence of ACoA aneurysms.[9A]

Distal ACA

Another common variant seen in approximately ten percent of all cases is the presence of a single pericallosal artery that supplies both cerebral hemispheres (Fig. 8-16). This particular variant is sometimes termed an **azygous ACA.** This anomaly may be associated with a higher than usual incidence of pericallosal artery aneurysms. In another uncommon variant, the **bihemispheric ACA,** two ACAs are present but only one supplies the majority of vessels to both hemispheres (Fig. 8-17A-C). A common normal variant is a **dominant callosomarginal artery.** Here, (Fig. 8-18), the ACA ends in a large callosomarginal artery. In another common variant a **hypoplastic callosomarginal artery** is present.

(Text continued on p. 204)

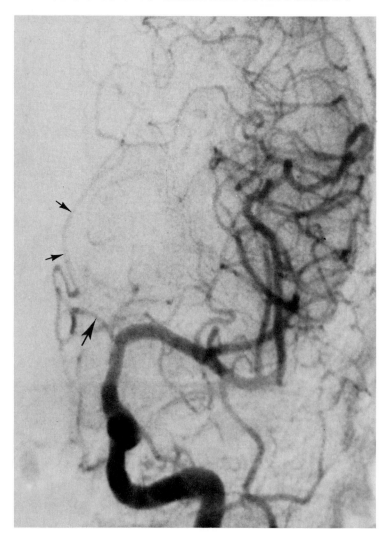

Fig. 8-14. Left common carotid angiogram (arterial phase, AP view). A hypoplastic A1 segment **(large arrows)** terminates in a frontopolar artery **(small arrows).**

Fig. 8-16. Left internal carotid angiogram (arterial phase, AP view). The study was performed with temporary cross-compression of the right common carotid artery. A single (azygous) ACA is present **(arrow).** This anomalous vessel supplies both cerebral hemispheres.

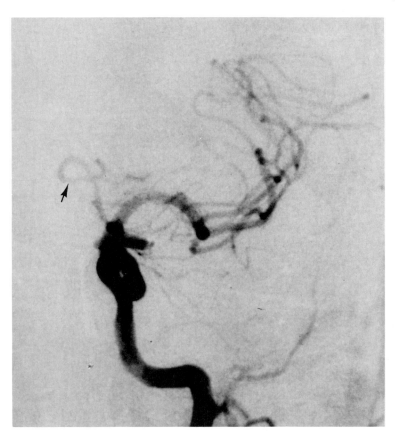

Fig. 8-15. Left common carotid angiogram (arterial phase, AP view). No horizontal ACA is seen. Injection of the contralateral internal carotid artery filled both ACAs. A small orbitofrontal artery **(arrow)** probably arises from the ICA.

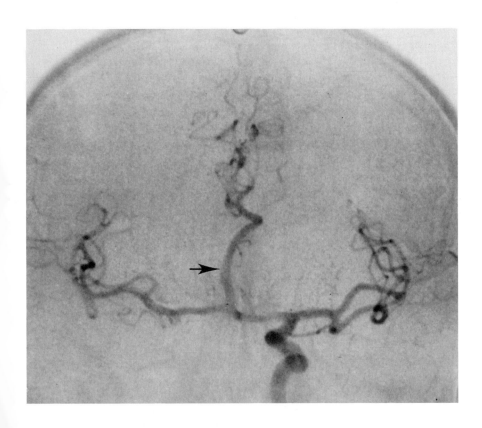

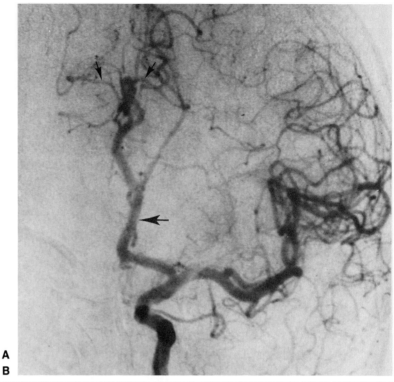

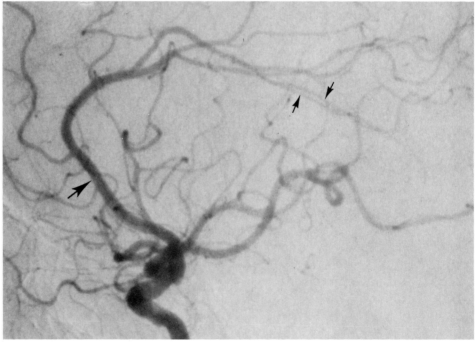

Fig. 8-17. Left common carotid angiogram (arterial phase). AP **(A)** and lateral **(B)** views show a large bihemispheric ACA **(large arrows)** supplying both hemispheres. Note the presence of two pericallosal arteries **(small arrows).** A right common carotid angiogram **(C)** in the same patient does not opacify a pericallosal artery. A moderately large anterior ACA branch **(arrows)** supplies the medial surface of the frontal pole.

(Fig. 8-17 continued on opposite page, top)

(Fig. 8-17 continued)   *The Anterior Cerebral Artery 203*

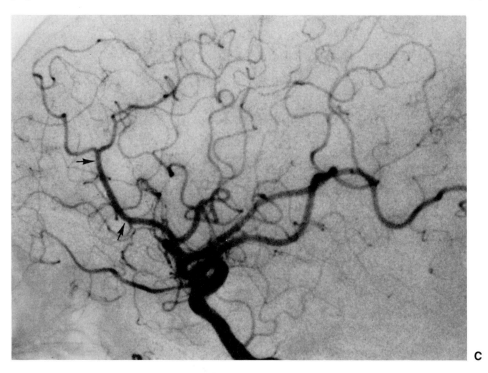

C

Fig. 8-18. Left common carotid angiogram (arterial phase, lateral view). The ACA ends in a large callosomarginal artery **(arrows).**

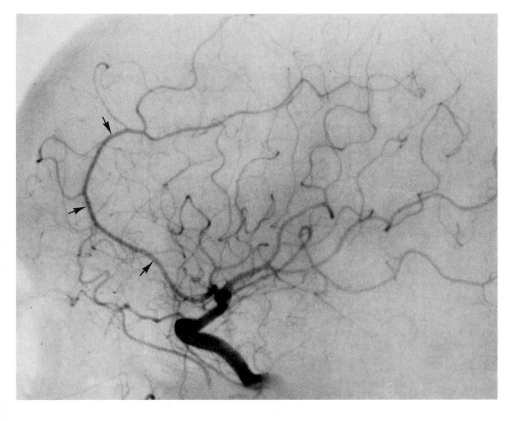

A large pericallosal artery supplies its usual area of distribution (see Fig. 8-4C).

Shallow *side-to-side undulations* of the pericallosal and callosomarginal arteries are frequently visible in the AP projection as these vessels dip into the sulci on the medial surface of the cerebral hemisphere (Fig. 8-19). Normal indulations appear gentle and short, returning to or even crossing the midline. In contrast, pathologic deviations of the ACA appear as displacements that persist across the midline (see below).

An anomalous but quite characteristic appearance of the ACA occurs in association with **corpus callosum agenesis.** In the frontal projection, the ACA branches wander in a somewhat disorganized, haphazard fashion within the large midline space due to absence of the corpus callosum (Fig. 8-20A). On the lateral view, instead of curving anteriorly around a nonexistent genu, the ACA and its branches course superiorly between the cerebral hemispheres (Fig. 8-20B).

Anomalous origin of the ACA is uncommon. Rarely the ACA arises from the intradural ICA near the ophthalmic artery origin (Fig. 8-21). In such cases it passes inferior to the optic nerve, then ascends in front of the chiasm. The incidence of associated berry aneurysm and other congenital vascular anomalies is high.[13]

ANTERIOR CEREBRAL ARTERY DISPLACEMENTS

Mass Lesions and Vascular Displacements

Whether intracerebral, intraventricular, subdural or extradural, intracranial space-occupying lesions usually produce displacement of the brain and its accompanying blood vessels. Pathologic vascularization of the lesion may also occur (see Chapter 9). A focal intracerebral mass may cause a localized rounded deformation of adjacent blood vessels which will consequently appear bowed,

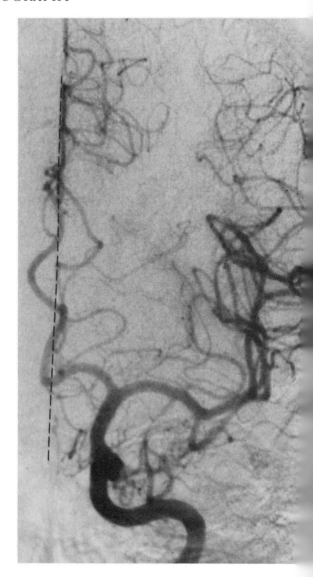

Fig. 8-19. Left internal carotid angiogram (arterial phase, AP view). The angiogram is normal. The ACA undulates from side to side across the midline **(dotted line).**

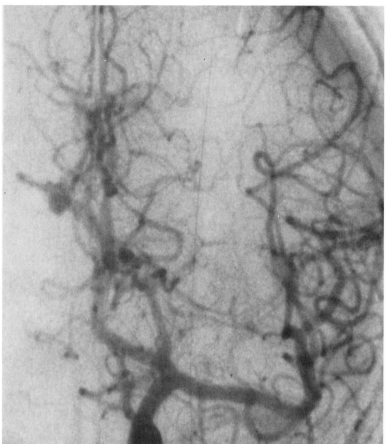

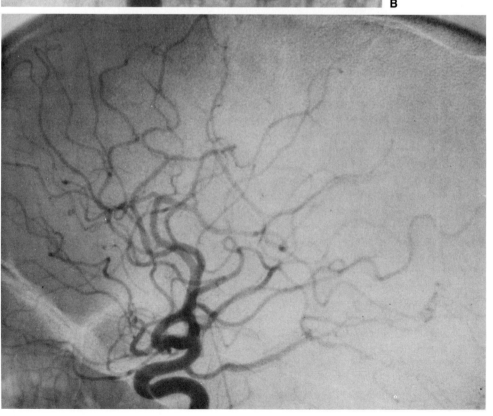

Fig. 8-20. Left common carotid angiogram (arterial phase) in agenesis of the corpus callosum. AP **(A)** and lateral **(B)** views. The ACA and its branches course directly superiorly.

A
B

205

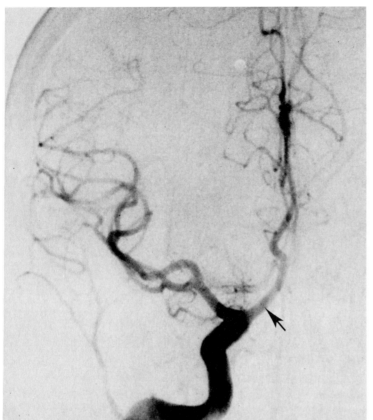

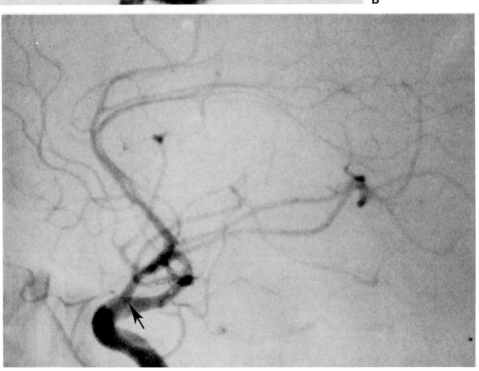

Fig. 8-21. Right common carotid angiogram (arterial phase) illustrating anomalous origin of the ACA **(arrows)** from the cavernous ICA. AP **(A)** and lateral **(B)** views.

A
B

stretched, and draped around the lesion. If the mass is sufficiently large it will also displace the cerebral hemisphere and its accompanying blood vessels across the midline under the relatively rigid falx cerebri. These cerebral subfalcine herniations or midline shifts are less accurate angiographic localizing signs than either focal displacement of otherwise normal vessels or tumor vascularity. Nevertheless, cerebral dislocations under the falx are general manifestations of an intracranial mass effect and are therefore helpful angiographic indicators.

The exact angiographic appearance of subfalcine herniations depends on the location of the mass lesion and the relationship of the ACA and its distal branches to the falx cerebri. The falx is a broad, sickle-shaped band of dura that extends from the crista galli anteriorly to the confluence of the tentorial leaves at the straight sinus and internal occipital protruberance posteriorly. The falx extends downward from the calvarial vault toward the corpus callosum in the sagittal plane between the two cerebral hemispheres (Fig. 8–22).

Fig. 8-22. Diagrammatic sketch of the ACA and its relationship to the falx cerebri and corpus callosum. Note that the distance between the pericallosal artery and the inferior or free edge of the falx decreases as the artery courses posteriorly. When a mass lesion is present, the relatively rigid falx will prevent significant midline displacement of brain and blood vessels posteriorly. But anteriorly, the height of the falx is attenuated. This permits considerable displacement of brain and vessels under its free edge.

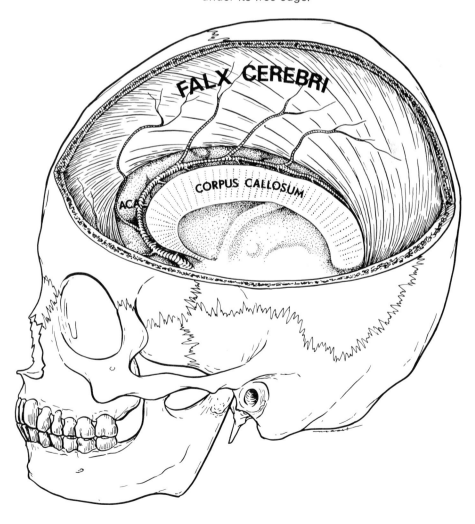

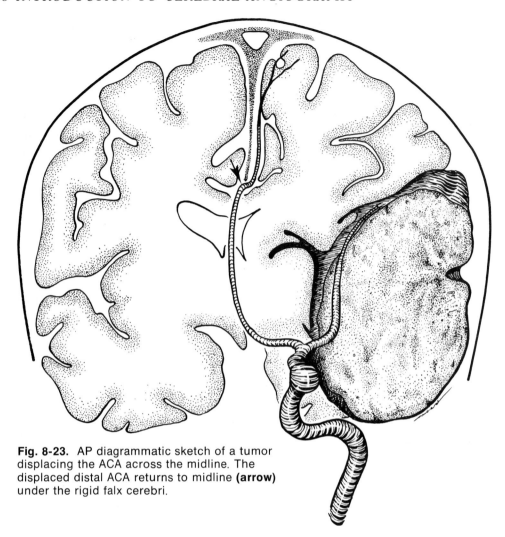

Fig. 8-23. AP diagrammatic sketch of a tumor displacing the ACA across the midline. The displaced distal ACA returns to midline **(arrow)** under the rigid falx cerebri.

The free or inferior margin of the falx is closer to the cranial vault superiorly; thus it is somewhat attenuated in its anterior portion while its height is greater in the parieto-occipital area. The very important relationship of the ACA to the anterior free edge of the falx cerebri is illustrated in Figure 8-22. Here the anterior aspect of the pericallosal artery lies at some distance from the anteroinferior free edge of the falx. However, the distance between the pericallosal artery and the falx decreases as this vessel courses posteriorly, thus reducing the space available for subfalcine herniation of the brain and ACA. Since the falx itself is a relatively rigid structure, its inferior margin does not bend or shift unless the mass effect is rather large.

Because of the relationship of the ACA to the falx cerebri, presence of a sufficiently large mass lesion will cause considerable displacement of the brain and its accompanying blood vessels under the free edge of the anterior falx. However, as the pericallosal artery courses posteriorly and distance between it and the falx diminishes, this artery is forced to return to the midline under the falx (Fig. 8-23).

Subfalcine Herniations of the ACA

Depending on their location, intracranial mass lesions may shift the entire ACA or only its proximal, middle, or distal portions. Subfalcine herniations or midline shifts of the ACA may be divided into four general categories: a round shift, a square shift, a proximal shift, and a distal shift. The manner is which the ACA is displaced provides important information regarding the general location of an intracranial mass.[3]

A **round shift** is caused by an anterior or frontal mass that lies adjacent to the ACA. Since the falx is some distance from the pericallosal artery anteriorly, large subfalcine herniations can occur in this location. With a round shift, the ACA and its branches are deviated across the midline in a smooth, rounded arc. Mid and posterior frontal masses can also produce such a rounded shift of the ACA (Figs. 8-24, 25). Occasionally, a mass located in the mid-frontal region will produce a peculiar distortion of the ACA that looks like a "3" or a reverse "3" (Figs. 8-26, 27). Because it must return under the free edge of the falx earlier than the pericallosal artery, the more superiorly located callosomarginal branch may cause medial tethering of the usually smooth curve of the shited ACA.

A **square shift** (Fig. 8-28) is caused by a mass effect primarily located behind the genu of the corpus callosum. It is less specific than a round shift and may be found with temporal, posterior frontal, or parietal lesions. A large mass of compressible brain lies between the lesions and the ACA. The intervening brain apparently acts to cushion the mass effect and the ACA is consequently shifted across the midline in a rather diffuse fashion. The proximal as well as distal portions of the pericallosal artery are equally displaced. As the ACA ascends and courses posteriorly it abruptly changes direction at nearly a right angle to return to the midline beneath the falx. This produces a well-delineated step or squared appearance of the ACA. With a square shift, the dislocated ACA may course straight upward

(Fig. 8-29) or return partially toward the midline between its two displaced segments (Fig. 8-30).

A **proximal shift** is caused by an inferior frontal, subfrontal, or anterior temporal mass (Fig. 8-31). It is of intermediate specificity in localizing a mass lesion. Here, the proximal or inferior portion of the ACA is displaced across the midline. As it ascends the distal ACA courses obliquely, gradually returning to the midline. Depending on the size of the lesion, the ACA may reach the midline by forming a definite subfalcine step (Fig. 8-32) or not (Fig. 8-33). Regardless, the distal ACA is less displaced than is its proximal segment.

A **distal shift** (Figs. 8-34, 9-15B) is also of intermediate specificity in localizing a mass lesion. The anterior or proximal portion of the ACA is either in the midline or appears less displaced than its mid or distal portion. The ACA and its branches gradually shift across the midline as they ascend and course posteriorly. A well-defined step is present where the dislocated vessels return to their paramedian position under the falx cerebri. As with other types of subfalcine herniation, a distal shift may be obvious or subtle (Figs. 8-35, 8-36). Distal midline shifts are caused by parietal, high posterofrontal, occipital, and mid or posterior temporal mass lesions.

Subfalcine ACA displacements of greater than 2 mm are usually considered significant. Slight but apparent displacements should be evaluated with caution. Either slight rotation of the head during filming or atherosclerotic tortuosity of the ACA and its branches may produce apparent but illusory displacement. Corrections for midline measurements as well as the lack of a subfalcine step are helpful in making the distinction between false and slight, but definite, ACA displacements.

Superior Displacement of the ACA

Sufficiently large juxta- or suprasellar masses may displace the horizontal ACA segment

(Text continued on p. 219)

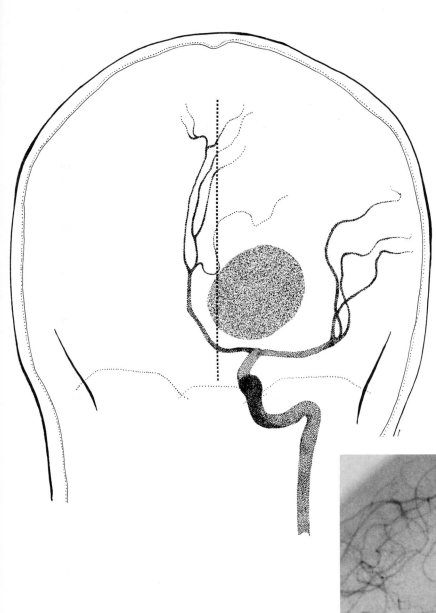

Fig. 8-24. Anatomic sketch of a left internal carotid angiogram (arterial phase, AP view) in a large mid-frontal mass lesion. The ACA and its branches are shifted across the midline **(dotted line)** in a smooth, rounded fashion. This is termed a *round shift* of the ACA.

Fig. 8-25. Right internal carotid angiogram (arterial phase, AP view) in a patient with a large round ACA shift caused by hypovascular frontal lobe neoplasm. The approximate midline is indicated **(dotted line)**.

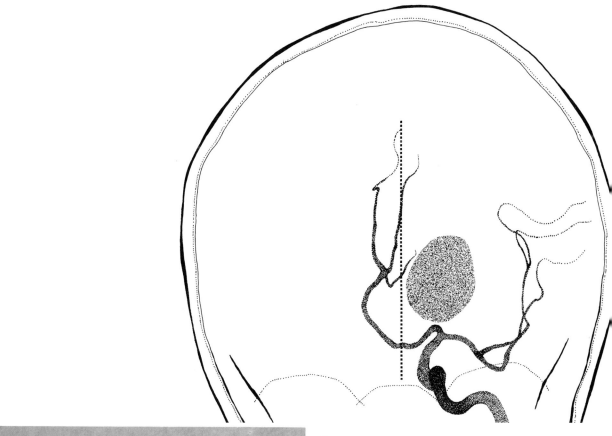

Fig. 8-26. Diagrammatic radiograph of a left internal carotid angiogram (arterial phase, AP view). A mid-frontal mass lesion has caused left-to-right subfalcine herniation of the ACA. The ACA is tethered medially by the callosomarginal artery.

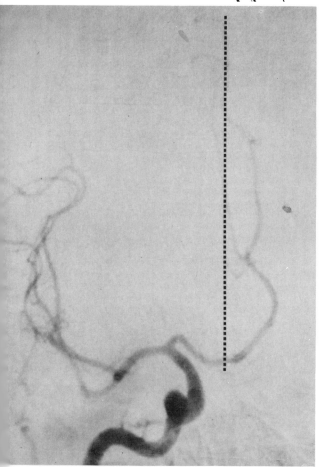

Fig. 8-27. Right internal carotid angiogram (arterial phase, AP view). This demonstrates a mid-frontal mass and a round ACA shift that is tethered in its midportion by the callosomarginal artery. Note the "3-shaped" appeareance of the displaced ACA.

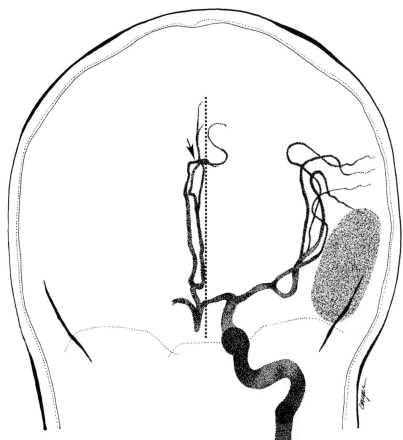

Fig. 8-28. Diagrammatic radiograph of a left internal carotid angiogram (arterial phase, AP view) of a large mass lesion in the temporal lobe. The ACA has been shifted across the midline **(dotted line)** in a diffuse, square fashion. The point where the displaced ACA returns to the midline under the falx cerebri is indicated **(arrow).**

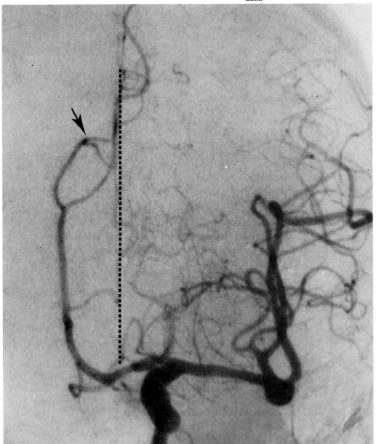

Fig. 8-29. Left internal carotid angiogram (arterial phase, AP view) in a temporal lobe neoplasm. The ACA shows a square-type subfalcine shift. The point where the herniated ACA returns towards the midline under the falx cerebri is indicated **(arrow).**

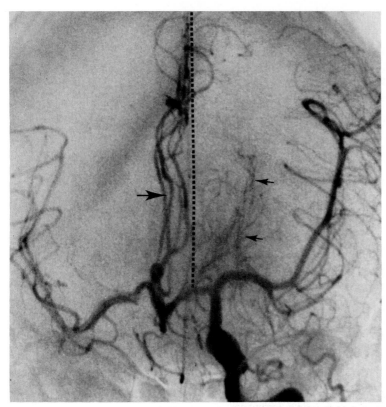

Fig. 8-30. Left internal carotid angiogram (arterial phase, AP view) in a large avascular left temporal lobe tumor. The neoplasm has extended into the insula, displacing the lenticulostriate arteries medially and reversing their normal laterally convex curve **(small arrows).** A square shift of the ACA is present. Note that while this vessel is displaced equally in both its proximal and distal segments. it tends to return slightly toward the midline **(large arrow)** between these two points.

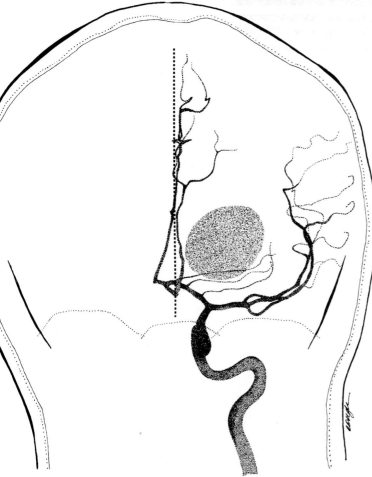

Fig. 8-31. Diagrammatic radiograph of a left internal carotid angiogram (arterial phase, AP view) in an inferior frontal mass lesion. A proximal shift of the ACA is present.

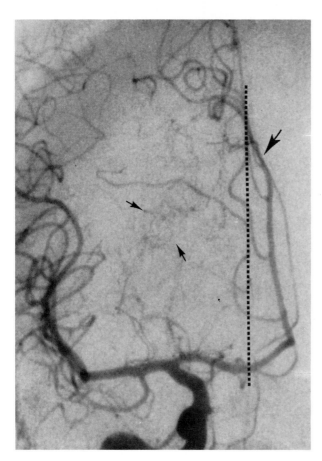

Fig. 8-32. Right internal carotid angiogram (arterial phase, AP view) in a deep mid-frontal neoplasm. A faint tumor stain is indicated **(small arrows).** Right to left proximal displacement of the ACA is present, along with a subfalcine step effect **(large arrow)** where the herniated ACA returns towards the midline.

Fig. 8-33. Right internal carotid angiogram (arterial phase, AP view). A right frontal epidermoid cyst has produced definite proximal displacement of the ACA. Since the mass effect is quite anterior and relatively small, the ACA has returned to the midline without a subfalcine step deformity.

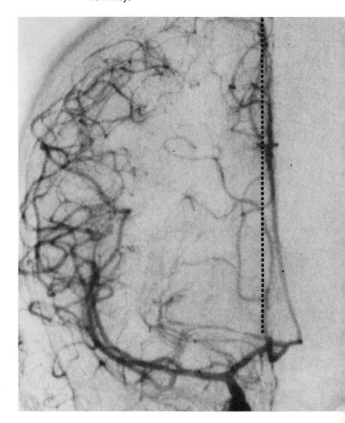

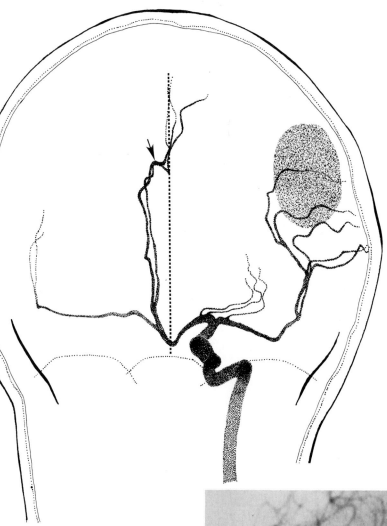

Fig. 8-34. Diagrammatic radiograph of a left internal carotid angiogram (arterial phase, AP view) in a parietal lobe tumor. The ACA displacement is maximal posteriorly, producing a distal type midline shift. A definite step-like deformity **(arrow)** is present where the displaced ACA must return to the midline under the falx cerebri.

Fig. 8-35. Right internal carotid angiogram (arterial phase, AP view) of a subtle but definite distal ACA shift **(arrows)**. Note the abrupt return of the ACA to the midline under the falx cerebri.

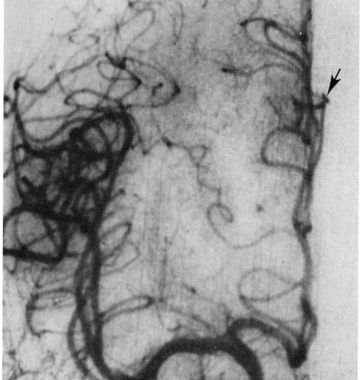

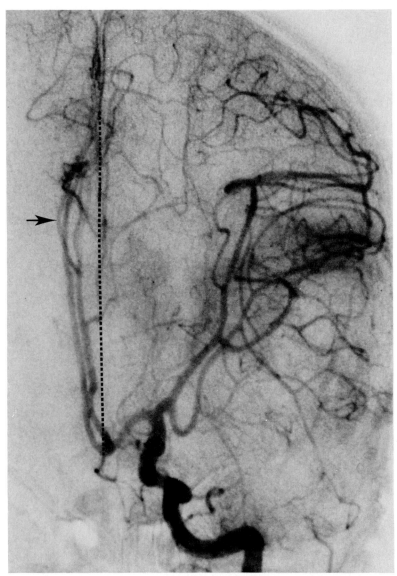

Fig. 8-36. Left internal carotid angiogram (arterial phase, AP view) in a huge temporal and posterior insular mass. The ACA is shifted across the midline in its entirety but the displacement is greatest posteriorly **(arrow)**.

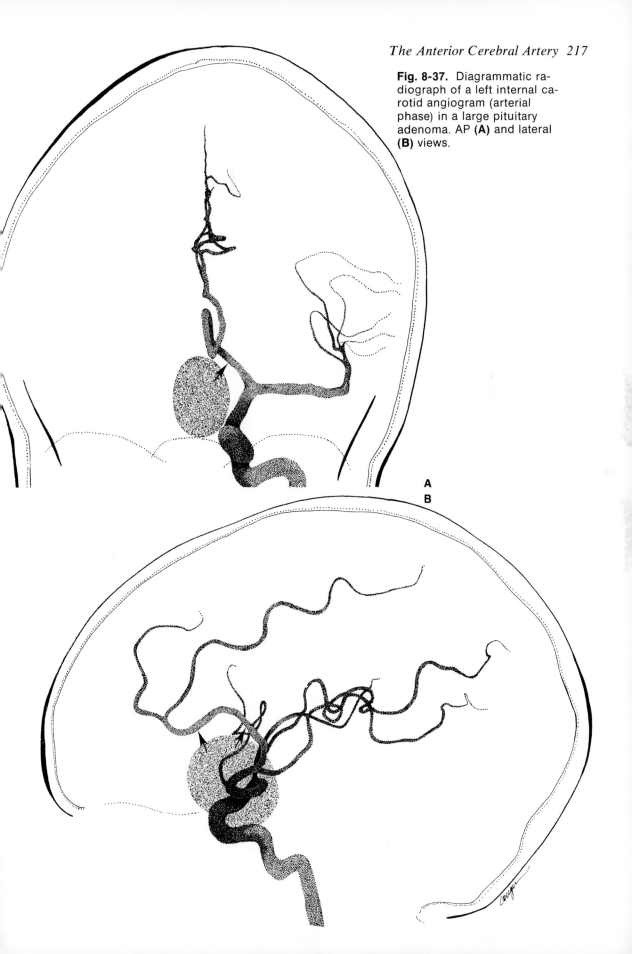

Fig. 8-37. Diagrammatic radiograph of a left internal carotid angiogram (arterial phase) in a large pituitary adenoma. AP **(A)** and lateral **(B)** views.

A
B

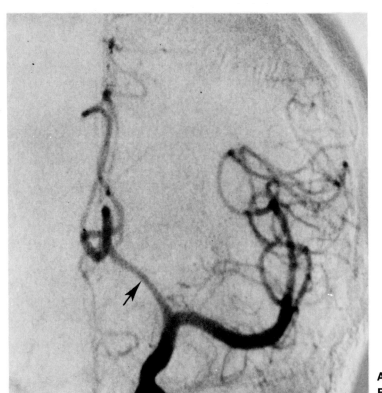

Fig. 8-38. Left internal carotid angiogram (arterial phase) in a large pituitary adenoma. The ACA is displaced upward and backward **(arrows).** AP **(A)** and lateral **(B)** views.

A

B

(Fig. 8-37). Upward and forward displacement of the horizontal ACA segment by a suprasellar or subfrontal mass is normally best seen in the frontal projection (Fig. 8-38A). If the mass is sufficiently large, posterosuperior displacement of the proximal ACA as it courses from the lamina terminalis to the corpus callosum genu may also be demonstrated (Fig. 8-38B). This angiographic appearance is found only when suprasellar extension of the mass is predominantly anterior. If the lesion extends straight up or grows posteriorly through the circle of Willis, the ACA may appear completely normal even in the presence of a large lesion.[15A] Only small vessels (*i.e.,* the anterior choroidal or thalamoperforating arteries) may show significant vascular displacement (see Fig. 7-17).

While the most common suprasellar mass effect is caused by superior extension of a pituitary adenoma through the diaphragm sellae, other lesions such as craniopharyngioma (Fig. 8-39), aneurysm (Fig. 8-40), glioma, or meningioma (Fig. 8-41) may produce identical ACA displacements.[10A] Also note that since the horizontal ACA may either ascend or curve downward as it passes medially toward the interhemispheric fissure, apparent elevation of the A1 segment may be a normal finding in younger patients. However, an A1 segment that appears elevated and shows a pronounced inferior concavity is usually abnormal.

Displacement of the Interhemispheric ACA Branches

An uncommon type of ACA displacement is caused by extra-axial fluid collections that extend into the interhemispheric fissure (Figs. 8-42, 8-43). Here the distal branches of the callosomarginal arteries are separated, leaving a wedge-shaped paramedian avascular area. Other interhemispheric masses such as falx meningioma may also produce displacement of these distal ACA branches away from the midline, as can marked cerebral atrophy.

(Text continued on p. 222)

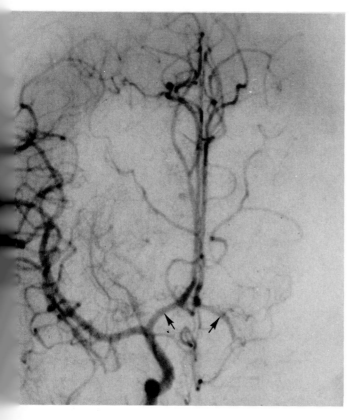

Fig. 8-39. Right common carotid angiogram (arterial phase, AP view) in a 4-year-old child with a craniopharyngioma. The horizontal segments of both ACAs are displaced superiorly **(arrows).**

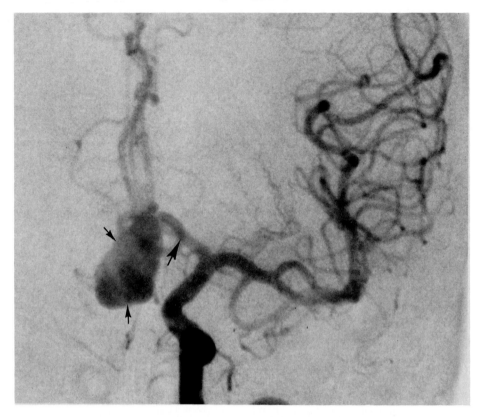

Fig. 8-40. Left internal carotid angiogram (arterial phase, AP view) in a giant ACoA aneurysm **(small arrows)**. The mass effect created by this partially thrombosed aneurysm has displaced the A1 segment superiorly **(large arrow).**

Fig. 8-41. Right internal carotid angiogram (arterial phase) in a meningioma **(small arrows)** arising from the chiasmatic sulcus. The ACA is displaced superiorly and posteriorly **(large arrows)** by the mass. AP **(A)** and lateral **(B)** views.

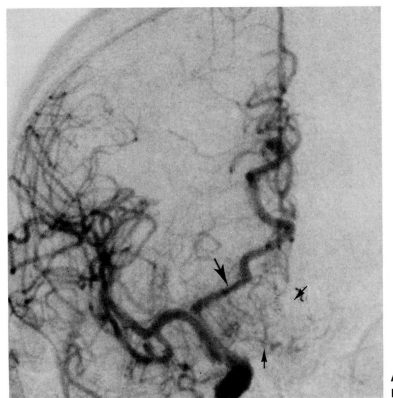

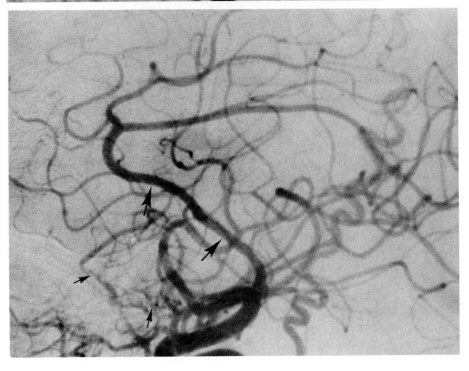

A
B

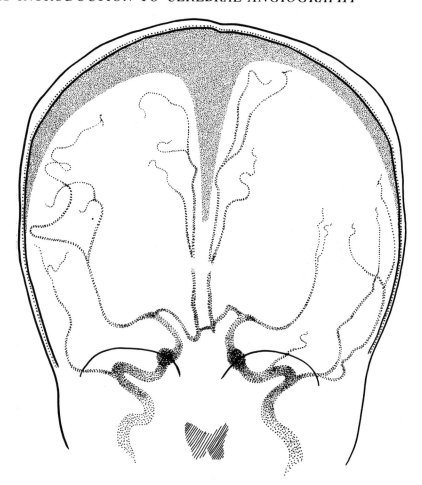

Fig. 8-42. Diagrammatic radiograph of a left internal carotid angiogram (arterial phase, AP view) in a large subdural hematoma that extends into the interhemispheric fissure **(arrows).**

Hydrocephalus

The most accurate angiographic indicators of ventricular enlargement are elongation and stretching of the subependymal veins (as illustrated in Chapter 11). Stretching of the cerebral arteries is a relatively insensitive angiographic indicator of hydrocephalus since these arteries usually appear normal in the presence of mild to moderate ventricular enlargement. With moderately severe ventricular dilatation the distance between the anterior and middle cerebral arteries appears increased on frontal projections because the enlarged lateral ventricles create a mass effect (Fig. 8-44). In the AP projection, the ACA and its branches appear taut and straightened; in the lateral view, they appear stretched and bowed superiorly (Fig. 8-45). The middle cerebral artery and its lenticulostriate branches are usually displaced laterally.

With symmetrical hydrocephalus the stretched ACA remains in the midline. A V-shaped appearance of the pericallosal pial plexus may also be detected during the capillary phase of the AP angiogram (Fig. 8-46). Asymmetrical ventricular dilatation, mass-producing porencephalic cysts, and encysted ventricles are avascular mass lesions and will

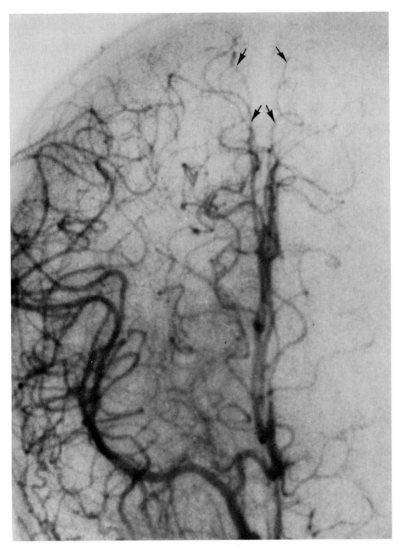

Fig. 8-43. Right common carotid angiogram (arterial phase, AP view) in an abused child with an interhemispheric subdural hematoma. Note the separation of the ACA branches, producing a wedge-shaped avascular area along the interhemispheric fissure **(arrows).**

produce appropriate displacements of the cerebral arteries.

As its branches extend into the pericallosal sulcus, the pericallosal pial plexus forms a "smile" during the capillary phase of angiography. Normally this plexal blush is symmetrical, curving very slightly upward (see Fig. 8-8A). With subfalcine herniation of the cingulate gyrus and accompanying distal branches of the ACA, the pericallosal sulcus and its plexus may become tilted or distorted (Fig. 8-47). Hence the blush will appear definitely asymmetrical.

Lack of ACA Displacement with Intracranial Masses

Occasionally the ACA and its distal branches may remain in their normal paramedian position despite the presence of an obvious intracranial mass effect. This can be seen with symmetrical contralateral space-occupying lesions. Typical examples of this entity would be bilaterally symmetrical subdural hematomas or bihemispheric cerebral metastases that are similar in size and extent. Infiltrating tumors may also fail to produce a significant ACA

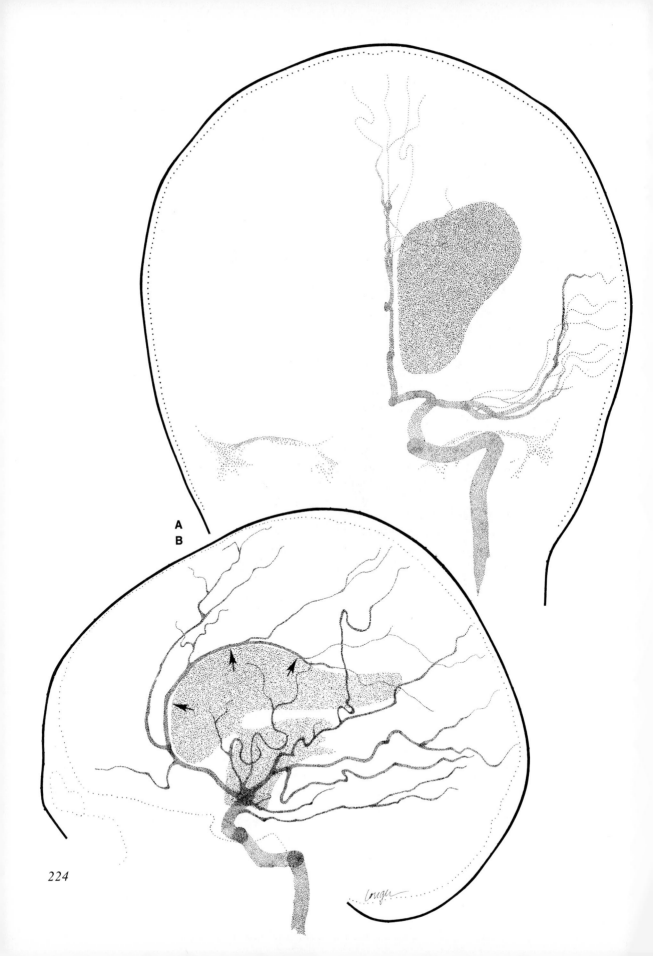

A
B

224

◀ Fig. 8-44. Diagrammatic radiograph of a left internal carotid angiogram (arterial phase) illustrating massive hydrocephalus secondary to ventricular enlargement. The huge lateral ventricles are indicated **(stippled areas)**. Note the marked straightening and stretching of the ACA on the AP view **(A)**. On the lateral view **(B)**, the ACA is bowed superiorly **(arrows)**.

midline shift. Mass lesions that are either deep (*i.e.*, within the thalamus) or located quite posterior to the free edge of the falx (*i.e.*, within the occipital lobe) may also fail to produce ACA displacement. Also, symmetrical midline tumors often occur in the presence of a normally positioned ACA. Corpus callosal neoplasms provide a striking example of this entity (Fig. 8-48).

OCCLUSIONS OF THE ACA

Radiographic Manifestations

The ACA is a relatively rare site of occlusion. Failure of this vessel to be visualized following injection of contrast into the carotid artery is most often due to hypoplasia of the horizontal segment rather than actual occlusion. Contralateral carotid injection may be necessary to demonstrate the filling of the ipsilateral ACA via the ACoA. If occlusion is actually present, the ACA will appear with neither carotid injection.

Once anomalous origin of the ACA has been excluded, ACA occlusion can be detected. Distal ACA occlusion is recognized angiographically as a tapering or abrupt termination of the contrast-filled vessel lacking distal opacification (Fig. 8-49). As with other arterial occlusions, delayed films may demonstrate collateral flow into the territory usually irrigated by non-occluded ACA branches or by ipsilateral branches of the middle and posterior cerebral arteries (see Chapter 9). Small interhemispheric infarctions usually occur without a significant mass effect. Persistent arterial opacification may last into the capillary phase with presence of an associated vascular stain or early draining veins.[7]

Clinical Sequelae

The clinical manifestations of ACA occlusion proximal to the ACoA are discussed in Chapter 6. ACA occlusion distal to the origin of Heubner's artery and the ACoA results in disordered mentation, retardation, emotional lability, and confusion. Motor aphasia may occur if the lesion is on the dominant side. Contralateral lower extremity hemiplegia and left-sided apraxia (regardless of which hemisphere is affected) may occur along with forced grasping and groping movements of the hemiplegic upper extremity.[15]

ANEURYSMS

The vast majority of ACA aneurysms arise from the anterior communicating artery (Figs. 8-40, 8-50). The ACoA is the single most common site of aneurysms associated with subarachnoid hemorrhage.[17B] ACA aneurysms distal to the ACoA are uncommon, constituting 2.5 to 9.8% of all intracranial arterial aneurysms.[8] Distal ACA aneurysms are usually found either adjacent to the genu of the corpus callosum or at the main pericallosal artery bifurcation (Fig. 8-51).[6, 8, 18] Aneurysms located at sites other than branching points are frequently secondary to trauma or inflammatory disease.[1A] Traumatic aneurysms of the pericallosal artery may occur where this vessel is anchored by the free edge of the falx.[13A]

ARTERIOVENOUS MALFORMATIONS

Congenital cerebrovascular malformations include capillary telangiectasias, cavernous angiomas, venous malformations, and arteriovenous malformations. (Capillary telangiectasias and cavernous angiomas are discussed in Chapter 3; venous malformations are discussed in Chapter 11.) Most intracranial telangiectatic malformations are asymptomatic although an occasional patient may present with subarachnoid hemorrhage or seizures (Fig. 8-52).

(Text continued on p. 233)

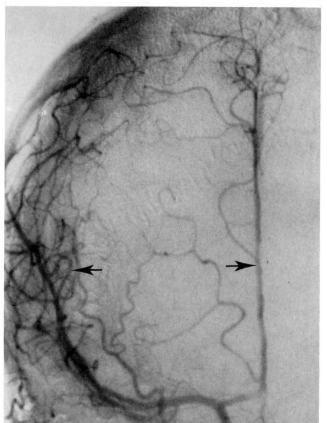

Fig. 8-45. Right common carotid angiogram (arterial phase, AP view). Massive hydrocephalus secondary to aqueductal stenosis is present. The ACA is straightened and the MCA and its branches are displaced laterally **(large arrows).**

Left internal carotid angiogram (**B,** arterial phase, lateral view) in another patient with aqueduct stenosis and obstructive hydrocephalus. The ACA is bowed superiorly **(large arrows).** Note incidental downward displacement of the posterior communicating artery **(small arrow)** secondary to the mass effect caused by the huge dilated ventricles.

A
B

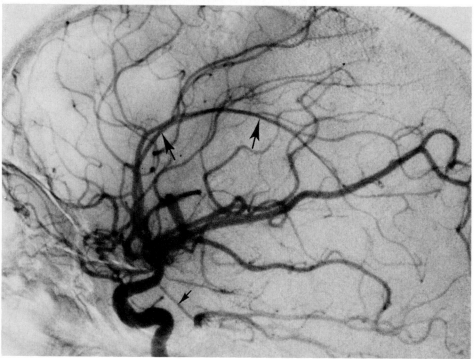

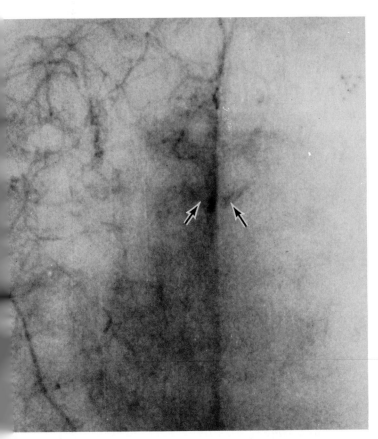

Fig. 8-46. Right common carotid angiogram (capillary phase, AP view) in a 2-year-old with severe hydrocephalus. The pericallosal pial plexus is displaced by the huge dilated ventricles, forming a "V" **(arrows).**

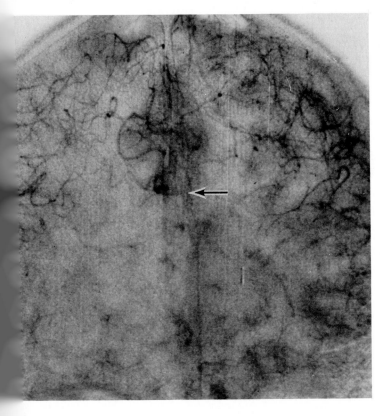

Fig. 8-47. Left internal carotid angiogram, performed with temporary cross compression of the right common carotid artery (late arterial phase, AP view). A large left hemisphere mass effect produced severe subfalcine ACA herniation. The pericallosal pial plexus is tilted and shifted across the midline **(arrow).**

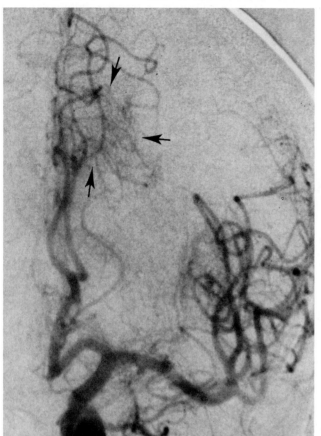

Fig. 8-48. Left internal carotid angiogram (arterial phase) in a patient with grade IV astrocytoma of the body and splenium of the corpus callosum. AP **(A)** and lateral **(B)** views. The vascular neoplasm is indicated **(arrows).**
Because the mass is symmetrical and involves both hemispheres equally there is a conspicuous lack of midline ACA displacement.

A
B

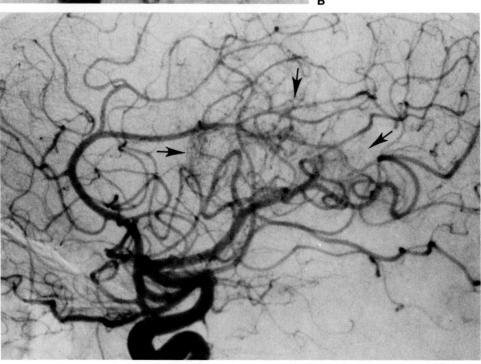

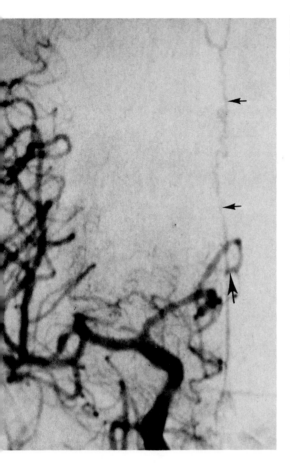

Fig. 8-49. Right common carotid angiogram (arterial phase, AP view) in occlusion of the ACA **(large arrow).** The smaller midline vessel **(small arrows)** is the anterior falx artery, a branch of the ophthalmic artery.

Fig. 8-50. Right internal carotid angiogram (arterial phase, oblique view). Temporary cross compression of the left common carotid artery was performed. A small lobulated aneurysm of the ACA is present **(arrow).**

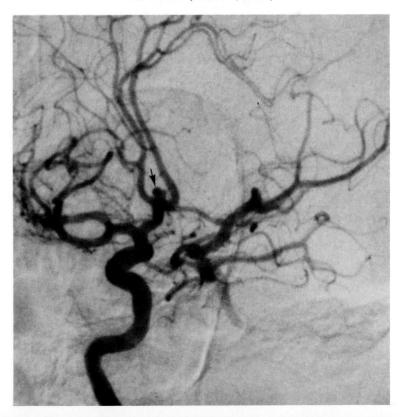

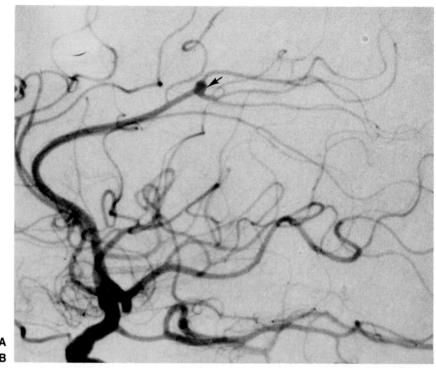

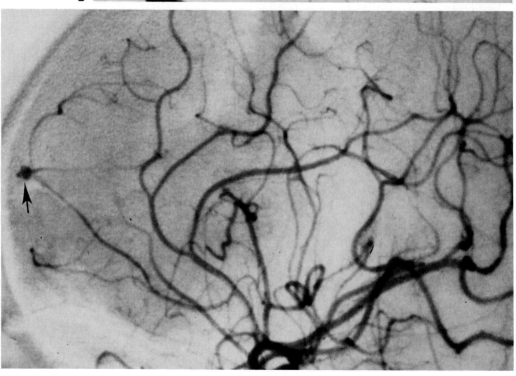

A
B

◀ **Fig. 8-51.** Left internal carotid angiogram (**A,** arterial phase, lateral view). A pericallosal artery aneurysm is identified **(arrow).** The lesion is probably developmental.

Left carotid angiogram (**B,** arterial phase, lateral view). This was seen in a patient with a post-traumatic aneurysm **(arrow)** of the frontopolar artery.

Fig. 8-52. Left internal carotid angiogram (arterial phase, lateral view) in a patient with a posterior frontal eliptogenic focus. A small telangiectatic vascular malformation is present **(arrows).**

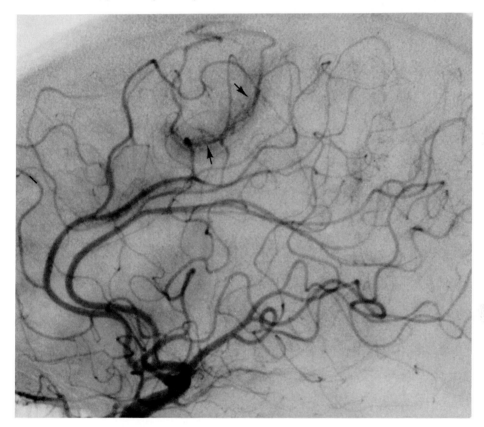

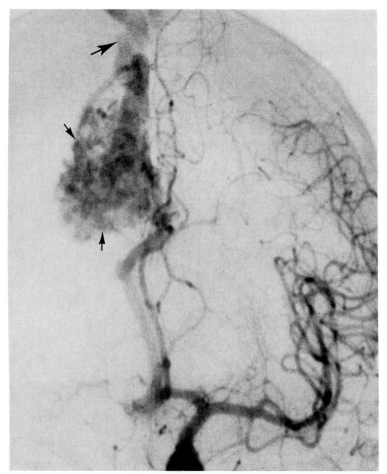

A
B

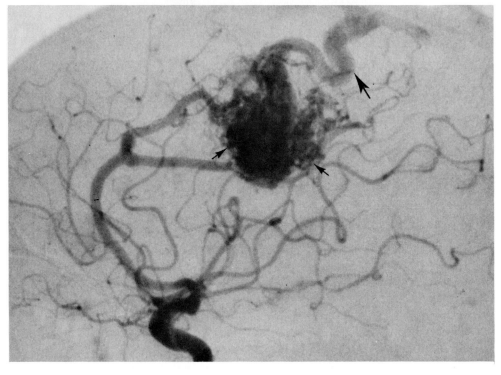

Arteriovenous malformations (AVMs) are the most common of the congenital vascular malformations and may involve any of the intracranial vessels. Some 88% are supratentorial and tend to occur at or adjacent to the "watershed" areas of the brain.[5]

Arteriovenous malformations may be pure pial, pure dural, or mixed pial-dural (see Chapter 3). The majority of arteriovenous malformations involving the ACA and its branches are pure pial, *i.e.,* no meningeal or dural vascular supply is present. However, perhaps as many as one-fifth of supratentorial AVMs will have some dural contribution demonstrated when complete selective examination of the internal and external carotid and vertebral arteries is performed (see Figs. 3-14, 5-23).[2A, 5]

Since AMVs are congenital lesions and *re*place rather than *dis*place normal brain there is no associated mass effect unless hemorrhage with edema or subsequent hematoma formation has occurred. The arteries supplying an AVM are usually dilated and are often somewhat tortuous. Also present is rapid shunting of blood into enlarged, tortuous draining veins (Fig. 8-53).

The angiographic appearance of a small arteriovenous malformation may occasionally be difficult to distinguish from that of a vascular neoplasm with arteriovenous shunting (such as a high grade astrocytoma). Although the afferent vessels supplying malignant neoplasms may increase in size, the degree of enlargement is less than that seen with arteriovenous malformations. AVMs also appear as tightly packed tangles of vessels with little or no interposed cerebral tissue. The close proximity of the dilated vessels to one another produces a "bag of worms" appearance (Fig. 8-53). In contrast, in malignant gliomas, neoplastic tissue is intercalated between scattered, widely spaced pathological vessels which often appear irregular and bizarre.[4] Also, an uncomplicated AVM usually exhibits no mass effect while a glioma tends to displace normal brain tissues. A word of caution: an infiltrating neoplasm may produce little or no mass effect while an AVM with an associated intracerebral hematoma may produce considerable vascular displacement (Fig. 8-54).

Occasionally, even careful angiography may fail to opacify AVMs. Varying degrees of thrombosis of the malformation and the resultant stagnant flow may prevent sufficient iodine accumulation for angiographic identification.[9, 10] Parenchymal hemorrhage can compress an AVM to such a degree that the draining veins are obliterated and only minimal residual enlargement of the efferent arteries remains.[12] An avascular mass effect secondary to cerebral edema or the hematoma may also be present (Fig. 8-55). Early opacification of draining veins can occasionally be identified in partially thrombosed AVMs. The feeding vessels may be somewhat irregular (on rare occasions) with focal areas of residual tortuosity and dilatation.[12] CT scans are often helpful in diagnosing angiographically occult cerebral vascular malformations.[17A]

Fig. 8-53. Left internal carotid angiogram (arterial phase, AP view) of an uncomplicated arteriovenous malformation of the corpus callosum and cirgulate gyrus. The enlarged right ACA supplies a tangle of tightly packed vessels **(small arrows)** representing the AVM. Rapid circulation with almost simultaneous appearance of a large, dilated draining vein **(large arrow)** is present. Note the lack of mass effect, characteristic for AVMs in the absence of intracerebral hemorrhage. AP **(A)** and lateral **(B)** views.

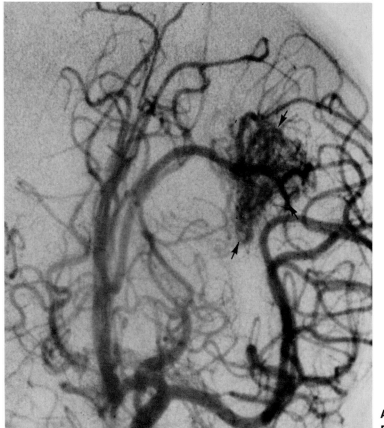

A
B

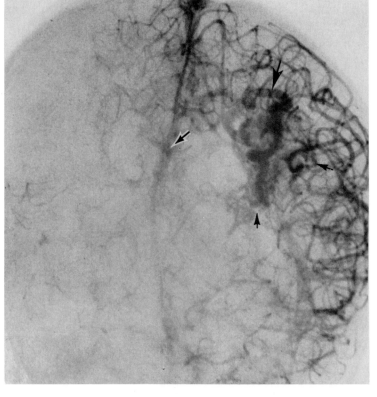

(Fig. 8-54 continued on opposite page)

(Fig. 8-54 continued)

The Anterior Cerebral Artery 235

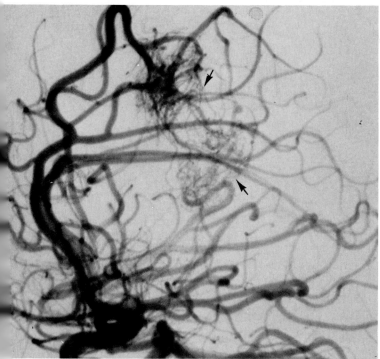

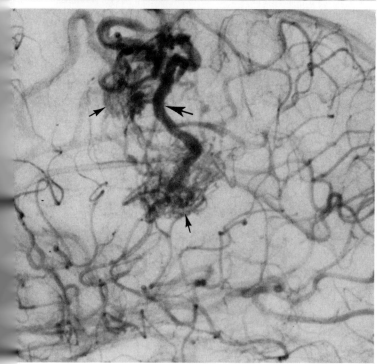

Fig. 8-54. Left internal carotid angiogram in a patient with a posterior frontal AVM. **(A)** AP view, mid-arterial phase; **(B)** AP view, late arterial phase; **(C)** Lateral view, mid-arterial phase; **(D)** Lateral view, late arterial phase. Enlarged ACA branches supply a tangle of abnormal vessels **(small arrows).** In the mid-arterial phase (8-53**A, C**) the lesion superficially resembles a glioblastoma multiforme. However, late arterial phase views (8-53**B, D**) show the lesion to be tightly packed with abnormal vessels. A dilated superficial vein **(large arrow)** drains the malformation. An associated hematoma has produced a left to right ACA midline displacement with tilting of the pericallosal pial plexus **(outlined arrow).**

C
D

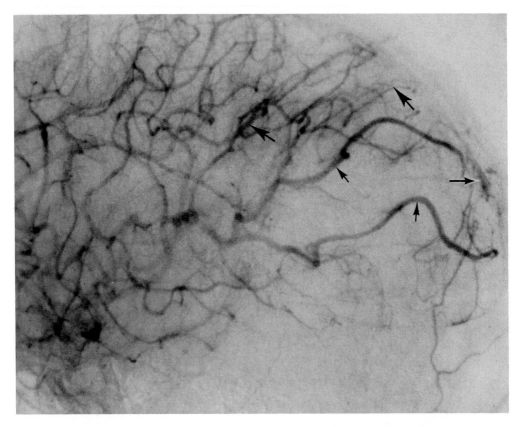

Fig. 8-55. Left common carotid angiogram (late arterial phase, lateral view) in a thrombosed parieto-occipital AVM. The posterior parietal and angular branches of the MCA are slightly enlarged **(small arrows).** A small residual portion of the AVM is seen posteriorly **(outlined arrow).** Note the associated mass effect and compressed gyri **(large arrows)** caused by hemorrhage and edema.

REFERENCES

1A. **Becker DH, Newton TH:** Distal anterior cerebral artery aneurysm. Neurosurg 6:495–503, 1979

1B. **Crowell RM, Morawetz RB:** The anterior communicating artery has significant branches. Stroke 8:272–273, 1977

2. **Dunker RO, Harris AB:** Surgical anatomy of the proximal anterior cerebral artery. J Neurosurg 44:359–367, 1976

2A. **Faria MA, Fleischer AS:** Dual cerebral and meningeal supply to giant arteriovenous malformations of the posterior cerebral hemisphere. J Neurosurg 52:153–161, 1980

3. **Galligioni F, Bernardi R, Mingrino S:** Anatomic variation of the height of the falx cerebri. Its relationship to displacement of the anterior cerebral artery in frontal space-occupying lesions. Am J Roentgenol 106:273–278, 1969

4. **Goree JA, Dukes HT:** The angiographic differential diagnosis between the vascularized malignant glioma and the intracranial arteriovenous malformation. Am J Roentgenol 90:512–521, 1963

5. **Houser OW, Baker HL Jr, Svien JH et al:** Arteriovenous malformations of the parenchyma of the brain. Radiology 109:83–90, 1973

6. **Kamisasa A:** Arteriography of the anterior communicating aneurysm. Neuroradiology 12:227–232, 1977

7. **Kitching GB, Hasso AN, Hieshima GB:** Interhemispheric infarction. Radiology 120:111–115, 1976

8. **Kondo A, Koyama T, Ishikawa J, Iwaki K, Yamasaki T:** Ruptured aneurysm of an azygous anterior cerebral artery. Neuroradiology 17:227–229, 1979

9. **Kramer RA, Wing SD:** Computed tomography of angiographically occult cerebral vascular malformations. Radiology 123:649–652, 1977

9A. **Kwak R, Niizuma H, Hatanka M et al:** Anterior communicating artery aneurysms with associated anomalies. J Neurosurg 52:162–164, 1980

10. **Leo JS, Lin JP, Kricheff II:** Pseudoaneurysm formation secondary to spontaneous thrombosis of a massive cerebral arteriovenous malformation. Neuroradiology 17:115–119, 1979

10A. **Miller JH, Peña AM, Segall HD:** Radiological investigation of sellar region masses in children. Radiology 134:81–87, 1980

11. **Moscow NP, Michoty P, Salamon G:** The anterior cerebral artery complex. Section II. Anatomy of the cortical branches of the anterior cerebral artery. In Newton TH, Potts DG (eds): Radiology of the Skull and Brain, Vol 2, pp 1411–1420. St. Louis, CV Mosby, 1974

12. **Newton TH, Troost BT:** Arteriovenous malformations and fistulae. In Newton TH, Potts DG (eds): Radiology of the Skull and Brain, Vol 2, pp 2490–2565. St. Louis, CV Mosby, 1974

13. **Nutik S, Dilenge D:** Carotid-anterior cerebral artery anastomosis. J Neurosurg 44:378–382, 1976

13A. **Parkinson D, West M:** Traumatic intracranial aneurysms. J Neurosurg 52:11–20, 1980

14. **Perlmutter D, Rhoton AL Jr:** Microsurgical anatomy of the anterior cerebral-anterior communicating-recurrent artery complex. J Neurosurg 45:259–272, 1976

15. **Perlmutter D, Rhoton AL Jr:** Microsurgical anatomy of the distal anterior cerebral artery. J Neurosurg 49:204–228, 1978

15A. **Richmond IL, Newton TH, Wilson CB:** Indications for angiography in the preoperative evaluation of patients with prolactin-secreting pituitary adenomas. J Neurosurg 52:378–380, 1980

16. **Ring BA, Waddington MM:** Roentgenographic anatomy of the pericallosal arteries. Am J Roentgenol 104:109–118, 1968

17. **Stephens RB, Stilwell DL:** Arteries and Veins of the Human Brain, pp 30–33. Springfield, IL, C C Thomas, 1969

17A. **Wilson CB, Usang H, Domingue J:** Microsurgical treatment of intracranial vascular malformations. J Neurosurg 51:446–454, 1979

17B. **Yock DH Jr, Larson DA:** Computed tomography of hemorrhage from anterior communicating artery aneurysms, with angiographic correlation. Radiology 134:399–407, 1980

18. **Yoshimoto T, Uchida K, Suzuki J:** Surgical treatment of distal anterior cerebral artery aneurysms. J Neurosurg 50:40–44, 1979

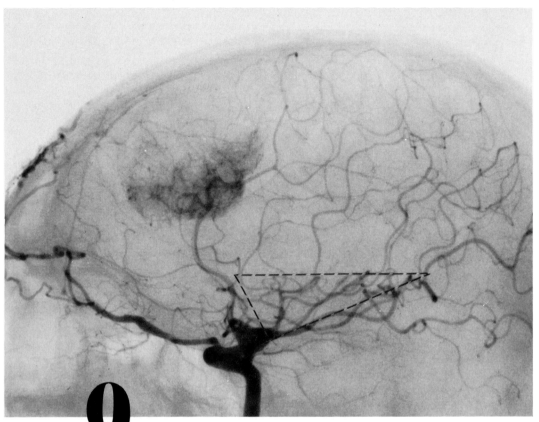

9 The Middle Cerebral Artery

A wide variety of intracranial pathologic processes such as tumors, aneurysms, and embolic and occlusive vascular disease affect the middle cerebral artery (MCA) and its branches. These important vessels supply a very extensive area that includes most of the lateral surfaces of the cerebral hemispheres. In addition, characteristic displacements of the MCA provide important clues pertaining to the location and extent of intracranial mass lesions. Hence, thorough knowledge of the normal gross and angiographic anatomy of the MCA is vital for complete, correct interpretation of cerebral angiograms.

NORMAL GROSS ANATOMY

The Proximal Middle Cerebral Artery

The MCA is the larger of the two terminal branches of the internal carotid artery (ICA). The proximal segment of the MCA extends laterally and horizontally in the lateral cere-

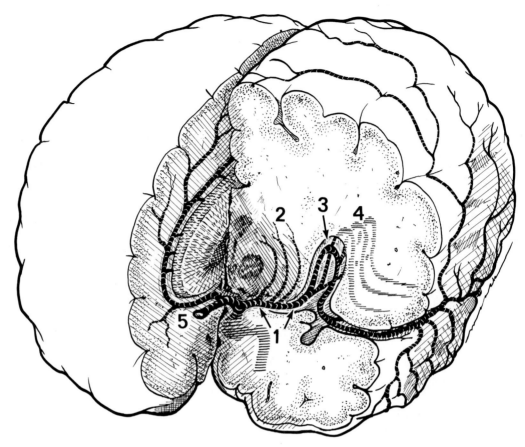

Fig. 9-1. Anatomic drawing of the middle cerebral artery (MCA) and its relationship to adjacent structures. The Sylvian fissure has been exaggerated so that the MCA loops over the insula can be more clearly depicted. **1.** M1 (horizontal) segment. The "genu" is where the MCA curves upwards into the Sylvian fissure. **2.** Lateral lenticulostriate arteries. **3.** Sylvian fissure. **4.** MCA within the depths of the Sylvian fissure. **5.** Left and right anterior cerebral arteries.

bral fissure beneath the anterior perforated substance to reach the Sylvian fissure (Fig. 9-1). This portion of the MCA is also termed the M1 segment, analogous to the initial or A1 segment of the anterior cerebral artery. Some six to 20 **lateral lenticulostriate arteries** arise from the superior aspect of the proximal MCA to supply portions of the basal ganglia, internal capsule, and caudate nucleus.[43B] The exact course of the proximal MCA segment varies with age. In children below the age of five or six years the horizontal MCA frequently courses somewhat superiorly. With increasing age it usually becomes horizontal or often convex inferiorly (See Fig. 8-5).

Near the limen insulae (a small gyrus located near the anteroinferior corner of the insula), the MCA turns upward in a gentle curve forming its so-called *genu* or "knee"

(Fig. 9-1). Turning around the island of Reil, the MCA then courses posterosuperiorly within the depths of the Sylvian fissure.[54]

The Sylvian Middle Cerebral Artery

The MCA divides into its major cortical branches approximately 1.5 cm from its ori-

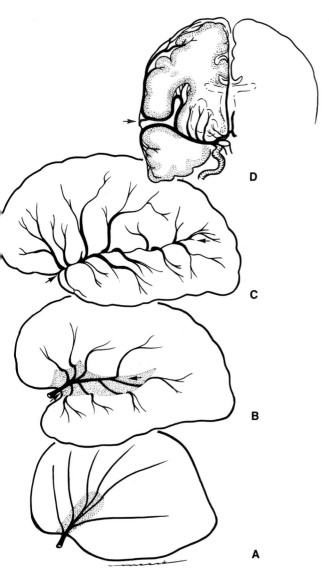

Fig. 9-2. Anatomic drawing depicting the development of the insula and Sylvian fissure **(arrows)** in the fetal brain. **A.** Fetal brain at 13-14 weeks. The middle cerebral vessels follow nearly a straight course over the surface of the brain. The insula is beginning to appear as a small fossa or depression on the cortical surface **(dotted area). B.** Fetal brain at 24 weeks. The Sylvian fissure deepens and begins to cover the insula **(dotted area).** The MCA branches, following the insula, begin to assume a more sinusoidal course. **C.** Brain at full term. The insula is buried in the depths of the Sylvian fissure. Branches of the MCA course over the insula, then must turn laterally to exit from the Sylvian fissure. **D.** Cut-away AP view of C. Note how the M1 segment courses laterally in the lateral cerebral fissure. When it reaches the limen insulae, its distal branches course superiorly over the surface of the insula. They then turn inferolaterally to exit from the Sylvian fissure **(arrow)** and course over the surface of the cortex.

gin. An understanding of the rather complicated tridimensional appearance of the MCA distal to the genu is dependent on an understanding of the intimate relationship between this artery and the embryological development of the insula and Sylvian fissure.

The insula (island of Reil) is a roughly triangular-shaped mound of cortex buried in the depths of the Sylvian fissure. The insula first appears in the third month of fetal development as a slight depression on the lateral surface of the cerebral hemisphere (Fig. 9-2A). Progressive deepening of this fossa leads to the formation of the insula with the frontal and parietal lobe operculae beginning to overlap the insula from above and the temporal lobe overlapping from below (Fig. 9-2B). Eventually, the frontoparietal and temporal operculae completely cover the insula (Figure 9-2C). This apposition of the superiorly located frontoparietal and the inferiorly located

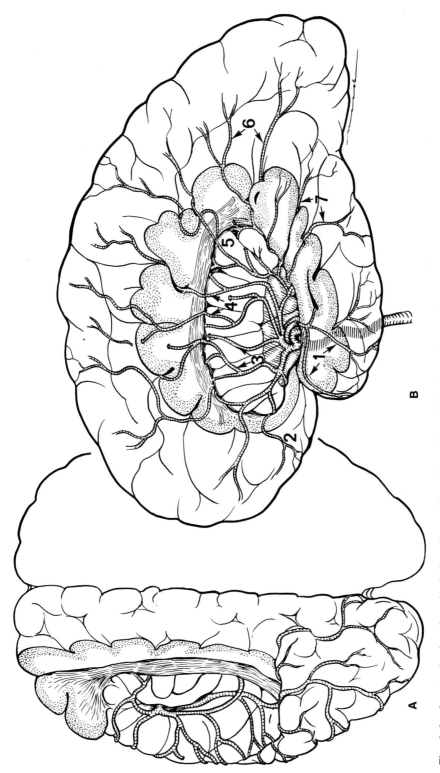

Fig. 9-3. Anatomic drawing depicting the relationship of the MCA branches to the insula, Sylvian fissure, and cerebral cortex. **(A)** Superior view. The Sylvian fissure and insula have been exposed by dissecting the frontoparietal operculae. **(B)** Lateral view. The insula is shown with the distal MCA branches coursing over its surface. **1.** Anterior temporal artery. **2.** Orbitofrontal artery. **3.** Operculofrontal arteries ("candleabra group"). **4.** Central sulcus arteries (rolandic group). **5.** Posterior parietal artery. **6.** Angular artery branches. **7.** Posterior temporal artery branches.

242

temporal lobe over the island ultimately forms the Sylvian fissure (Fig. 9-2D).

Early in fetal development before the insula and Sylvian fissure are formed, cortical branches of the MCA ramify directly over the cerebral hemispheres. The cortical branches appear only slightly curved and course almost vertically over the smooth cerebral hemispheres. Progressive infolding of the cerebral cortex to form the insula carries with it the peripheral branches of the MCA. As the insula develops, the MCA changes from a relatively linear to a more tortuous pattern. By 28 to 32 weeks of gestation, the MCA cortical branches assume a configuration which begins to approximate the adult pattern (Fig. 9-2).[19]

The normal MCA in an adult is depicted in Figures 9-1 and 9-3. Near the anterior aspect of the limen insulae the horizontal MCA divides into its major cortical branches. Buried in the depths of the Sylvian fissure, these branches first course superiorly over the convex surface of the insula. At the superior limit of the insula, they turn inferiorly then laterally under the frontoparietal operculum. After reaching the lateral aspect of the Sylvian fissure, the cortical branches of the MCA loop around and over the opercula to ramify on the surface of the cerebral hemispheres.

Cortical Branches of the Middle Cerebral Artery

The origin and course of the cortical MCA branches are so variable that the only truly constant anatomic finding is in their terminal distribution. However, a discussion of the most common patterns of distal branching is usually helpful.

The Anterior Temporal Artery. This is a small branch of the MCA that frequently arises before the main MCA bifurcation, passing anteriorly and inferiorly over the temporal tip. The anterior temporal artery arises from the main MCA trunk at approximately the same level as the lenticulostriate vessels and does not usually enter the Sylvian fissure (Fig. 9-3B, arrow 1).

Anterior Branches. The main MCA trunk usually bifurcates into anterior and posterior groups. The anterior or ascending frontal artery complex includes both the operculofrontal arteries and the central sulcus arteries.

The ascending frontal complex occasionally arises as a single trunk but more often originates as two or three separate vessels. The first branch of this complex is usually the **orbitofrontal artery** (which occasionally arises from the horizontal MCA). The orbitofrontal artery courses anteriorly and slightly superiorly to supply the inferolateral portions of the frontal lobe (Fig. 9-3B, arrow 2).

The next branches of the ascending frontal complex, the **operculofrontal arteries,** are frequently nicknamed the "candelabra" group because of their occasional resemblance to candlesticks. This group includes all the branches anterior to the central sulcus arteries. The operculofrontal arteries supply most of the middle and inferior frontal gyri including Broca's and the premotor areas (Fig. 9-3B, arrow 3).

One or two **central sulcus arteries** (rolandic group) arise posterior to the operculofrontal group and ascend over the cerebral convexity to supply the motor and sensory strips (Fig. 9-3B, arrow 4).

Posterior Branches. The posterior division of the MCA usually has three major branches. These posterior branches arise within the depths of the Sylvian fissure, loop upward over the insula and then turn posterolaterally to exit from the Sylvian fissure and ramify over the cerebral hemisphere.

The first major posterior branch of the MCA is the **posterior parietal artery.** This vessel exits from the Sylvian fissure and courses posterosuperiorly to supply the parietal lobe immediately behind the sensory strip. The posterior parietal artery and the angular artery often arise from a common trunk (Fig. 9-3B, arrow 5).

The **angular artery** is the terminal continuation and usually the largest cortical branch of the MCA. The proximal portion of the angular artery initially lies within and runs parallel to the axis of the Sylvian fissure. Emerging from the apex of the Sylvian fissure, the angular artery courses posteriorly and superiorly to supply a variable area that includes the posterolateral parietal and lateral occipital lobes, and the superior temporal gyri (Fig. 9-3B, arrow 6).

The third major posterior branch of the MCA is the **posterior temporal artery**. This artery descends over the lateral aspect of the temporal lobe. Its size and area of distribution vary widely, often including virtually the entire temporal lobe except for its anterior portion (Fig. 9-3B, arrow 7).

Figure 9-4 is a lateral sketch of the left cerebral hemisphere. The branches of the MCA and their most common zones of vascular distribution are summarized. Although the exact branching pattern of the MCA may vary widely, the area supplied by the major cortical branches is quite constant. Understanding these terminal areas of distribution is an important prerequisite for the recognition of vessel occlusions and displacements.[34, 44, 60]

NORMAL RADIOGRAPHIC ANATOMY

Angiographic Appearance of the Middle Cerebral Artery

The proximal MCA segment is best visualized in either the AP or submentovertex view. It usually follows a relatively straight horizontal course from its origin to the Sylvian fissure (Fig. 9-5A, arrow 1). However, in neonates or very young patients, the proximal MCA may course quite superiorly while in older patients it often describes a marked inferior oblique curvature (Fig. 8-5).

The lateral lenticulostriate arteries arise from the proximal portion of the MCA. In the AP projection, they initially course superomedially, then turn laterally around the basal ganglia in a gentle, convex, lateral curve (Fig. 9-5A, arrow 2). In the lateral projection (Fig. 9-5B, arrow 1), the lenticulostriate arteries assume a fan-shaped distribution that is partially obscured by superimposed cortical branches of the MCA (Fig. 9-36A). Late arterial phase films may demonstrate prominent lenticulostriate arteries and a dense vascular stain in the basal ganglia area (Fig. 9-21). This is a normal finding and should not be mistaken for a neoplasm.

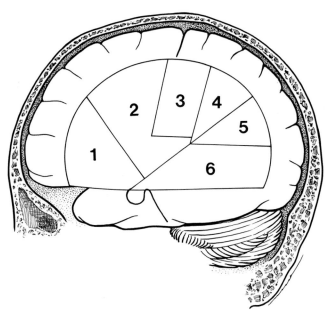

Fig. 9-4. Anatomic drawing of the left cerebral hemisphere. The approximate zones of vascular distribution of the MCA branches are depicted. **1.** Orbitofrontal artery. **2.** Operculofrontal arteries. **3.** Central sulcus arteries supplying motor and sensory areas. **4.** Posterior parietal artery. **5.** Angular artery. **6.** Posterior temporal branches. *(Adapted from M. M. Waddington.)*[34]

The anterior temporal artery, the first cortical branch of the MCA, is usually small and sometimes difficult to identify angiographically. However, in the lateral projection (Fig. 9-5B, arrow 2) it can occasionally be seen descending immediately posterior and parallel to the greater wing of the sphenoid (anterior border of the middle fossa).

Distal to the genu of the MCA, the cortical branches course superiorly over the insula. In the AP projection, these vessels have a slight lateral convexity as they ascend over the insula (Fig. 9-5A, arrow 4). At the top of the insula (Fig. 9-5A, arrow 5), the MCA branches turn inferolaterally within the Sylvian fissure to reach the surface of the cortex. The more anterior MCA cortical branches appear somewhat lower in the routine (+15°) AP projection while posterior branches are higher. The highest and most medial point where the last cortical MCA branch (usually a branch of the angular artery) turns inferolaterally is termed the *angiographic Sylvian point* (Fig. 9-5). This point approximates the apex of the insula and represents the posterior limit of the Sylvian fissure.

In the lateral projection, the tops of the insular loops form a relatively straight line demarcating the top of the insula. The Sylvian point in the lateral view is indicated by the top of the most posterior intrasylvian loop. The *angiographic Sylvian triangle* is demarcated by the superior insular line (a line tangent to the tops of the intrasylvian loops), the main trunk of the MCA (which forms the posterior-inferior margin of the triangle), and the most anterior branch of the ascending frontal complex (which forms the anterior border of the triangle).

The angiographic Sylvian triangle is clearly seen in Figure 9-6. Complete occlusion of the ICA is present and the MCA has filled via collaterals. The anterior cerebral artery (ACA) and opercular branches of the MCA are not opacified, permitting delineation of the Sylvian triangle without overlapping vessels. Angiographically, the *Sylvian fissure* is indicated by the point where the insular loops, having turned inferiorly, course laterally to curve over the opercula (Fig. 9-6, dotted line).

The individual opercular branches of the MCA vary widely in their origin and course. However, their terminal area of distribution is relatively constant (see above) and can be depicted by a variety of templates devised for superimposition on routine nonmagnified lateral cerebral angiograms (Fig. 9-7).[34, 44, 60]

Normal Measurements

A variety of normal measurements have been devised for the MCA complex. These measurements can help detect slight displacements of the MCA caused by intracranial mass lesions.

The angiographic Sylvian point normally lies from 30 to 43 mm from the inner table of the skull on routine nonmagnified AP films (Fig. 9-8A, line c to d). If a line is also constructed tangent to the inner table of the skull (Fig. 9-8A, line a to b) the angiographic Sylvian point should lie approximately halfway between this line and the orbital roof or top of the petrous temporal bone (whichever is lower). The lateral margin of the insula should be within 20 to 30 mm from the inner table of the skull (Fig. 9-8A, line e to f).

A simple method for measuring the Sylvian triangle on lateral carotid angiograms has been described. The superior insular line (Fig. 9-8B, line a to b) should be within 5 mm of the midpoint of a line extending vertically from the superior border of the external auditory meatus to the inner table of the skull (Fig. 9-8B, line f to o).[34, 50, 56]

A line drawn between the anterior clinoid processes and the inner table of the skull (9 cm above the internal occipital protuberance) is called the clinoparietal line (Fig. 9-8B, line c to d). The main axis of the MCA within the Sylvian fissure should lie no more than 1 cm above this line in adults (1.5 cm in children and 1.8 cm in infants) at a point on the line 2 cm posterior to the carotid siphon. The angiographic Sylvian point (where the last main branch of the MCA leaves the Sylvian fissure to reach the surface of the brain) is never more than 3.1 mm anterior or 14.4 mm posterior to the midpoint of the clinoparietal line. It also

(Text continued on p. 251)

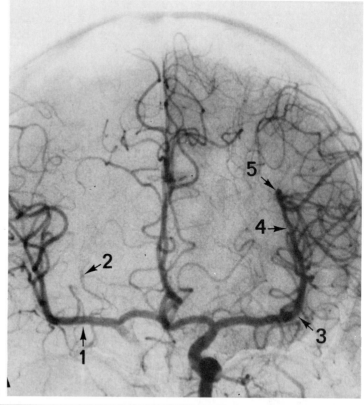

A
B

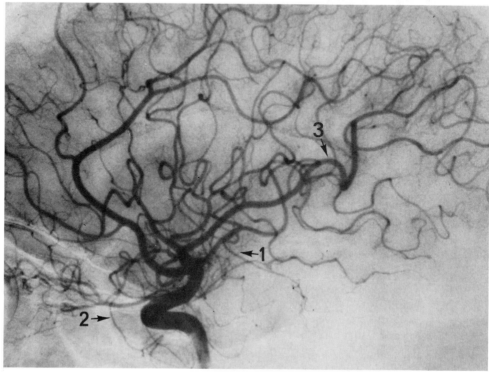

◀ **Fig. 9-5. (A)** Normal left internal carotid angiogram (arterial phase, AP view). Temporary cross compression of the right common carotid artery has permitted filling of both ACAs and MCAs. **1.** M1 (horizontal) MCA segment. **2.** Lateral lenticulostriate arteries. **3.** MCA genu. **4.** MCA as it courses over the insula. **5.** Sylvian point (top of the insula). **(B)** Normal left internal carotid angiogram (arterial phase, lateral view). **1.** Lenticulostriate arteries. **2.** Anterior temporal arteries. **3.** Sylvian point.

Fig. 9-6. Left common carotid angiogram (late arterial phase, lateral view). This was seen in a patient with complete occlusion of the ICA. Retrograde filling of the distal ICA has occurred via external-internal carotid collaterals through the ophthalmic artery. The insular branches of the MCA are clearly seen. The insula (Sylvian triangle) is demarcated by the superior insular line **(solid line, a to b),** a line along the main MCA axis **(solid line, b to c),** and the most anterior MCA branch **(solid line, a to c).** The Sylvian fissure **(dotted line, a to b)** is demarcated by the inferolateral insular loops.

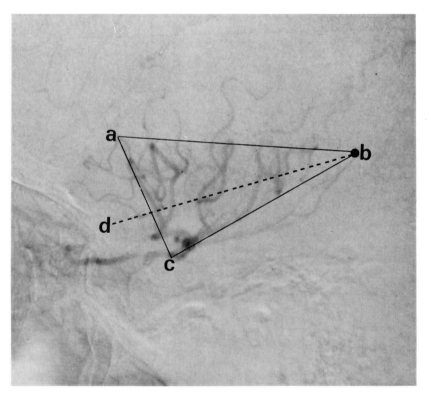

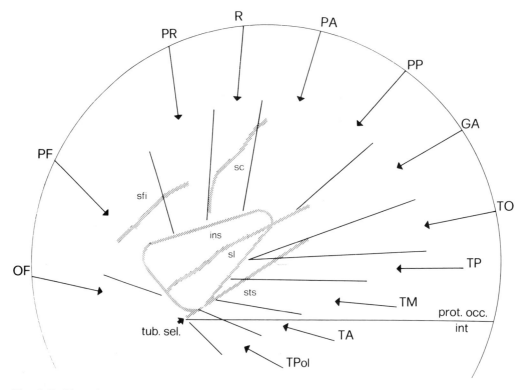

Fig. 9-7. Template used to identify cortical branches of the MCA. *(Michoty P, Moscow NP, Salamon G: Anatomy of the cortical branches of the middle cerebral artery. In Newton TH and Potts DG (eds), Radiology of the Skull and Brain, Vol. 2, pp 1476, CV Mosby, St. Louis, 1974.)* Tuberculum sellae **(tub sel).** Internal occipital protuberance **(prot occ int).** Orbitofrontal artery **(OF).** Prefrontal artery **(PF).** Precentral or prerolandic artery **(PR).** Central or rolandic artery **(R).** Anterior parietal artery **(PA).** Posterior parietal artery **(PP).** Angular artery **(GA).** Temporo-occipital artery **(TO).** Posterior temporal artery **(TP).** Middle temporal artery **(TM).** Anterior temporal artery **(TA).** Temporal polar artery **(TPol).** Inferior frontal sulcus **(Sfi).** Central sulcus **(SC).** Insula **(INS).** Lateral sulcus **(SI).** Superior temporal sulcus **(Sts).**

Fig. 9-8(A). Right internal carotid angiogram (arterial phase, AP view) with temporary ▶ cross-compression of the left ICA. Reflux into the left MCA has opacified its main branches. The angiographic Sylvian points are indicated **(large dots).** The height of the normal Sylvian point should be approximately halfway along a line **(b** to **g)** constructed between the roof of the orbit or petrous ridge (whichever is lower) and a second line **(a** to **b)** drawn tangential to the inner table of the skull. The normal Sylvian point should also lie between 30 and 43 mm from the inner table of the skull **(c** to **d).** The lateral margin of the insula **(e)** should be 20-30 mm from the inner table of the skull **(e** to **f). (B)** Normal left internal carotid angiogram (early arterial phase, lateral view). The superior insular line **(a** to **b)** should lie within about 5 mm of the midpoint of a line (**f** to **o)** drawn perpendicularly between the external auditory meatus and inner table of the skull. The main MCA axis should be no more than 1 cm away from a line drawn from a point 9 cm above the internal occipital protuberance **(e)** to the anterior clinoid process **(c** to **d).** This is called the *clinoparietal line.* The angiographic Sylvian point **(large black dot, b)** should be near the clinoparietal line (see text).

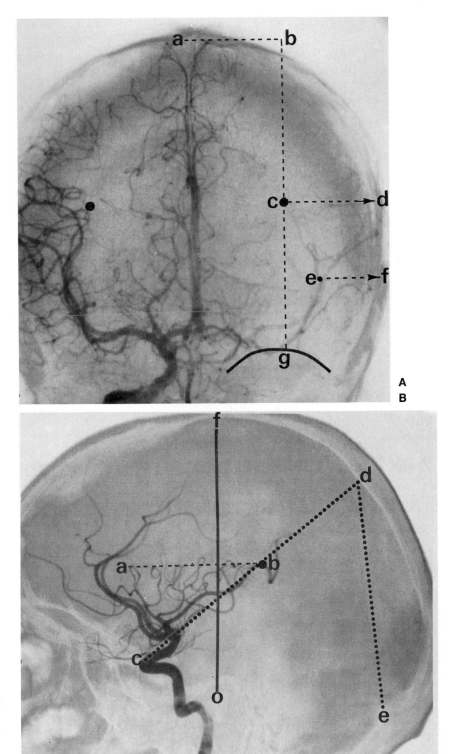

A
B

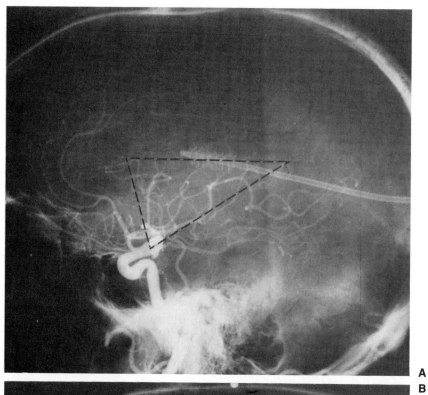

A

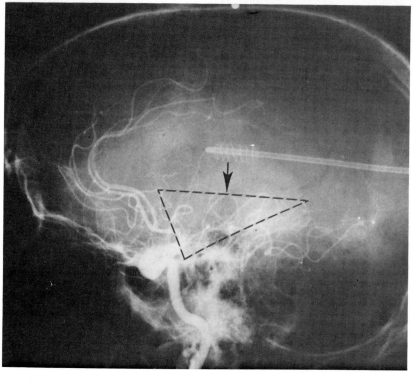

B

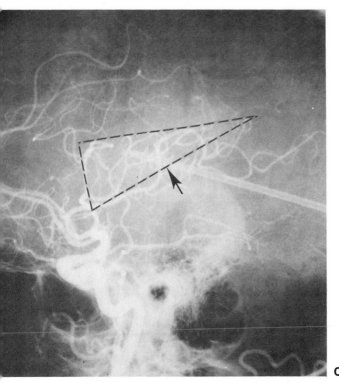

Fig. 9-9. Series of left common carotid angiograms (mid-arterial phase, lateral view). Correct head position **(A).** The Sylvian triangle appears normal. Same patient as **A (B).** The head is angled towards the film changer, producing the false impression of an inferiorly displaced Sylvian triangle **(arrow, dotted lines).** Same patient **(C)** as **A, B.** The head is angled away from the film changer, giving the erroneous impression of an elevated Sylvian triangle **(arrow, dotted lines).**

C

lies within 8 mm above or below this point in normal angiograms.[26]

In borderline or questionable abnormal cases, the relative position of the MCA branches can be compared with those on the contralateral side. AP films with temporary manual cross-compression of the contralateral common carotid artery during contrast injection will allow comparison of both Sylvian points (Figs. 9-5A, 9-8A). Minimal side-to-side discrepancies will be readily apparent although no maximum differences in symmetry for normal variation have been established.

It should be emphasized that tilting or angulation of the head during filming changes the relationship between the Sylvian triangle and skull landmarks, rendering the usual measurements inaccurate (Fig. 9-9).

NORMAL VARIATIONS AND ANOMALIES OF THE MIDDLE CEREBRAL ARTERY

Branching patterns of the MCA are highly variable. In most patients the MCA bifurcates (50% of cases) or trifurcates (25% of cases) near the insula (Figs. 9-5A, 9-10).[26] However, early division of the M1 segment is not unusual (Fig. 9-10A, C).

Anomalies of the MCA are uncommon. However, occasional anomalies include hypoplasia of the M1 segment (Fig. 9-11), duplication, accessory artery (Fig. 9-10D), and fenestration of the main MCA trunk.[15, 16, 58]

DISTORTIONS OF THE MIDDLE CEREBRAL ARTERY CAUSED BY INTRACRANIAL MASS LESIONS

The MCA has been described as the single most important vascular configuration in the angiographic localization of supratentorial mass lesions. Because the MCA branches which course over the insula and constitute the angiographic Sylvian triangle lie in a relatively constant position deep within the cerebral hemispheres, subtle distortions in their configuration may provide an early indication of a space-occupying process.[14, 21, 30]

Intracranial mass lesions involve the MCA

(Text continued on p. 254)

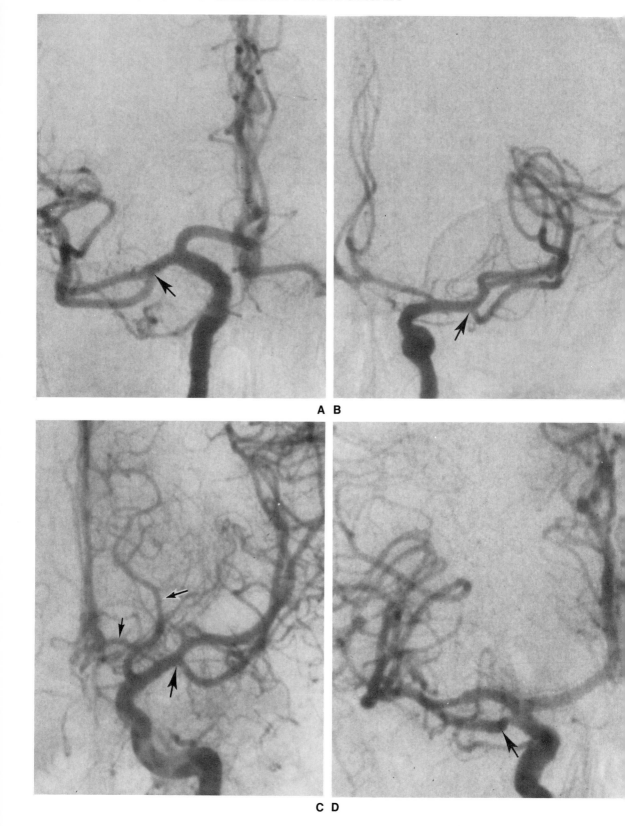

A B

C D

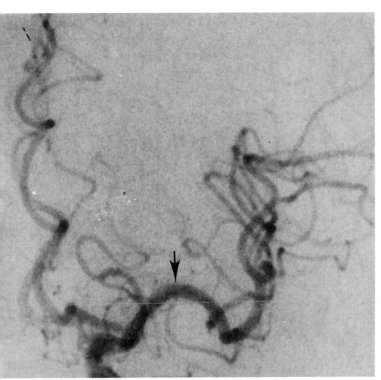

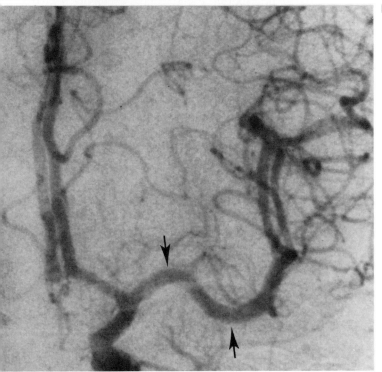

E
F

Fig. 9-10. Normal variations in course and branching patterns of the middle cerebral artery (arterial phase, AP views). Early bifurcation **(A) (arrow)**. Early trifurcation **(B) (arrow)**. Early MCA division **(C) (large arrow)** in a patient with a hypoplastic A1 **(small arrow)** and fetal origin of the posterior cerebral artery **(outlined arrow)**. Accessory MCA **(D) (arrow)** arising from the ICA. Superiorly convex M1 segment **(E) (arrow)**. Biconvex segment **(F) (arrows)**.

either by deriving abnormal vascular supply from its branches or by displacing vessels that are otherwise normal. A focal intracerebral mass may cause a localized rounded deformation of adjacent blood vessels. These vessels will appear bowed, stretched, and draped around the lesion. If the mass effect is sufficiently large it will also displace part or all of the Sylvian triangle.

The Sylvian triangle can be displaced in several directions:

1. anterior or posterior
2. superior or inferior
3. medial or lateral

The exact displacement present in any given abnormal angiogram will be determined by the size of the mass and its relationship to the insula. Supratentorial mass lesions in different locations are considered below.

Anterior Masses

Frontal masses displace the Sylvian triangle posteriorly in the lateral view. Vessels directly adjacent to the mass appear stretched and bowed while the Sylvian triangle is compressed and displaced posteriorly. A typical posterior shift of the Sylvian triangle is depicted diagrammatically in Figure 9-12A. In Figure 9-12B, an avascular astrocytoma has displaced the Sylvian triangle posteriorly, compressing and crowding the insular loops together.

Retrosylvian Mass Lesions

The insula is displaced forward by masses posterior to the island of Reil. The Sylvian MCA branches are compressed and displaced anteriorly in the lateral view (Fig. 9-13A). In Fig. 9-13B, a huge vascular tumor orginating in the atrium of the lateral ventricle has displaced the Sylvian triangle anteriorly. The posterior parietal, angular, and posterior temporal MCA branches are markedly stretched and draped around the mass. In the AP view, the Sylvian point can be displaced either medially or laterally depending on the exact location of the mass within the cerebral hemisphere.

Suprasylvian Masses

These lesions displace the Sylvian point inferiorly in the AP view (Fig. 9-14A, B). Note the marked inferior displacement of the Sylvian point as well as the large distal shift of the ACA. Depending on the precise location of the mass, part or all of the superior insular line is bowed downward in the lateral view (Fig. 9-15A, B) and the adjacent opercular branches are splayed around the mass (Fig. 9-15B). Suprasylvian masses may also displace the opercular branches and Sylvian point laterally. Mid or posterior convexity masses can also produce inferior displacement of the Sylvian point in the AP view.[22]

Temporal Lobe Masses

Middle cranial fossa masses usually displace the MCA vessels and angiographic Sylvian point superiorly or medially. A holotemporal avascular mass is illustrated in Figures 9-16A and 9-17A. The entire Sylvian triangle is elevated and the angiographic Sylvian point displaced superomedially compared to the contralateral normal side. AP and lateral arterial phase films of a very vascular temporal lobe glioma are shown in Figures 9-16B and 9-17B. Note the gross elevation of the Sylvian point and entire Sylvian triangle. In the AP view, the genu of the MCA is also markedly elevated. Masses in or adjacent to the anterior temporal lobe also elevate the horizontal segment and genu of the MCA. Posterior temporal mass lesions may also crowd the Sylvian vessels anteriorly as seen on the lateral view (Fig. 9-13).

Centrosylvian Masses

Lesions deep to the insula arise in the basal ganglia, lateral ventricles, and internal or external capsule. Consequently, as the insula is displaced laterally the Sylvian vessels are bowed outwardly. The distance between the insula and inner table of the skull is therefore diminished (Fig. 9-18A). If the mass effect is located within the lateral ventricles or basal ganglia, the lenticulostriate arteries are also displaced laterally (Fig. 9-18B).[1] However, if the epicenter of the mass lies within the claustrum or external capsule (as often occurs with infiltrating neoplasms or hypertensive intracerebral hemorrhage), the lenticulostriate arteries will appear displaced medially (Fig. 9-18C).

(Text continued on p. 263)

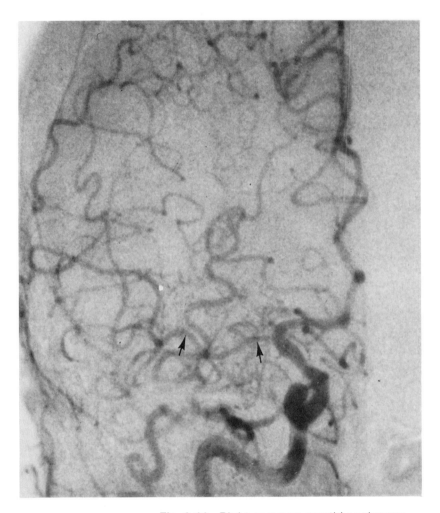

Fig. 9-11. Right common carotid angiogram (mid-arterial phase, AP view) showing hypoplasia of the M1 segment **(arrows).**

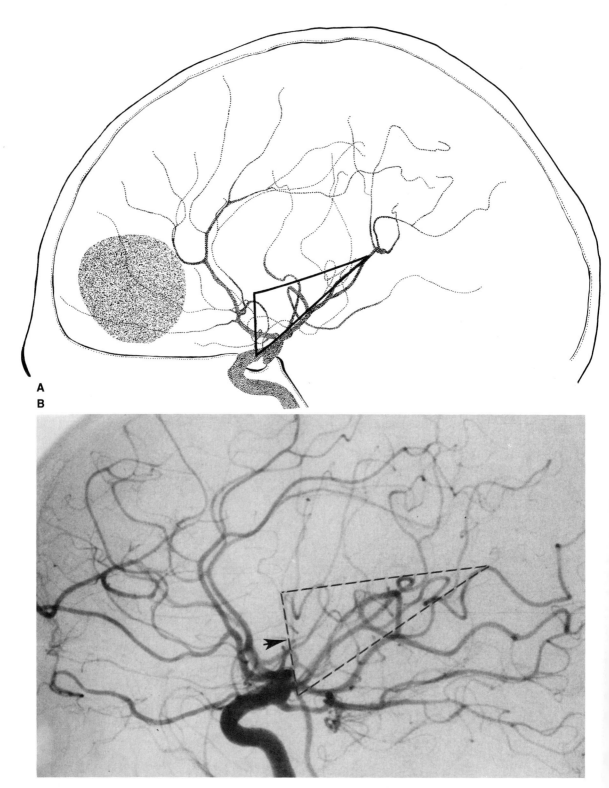

Fig. 9-12. Diagrammatic radiograph **(A)** of a left internal carotid angiogram (lateral view) of a large frontal mass. The Sylvian triangle **(solid lines)** is compressed and displaced posteriorly. Left internal carotid angiogram **(B,** arterial phase, lateral view). This was seen in a patient with a large avascular astrocytoma in the frontal lobe. The insular vessels **(dotted triangle)** are displaced posteriorly.

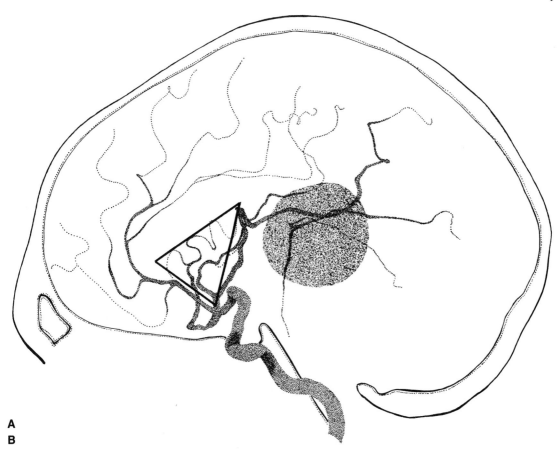

A

B

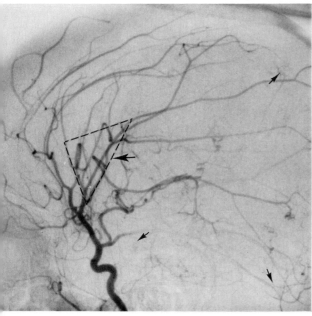

Fig. 9-13. Anatomic diagram of a left carotid angiogram (**A,** arterial phase, lateral view) of a retrosylvian mass. The insula **(solid triangle)** is displaced anteriorly. Left common carotid angiogram (**B,** arterial phase, lateral view). This was seen in a four-month-old child with huge intraventricular tumor **(small arrows)** originating in the atrium. The Sylvian triangle **(dotted lines)** is displaced anteriorly.

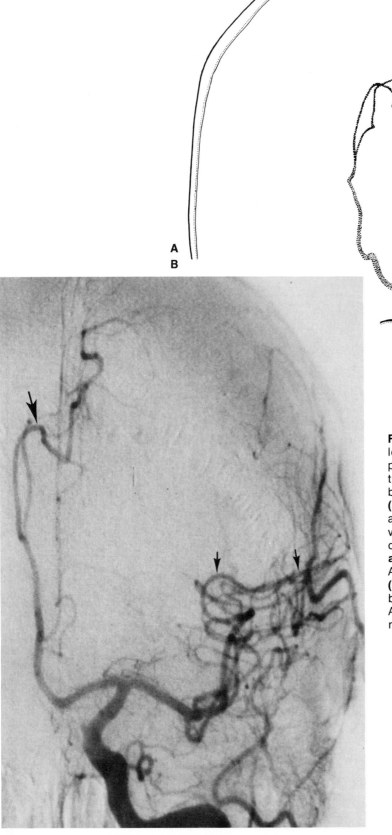

Fig. 9-14. Anatomic diagram of a left carotid angiogram (**A,** arterial phase, AP view) of a large parietal tumor. The Sylvian point and MCA branches are displaced inferiorly **(arrow).** Left common carotid angiogram (**B,** arterial phase, AP view). A large parietal tumor has depressed the MCA vessels **(small arrows).** Note the pronounced distal ACA shift and subfalcine "step" **(large arrow)** where the herniated brain and its accompanying distal ACA branches return toward the midline.

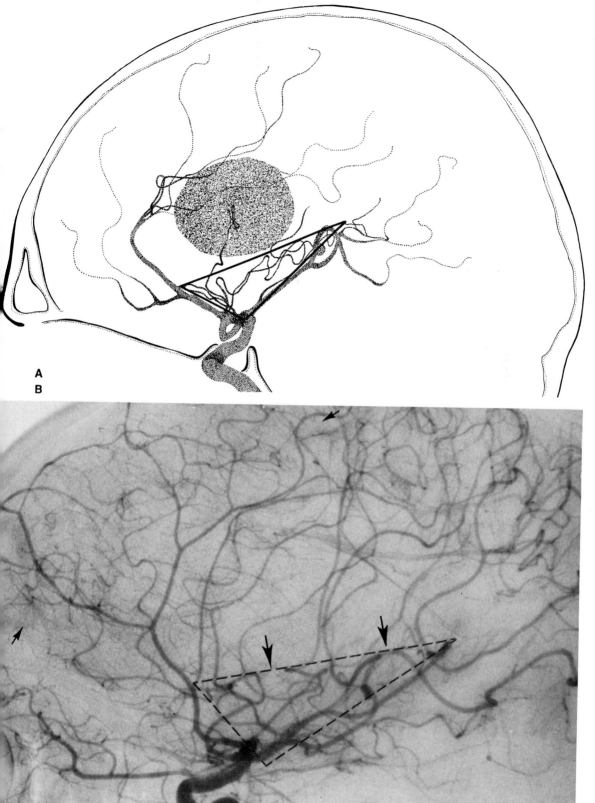

Fig. 9-15. Anatomic drawing of a left carotid angiogram (**A,** arterial phase, lateral) of a large suprasylvian mass. The insula **(solid triangle)** is compressed and displaced inferiorly. Left internal carotid angiogram (**B,** arterial phase, lateral view) of a huge astrocytoma **(small arrows)** involving the entire frontal and part of the anterior parietal lobes. The Sylvian triangle **(dotted lines)** is displaced inferiorly.

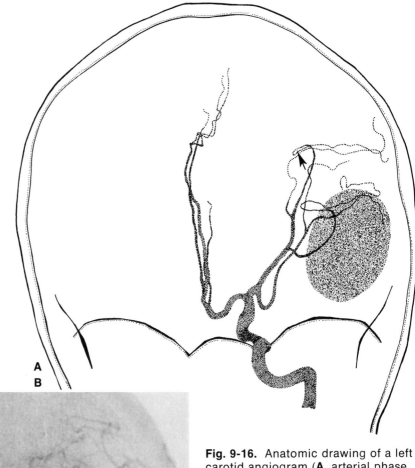

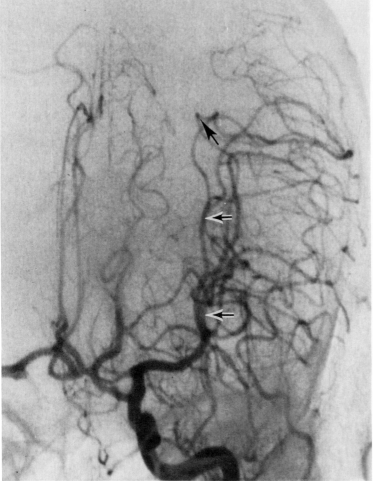

Fig. 9-16. Anatomic drawing of a left carotid angiogram (**A,** arterial phase, AP view) of a temporal lobe mass. The horizontal MCA is elevated and the angiographic Sylvian point is displaced superiorly **(arrow).** Left internal carotid angiogram (**B,** arterial phase, AP view) of a large holotemporal avascular mass. The Sylvian point is elevated **(black arrow)** and the insula is displaced medially **(outlined arrows),** increasing the distance between it and the calvarium.

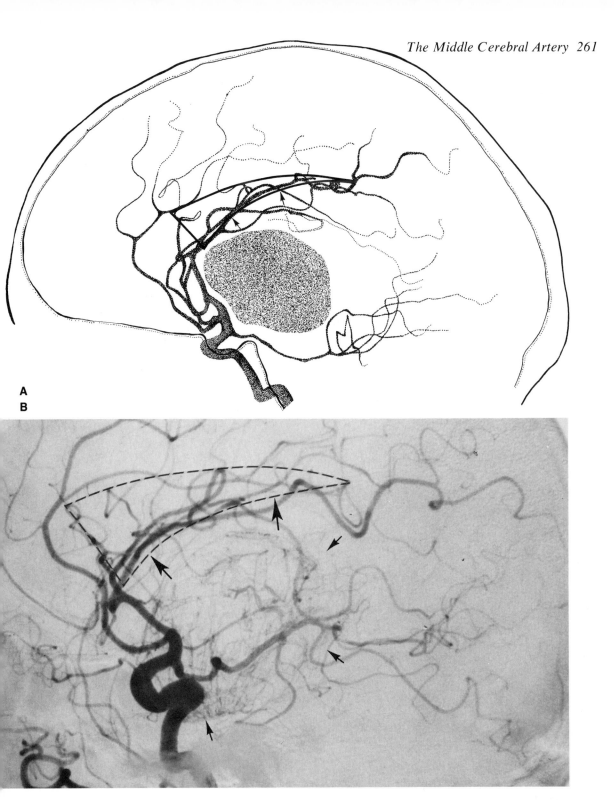

Fig. 9-17. Anatomic drawing of a left carotid angiogram (**A,** arterial phase, lateral view) of a temporal lobe mass. The Sylvian triangle **(solid lines)** is markedly elevated. Left common carotid angiogram (**B,** arterial phase, lateral view) of a large temporal high grade astrocytoma **(small arrows).** The Sylvian triangle **(dotted lines)** is markedly elevated.

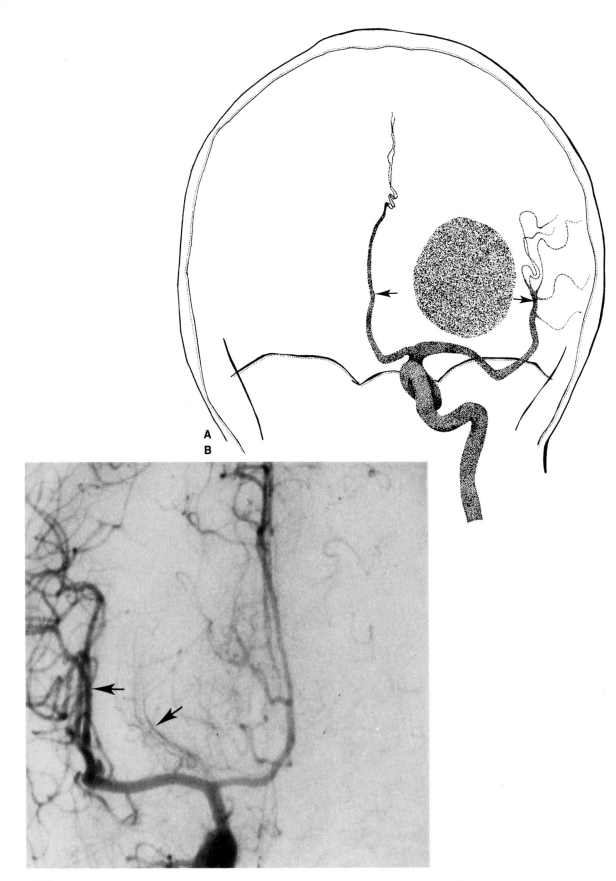

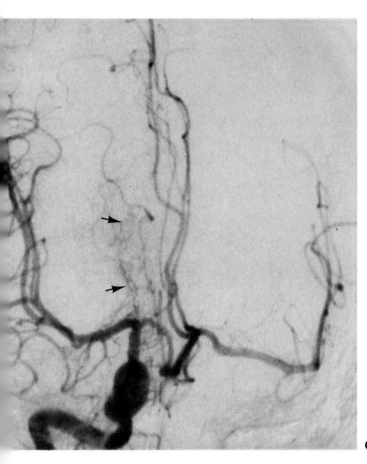

Fig. 9-18. Anatomic drawing of a left internal carotid angiogram (**A,** arterial phase, AP view) of a large mass deep to the insula. The MCA vessels are displaced laterally and the ACA is herniated across the midline **(arrows).** Right internal carotid angiogram (**B,** arterial phase, AP view) of a giant-celled astrocytoma in the right frontal lobe and basal ganglia. The lenticulostriate and MCA arteries are displaced laterally **(arrows).** Note the proximal ACA shift. Right internal carotid angiogram (**C,** arterial phase, AP view) of a posterior temporal lobe tumor that has also infiltrated the insula and external capsule. The lenticulostriate arteries are displaced medially **(arrows).**

C

ABNORMAL VASCULARITY

Tumor Circulation

The diagnosis as well as the localization of intracranial neoplasms is based not only on the displacement of otherwise normal vessels but on circulatory alterations within the tumor itself. Circulatory abnormalities in intracranial neoplasms are of three general types: abnormal new vessels or "neovascularity"; diffuse or focal hypervascularity; alterations in circulation time (either delayed circulation or arteriovenous shunting).[61] With the possible exception of genuine neovascularity, none of these findings is definitely indicative of a cerebral neoplasm; circulatory abnormalities are non-specific and have been identified in both benign and malignant neoplasms as well as in a variety of non-neoplastic processes (see below).

"Neovascularity" or Tumor Vessels. The abnormal vessels identified in intracranial neoplasms are usually large capillaries or sinusoids that do not contain smooth muscle elements in their walls.[10] Striking vascular endothelial proliferation is present in 95% of all glioblastomas, other malignant gliomas, and in some metastatic carcinomas. The endothelial proliferation mainly affects the capillaries and is accompanied by an actual numerical increase in these vessels.[46] Histologically, most malignant neoplasms contain large endothelial-lined vascular spaces with surrounding fibrous connective tissue. Few, if any, normal arteries are seen within the tumor parenchyma itself.[52, 61]

Angiographically, the abnormal vessels within the interstices of the tumor often appear tortuous and irregular in caliber with areas of localized constriction and dilatation

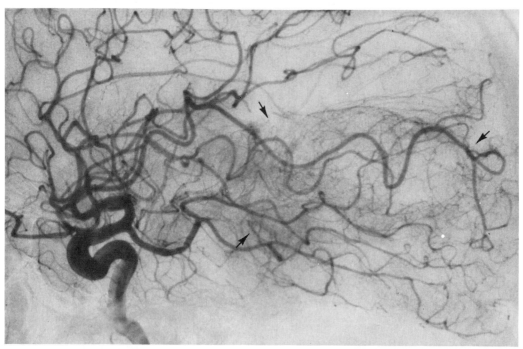

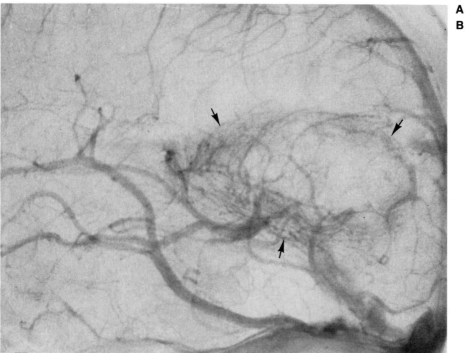

A
B

Fig. 9-19. Left internal carotid angiogram (lateral view) of a large occipital astrocytoma. Numerous small tumor vessels are seen in the arterial phase study
(A). Venous films **(B)** show a ring-like area of neovascularity.

instead of the normal gradual, distal tapering. Puddling and vascular staining representing contrast accumulation in the proliferating capillaries or sinusoids are often seen. Neovascularity may appear either as discretely identifiable vessels (Fig. 9-19) or as an area of rather homogeneous opacification.[61] Neovascularity can be seen with both primary and metastatic lesions (see below).

Diffuse Hypervascularity: Differential Diagnosis.
A diffuse homogeneous blush or vascular stain may indicate an infiltrating **neoplasm** (Fig. 9-20). However, this angiographic finding is non-specific. A variety of **normal structures** as well as numerous non-neoplastic lesions may demonstrate an area of angiographic hyperemia. Certain intracranial structures, such as the choroid plexus (Fig. 7-5) and basal ganglia

(Fig. 9-21), may normally show dramatic vascular staining. Cerebral infarction, a variety of inflammatory processes, contusions, resolving hematoma, epileptogenic foci, and toxic encephalopathy may present with the angiographic pattern of hypervascularity.

In addition to identifiable arterial occlusions, the angiographic findings in **cerebral ischemic disease** may also include a diffuse or focal mass effect, a vascular blush, and early draining veins (see Chapter 11). The increased vascular staining occasionally identified in infarction can be quite striking (Fig. 9-22). This probably results from both the loss of vascular autoregulatory mechanisms within the ischemic area as well as increased blood flow in adjacent areas that occurs in response to acute metabolic acidosis.[57]

(Text continued on p. 269)

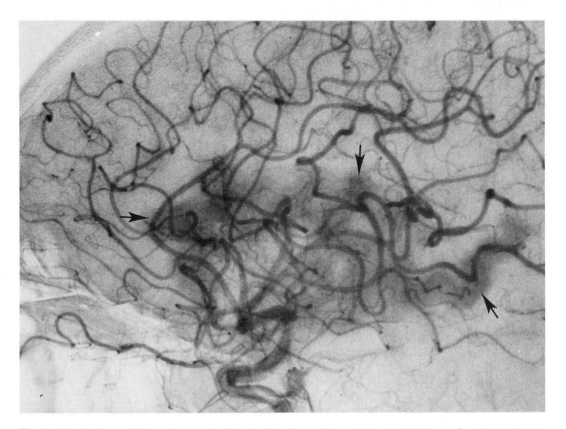

Fig. 9-20. Left carotid angiogram (mid-arterial phase, lateral view). A high grade astrocytoma has infiltrated along the cortical gyri of the insula. Although no discrete tumor vessels are seen, serpiginous areas of homogeneous hypervascular stain are present **(arrows).**

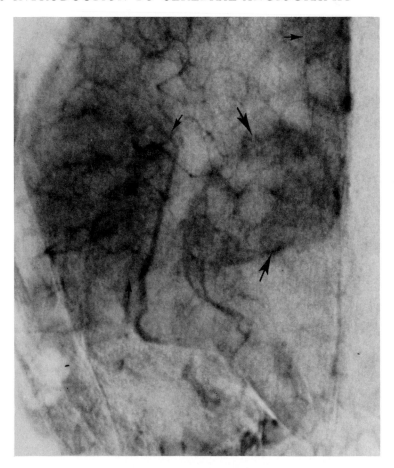

Fig. 9-21. Normal right internal carotid angiogram (capillary phase, AP view). Striking but normal contrast accumulation is present in the basal ganglia **(large arrows).** Several areas of cortical gray matter (*e.g.* insular and cingulate gyri) also show a prominent but normal vascular blush **(small arrows).**

Fig. 9-22. Left carotid angiogram (lateral view) of an MCA infarction. Arterial phase films **(A)** show a prominent, homogeneous vascular blush ("luxury perfusion") in the area adjacent to the infarct **(arrows).** Capillary phase films **(B)** show multiple early draining veins **(large arrows)** and slow flow in the posterior temporal and parietal branches **(small arrows).**

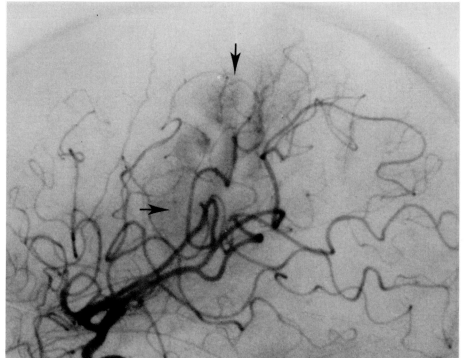

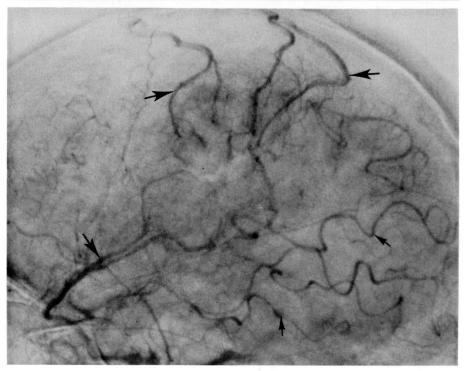

A
B

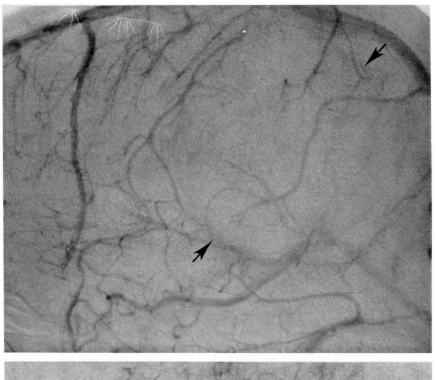

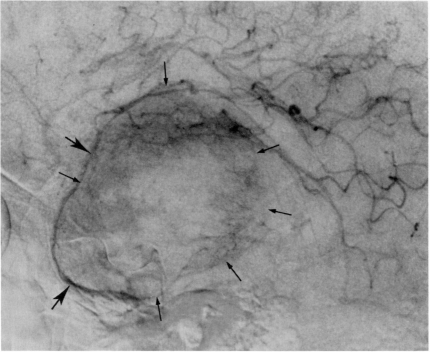

A

B

Fig. 9-23. Left internal carotid angiogram (lateral view, venous phase). A large parietal mass with a faint ring blush **(arrows)** is present. A thin-walled abscess was found at surgery. Left internal carotid angiogram (**B,** late arterial phase, lateral view) of a large necrotic temporal lobe astrocytoma. A ring-like vascular blush with an irregular central avascular area is present. Note the early draining vein **(large arrows)** and elevation and draping of the MCA arteries over the mass.

Inflammatory processes may also be a cause of angiographically detectable hyperemia. The most common findings in focal **cerebral abscess** include displaced vessels (45%), an avascular area indicating a focal mass lesion (82.5%), and segmental arterial constrictions or branch occlusions (82.5%).[38] A parenchymal abscess may also occasionally have enough vascularity in its reactive capsule to be identified (particularly with the use of subtraction films) as a hypervascular blush with a translucent center (Fig. 9-23A). When present, the hyperemic ring of a true abscess capsule usually appears in the capillary phase and persists into the late venous phase.[62] The appearance of a ring-like "pseudocapsule" may also be caused by the compression of blood vessels in adjacent gyri surrounding the abscess.[38] A capsular blush and the so-called "ripple sign," caused by perifocal edema and compressed gyral arteries, are seen in a minority of cases (47.5% and 25% respectively). The angiographic pattern of a vascular ring is also not pathognomonic of cerebral abscess. Metastases, primary neoplasms with central necrosis, resolving hematomas, cerebral infarcts, and a variety of other lesions may all

appear as a distinct ring-like region of hypervascularity (Fig. 9-23B).

Acute necrotizing **encephalitis,** commonly caused by herpes simplex virus, is a sporadic but fulminant, often fatal infection predominantly affecting the temporal lobe and, less frequently, the parietal cortex and frontal lobe.[5] While the most commonly identified angiographic abnormality is an avascular mass effect, a rather diffuse hypervascular blush conforming to the cortical gyri can be observed on occasion (Fig. 9-24). Premature filling of regional veins is not uncommon. Rarely, focal encephalitis produces a vascular stain with early venous filling and angiographic findings that are indistinguishable from neoplasm (Fig. 9-25).[43]

Other forms of intracranial inflammatory disease can produce distinct angiographic abnormalities. Tuberculous and bacterial **meningitis** often show marked spasm of the vessels at the base of the brain (See Chapter 5). Multiple stenoses or occlusions of small arteries secondary to perivasculitis and cortical and dural vein thromboses secondary to septic phlebitis are also occasionally observed. Hypervascularity may be present as a manifesta-

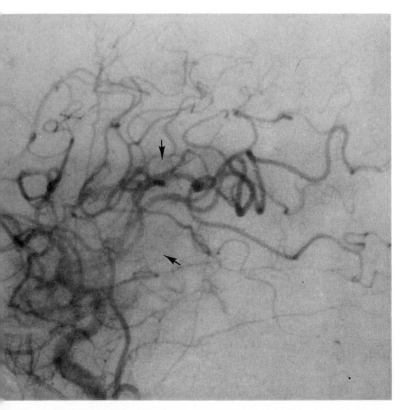

Fig. 9-24. Left common carotid angiogram (lateral view, mid-arterial phase) of herpes encephalitis. A homogeneous diffuse vascular blush is present in the cortex of the insula and temporal lobe **(arrows).** Note the similarity to Figures 9-20 and 9-22A.

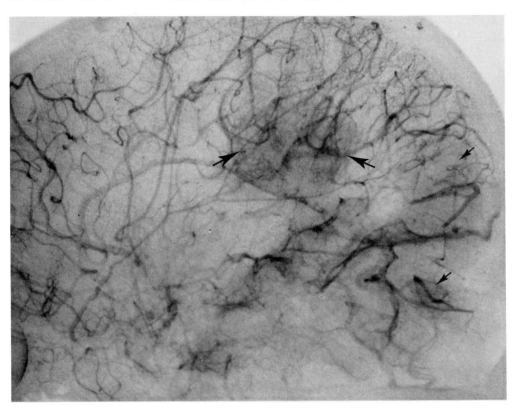

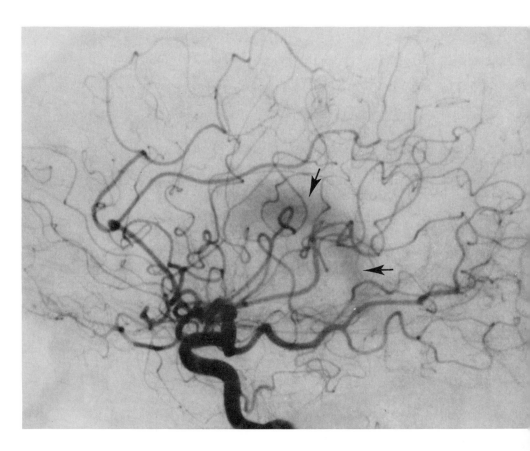

Fig. 9-25. Left common carotid angiogram (late arterial phase, lateral vein). This is a case of autopsy-proven herpes encephalitis. A focal vascular lesion is present in the parietal lobe **(large arrows).** Note other, more diffuse areas of hyperemia **(small arrows).**

tion of increased blood flow to the subarachnoid vasculature. Arteriovenous shunting in such cases has also been reported.[9, 49]

Focal areas of vascular hyperemia have also been reported with **miscellaneous lesions:** Epileptogenic foci, cerebral contusions, intracerebral hematomas, and toxic encephalopathy.[25, 27] Artifactual smudges on subtraction films can resemble a vascular blush. These artifacts are produced by dirty screens, emulsion defects on the films, static electricity, fingerprints resulting from improper handling of the film, cassette light leaks or film fogging, and poor film-screen contact (Figs. 9-26, 9-27). Faulty subtraction technique due to improper density range in the mask, mismatches between the film and mask, patient motion, or anatomic movement (swallowing during the film series often results in an artifactual smudge in the nasopharyngeal area) can also produce artifacts on the final subtraction print. Most of these artifacts can be recognized as such. It is essential that the subtraction masks and entire film series be carefully examined before an ill-defined stain

Fig. 9-26. Normal left carotid angiogram (lateral view). Subtraction artifact **(arrows)** probably caused by an emulsion defect in the initial mask.

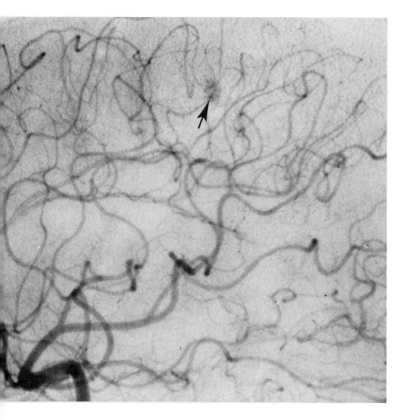

Fig. 9-27. Normal left carotid angiogram (lateral view). Subtraction artifact **(arrow)** should not be mistaken for a lesion.

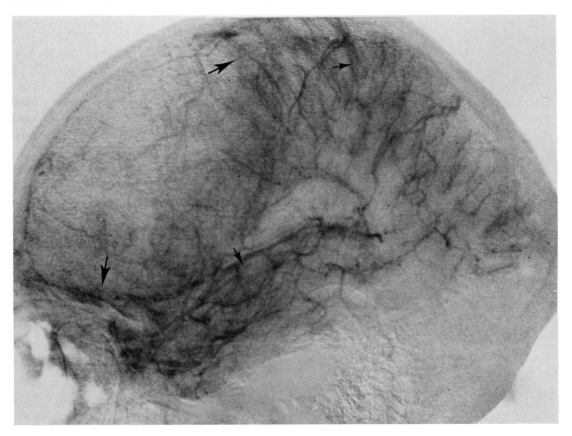

Fig. 9-28. Left carotid angiogram (capillary phase, lateral view of a huge frontal abscess **(large arrows)**. The avascular mass compresses the adjacent gyri which appear hypervascular because of the crowded, compressed gray matter **(small arrows)**.

Fig. 9-29. Left internal carotid angiogram (capillary phase, lateral view) of a large vascular glioma **(large arrows)**. Arteriovenous shunting with multiple early draining veins **(small arrows)** is present.

or odd density is interpreted as abnormal. It may be necessary on occasion to repeat the whole subtraction process or use double order subtraction to eliminate bothersome artifacts.

Alterations in Circulation Time are evidenced by generalized or focal circulatory slowing or arteriovenous shunting with the presence of early draining veins. Generalized **decrease in intracranial blood flow** may be present in patients with severe, diffuse cerebral edema or increased intracranial pressure (Fig. 4-12). Focal slowing or actual diminution of blood flow may be present in areas of devascularized or compressed brain secondary to vascular occlusion (Figs. 9-22, 9-36A), brain tumors, abscesses, hematomas, and other localized lesions. Angiographically, this is usually represented by delayed flow in regional vessels but occasionally is seen as a "hole" in the capillary phase of angiography (Fig. 9-28). Compression of adjacent cortical gyri by a large mass may produce the appearance of increased vascular staining.

When present, **arteriovenous shunting** with early venous opacification is not pathognomonic of any particular lesion (see Chapter 11). Primary (Fig. 9-29) and metastatic lesions (Fig. 9-30), arteriovenous malformations (Fig. 9-31), cerebral infarction or ischemia (Fig. 9-22B), epileptogenic foci, trauma, toxic processes, and certain inflammatory lesions may be associated with early opacification of draining veins.[27] Early filling of veins in the parietal region has also been reported in some normal cases.[2, 3]

The abnormal vessels present within neoplasms often have impaired autoregulatory mechanisms and are relatively refractory to the normal vasoconstriction associated with hypocapnia. Hence, tumor vessels tend to respond less to changes in arterial CO_2 levels than do normal vessels. Hyperventilation during angiography can increase tumor circulation relative to the normal diminished blood flow in adjacent normal tissue. Occasionally, this may enhance angiographic visibility of the neoplasm.

Vascular Patterns in the Differential Diagnosis of Cerebral Neoplasms

While angiography is extremely helpful in the localization and diagnosis of intracranial neoplasms, the finding of abnormal vascularity is often nonspecific. Caution should be exercised when attempting to establish a histologic diagnosis based on the cerebral angiogram alone. A precise description of the nature and exact extent of the neoplasm together with an appropriate differential diagnosis should be the neuroradiologist's goal. Nevertheless, certain general characteristics of each type of neoplasm can be outlined.[48]

Metastases. Approximately 50 percent of intracranial metastases are hypervascular. These lesions display a spectrum of vascularity rang-

(Text continued on p. 276)

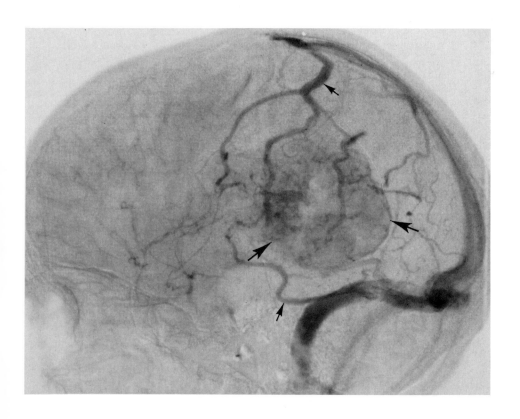

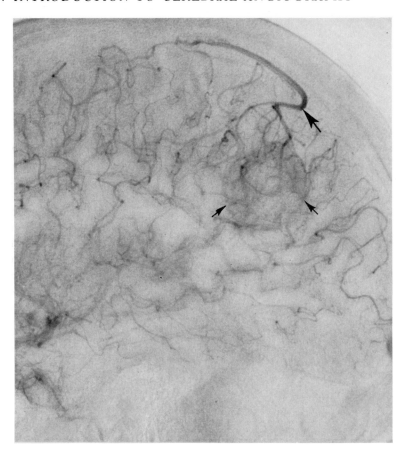

Fig. 9-30. Left internal carotid angiogram (late arterial phase, lateral view). A solitary vascular metastasis **(small arrows)** from a lung carcinoma is present. Note the prominent early draining vein **(large arrow).**

Fig. 9-31. Left common carotid angiogram (arterial phase, lateral view) illustrating a temporal lobe AVM **(A, arrows).** Capillary phase films show multiple tortuous early draining veins **(B, arrows).**

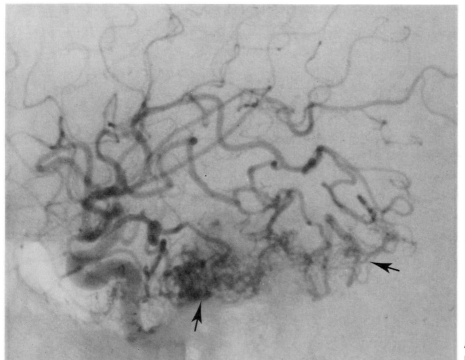

A
B

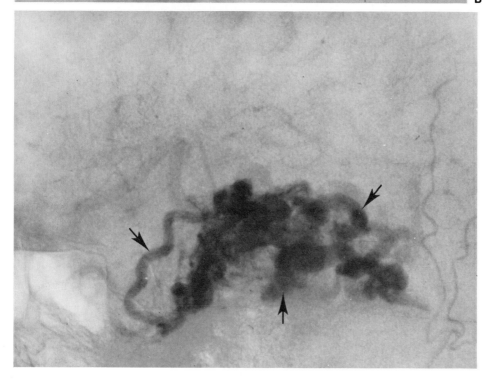

ing from a small stain or tangled network of vessels (Fig. 9-32) to larger, cloudlike areas, to "target"-like lesions with a central avascular zone and a peripheral vascular rim. Metastases are often round and are usually associated with considerable edema. As with primary neoplasms their vascular supply may be pial, dural, or mixed. Metastases can show arteriovenous shunting and tend to drain primarily via the superficial cortical veins (Fig. 9-30).

The most common vascular metastases are from lung, breast carcinomas, or hypernephroma. In general, the degree and type of vascularity of intracranial metastases correlates poorly with the vascularization of the primary lesion. The presence of multiple small, round vascular lesions favors metastatic disease. However, metastases may sometimes be indistinguishable from multifocal glioma or meningioma, or multiple abscesses.[3, 48]

Astrocytoma. The angiographic appearance of astrocytoma varies from an avascular mass effect (Fig. 9-16B) to a highly vascular neoplasm with bizarre, irregular vessels and arteriovenous shunting into dilated deep medullary (as well as cortical) veins (Figs. 9-17B, 9-19, 9-29). There is a rough angiographic correlation between the degree of neovascularity and the degree of tumor malignancy. Most astrocytomas with moderate to marked tumor circulation are grade III or IV while those lesions with sparse or no angiographically detectable abnormal vascularity tend to be grade I or II. However, it should be noted that the absence of neovascularity does not preclude the possibility of a highly malignant lesion, particularly of the widely infiltrating variety. Occasionally, non-neoplastic lesions such as cerebral infarcts or the rare hypervascular cavernous angioma may mimic an astrocytoma.[43A]

Meningiomas are discussed in detail in Chapter 3. The degree and type of vascularization in these lesions often seems to be related to their location. Meningiomas at the skull base, such as those growing *en plaque* along the sphenoid wing or sella, sometimes appear poorly vascularized. Convexity, falx, and parasagittal meningiomas tend to appear more vascular. In these lesions, the afferent arteries are usually of uniform caliber. Diffusely homogeneous contrast accumulation persisting into the venous phase of angiography is common. Vascular encasement may be present, particularly at the skull base. Because early draining veins have been reported in up to 40% of all meningiomas, their presence should alert the angiographer to a possible angioblastic meningioma.

Other Intracranial Neoplasms that may be hypervascular include such lesions as neurinoma, chemodectoma, pinealoma, lymphoma, medulloblastoma or ependymoma, hemangioblastoma, choroid plexus papilloma, pituitary adenomas, etc.

ANEURYSMS OF THE MIDDLE CEREBRAL ARTERY

Most congenital or atherosclerotic aneurysms arise from the circle of Willis (see Chapter 6). However, the initial MCA bifurcation is the third most common site of origin for congenital aneurysms (Fig. 9-33A). Approximately one-fifth of all intracranial aneurysms arise in this location. With the exception of MCA aneurysms and those located at the origin of the frontopolar or callosomarginal arteries, aneurysms distal to the circle of Willis are more often mycotic or traumatic. Rarely, tumor emboli produce peripherally located aneurysms.[18, 40] Fusiform aneurysms secondary to atherosclerotic disease are usually located in the proximal MCA (Fig. 9-33B). Traumatic MCA aneurysms are commonly adjacent to the sphenoid ridge.[41A]

Occasionally, a large aneurysm may present as a space-occupying lesion without evidence for subarachnoid hemorrhage. The most common clinical manifestations of giant MCA aneurysm are seizures and hemiparesis. The

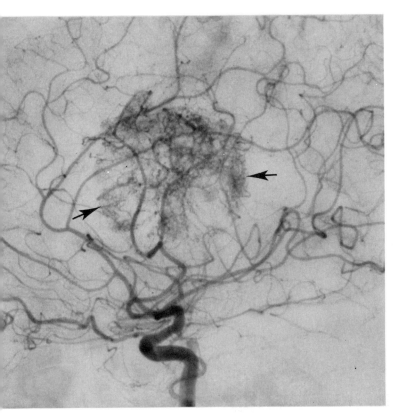

Fig. 9-32. Left internal carotid angiogram (arterial phase, lateral view). A solitary hypervascular metastasis from a renal cell carcinoma is present **(arrows).**

clinical course resembles that of a slow-growing temporal lobe mass.[33] Giant aneurysms are often partially or completely thrombosed; a bizarre tortuous vascular channel coursing through the aneurysm thrombus is a classical, diagnostic appearance (Fig. 9-34).[42] CT scans are helpful in delineating the precise extent of the thrombotic aneurysm.[47, 48A]

OCCLUSIONS OF THE MIDDLE CEREBRAL ARTERY

Angiographic Findings

The angiographic findings with MCA occlusion vary. Local cerebral circulation time is frequently altered with absent or slow flow in the affected arterial bed. Abrupt termination or tapering of the affected vessel (Fig. 9-35) with focal areas of absent perfusion may be

seen (Fig. 9-36A).[20] A frequent finding is slow retrograde filling of distal branches of the occluded vessels via collateral channels (Figs. 9-36B, 9-37).[35, 57]

Cortical ischemia or cerebral infarction can also be accompanied by strikingly increased blood flow ("luxury perfusion") in or adjacent to the affected area. Definite capillary staining or a distinct vascular blush with early draining veins may be present (Fig. 9-22B). Occasionally, both the angiographic and CT findings in ischemic vascular disease will be indistinguishable from an infiltrating neoplasm (see below).

Collateral Flow in Vascular Occlusions

The major source of collateral blood flow in the human cerebral cortex is via the circle of Willis. The numerous external to internal ca-

(Text continued on p. 285)

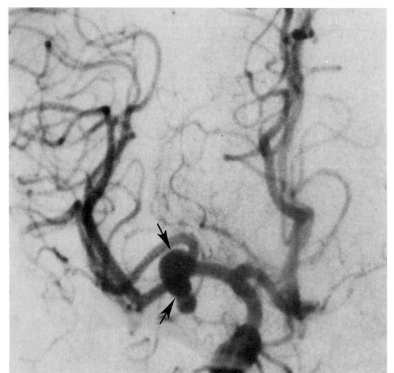

Fig. 9-33. Right internal carotid angiogram (**A,** arterial phase, AP view). A lobulated aneurysm **(arrows)** at the MCA bifurcation is present. Left internal carotid angiogram (**B,** arterial phase, AP view) illustrating diffuse atherosclerotic disease. Elongation and fusiform dilatation of the proximal MCA is present **(arrows).**

A

B

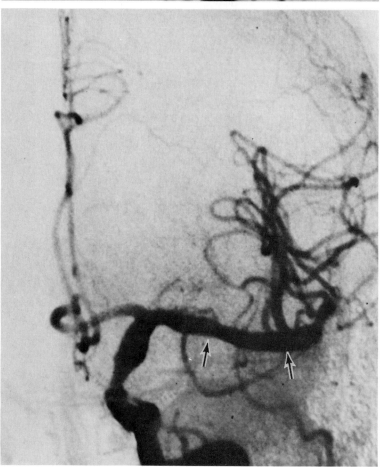

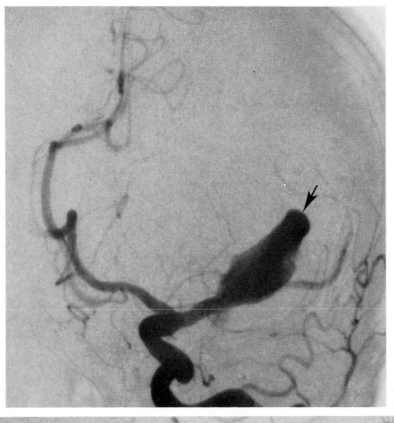

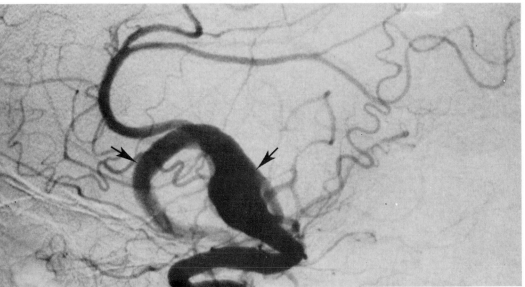

A
B

Fig. 9-34. Left common carotid angiogram (arterial phase). Seen here is a huge, partially thrombosed MCA aneurysm **(arrows).** The size of the associated mass is larger than the opacified vascular channel, indicating that significant thrombus is present in the lesion. AP **(A)** and lateral **(B)** views.

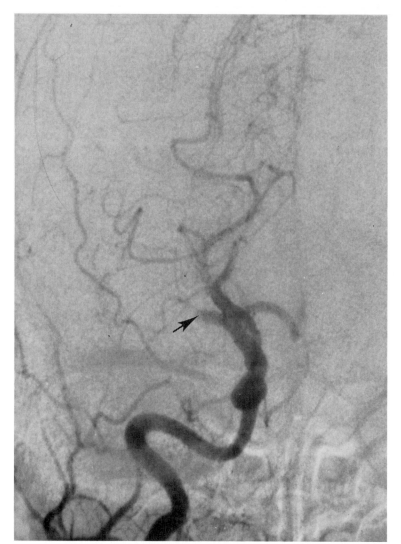

Fig. 9-35. Right common carotid angiogram (arterial phase, AP view). A young comatose patient is presented with occluslon just distal to the MCA origin **(arrow).**

Fig. 9-36. Left common carotid angiogram (lateral view) depicting complete MCA occlusion. Early arterial phase film **(A)** shows no MCA vessels distal to the lenticulostriate arteries **(arrows).** Later films **(B)** show filling of the distal MCA branches **(arrows)** via leptomeningeal collaterals from the anterior and posterior cerebral arteries.

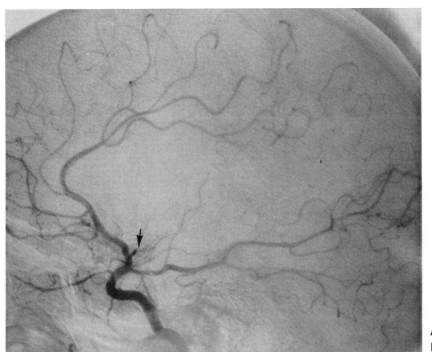

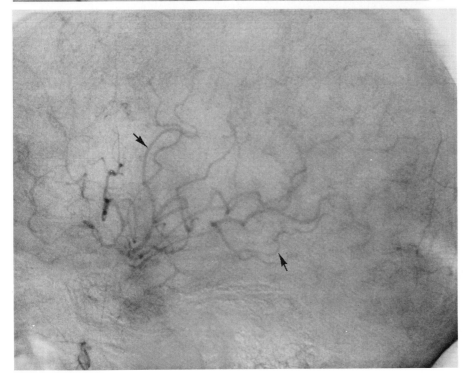

A
B

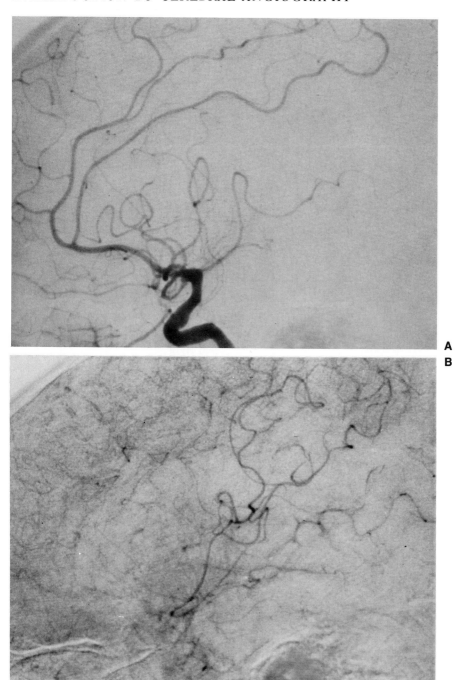

A
B

Fig. 9-37. Left carotid angiogram (lateral view) This patient has occlusion of the posterior MCA division. Early films **(A)** demonstrate lack of opacification (note the *"bare area"*) of the parietal, angular, and posterior temporal branches while later films **(B)** show retrograde filling of these vessels via pial and leptomeningeal collaterals.

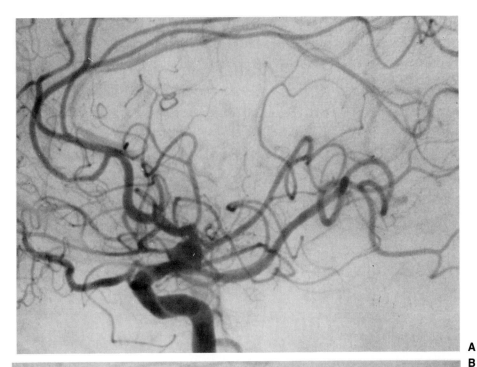

A
B

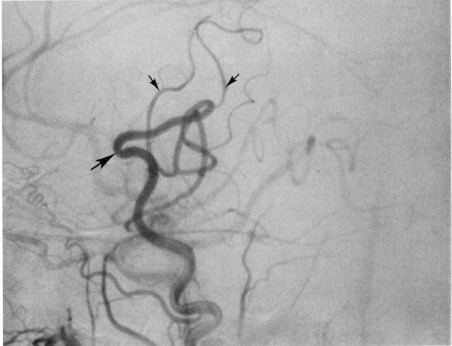

Fig. 9-38. Left carotid angiogram (lateral view) showing occlusion of the central sulcus (rolandic) artery **(A).** A superficial temporal–MCA bypass graft was performed. A post-operative external carotid study **(B)** shows excellent filling of the rolandic vessels **(small arrows)** via the superficial temporal anastomosis **(large arrow).**

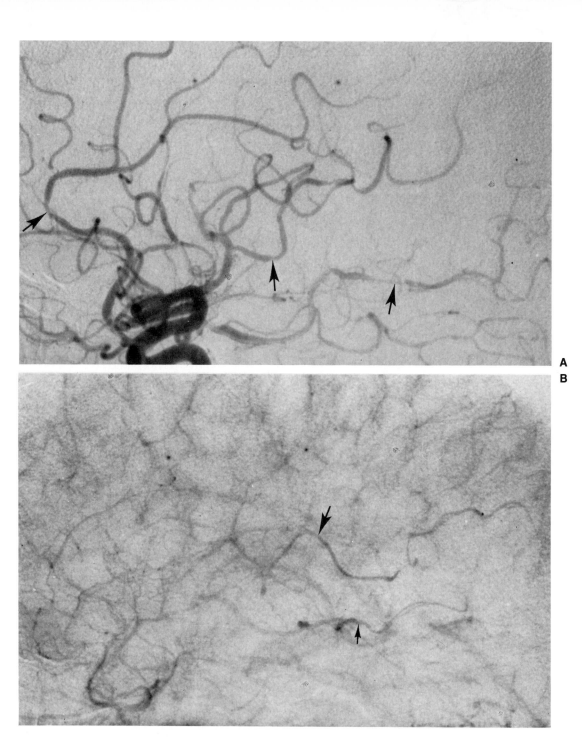

Fig. 9-39. Left internal carotid angiograms (lateral view) from a young patient with intracranial arteritis of unknown etiology. Early arterial phase film **(A)** shows multiple segmental stenoses alternating with areas of focal dilatation involving branches of all three major cerebral vessels **(arrows)**. Late arterial phase film **(B)** shows delayed flow in angular and occipital branches **(arrows)**.

rotid artery anastomoses also provide potential pathways for collateral flow (see Chapter 3). When occlusion occurs distal to the circle of Willis a number of other pre-existing potential collateral channels may provide significant (although delayed) retrograde flow through the various anastomoses into vessels deprived of their normal blood supply.[35]

A number of small anastomotic channels are present between the terminal branches of the three major cerebral arteries. These leptomeningeal collaterals are in the so-called "watershed areas" (*i.e.,* the borders between the anterior, middle, and posterior cerebral artery territories). They may enlarge sufficiently to permit significant flow from one arterial system to another and represent the major collateral system distal to the circle of Willis.[20] Anastomotic vascular channels between adjacent branches of a single cerebral artery also represent pial or leptomeningeal arterial collateral flow. Less commonly, meningeal vessels of the dura mater may cross the subdural space to anastomose with cortical vessels and provide an additional source of collateral circulation (Fig. 3-14).[12, 35]

If the naturally-occurring sources of collateral flow are inadequate, surgical anastomosis between a branch of the ECA (usually the superficial temporal artery) and a cortical branch of the MCA may enhance collateral flow (Fig. 9-38).[22A]

Clinical Manifestations

The syndromes associated with MCA occlusions vary according to the site obstructed, the number of branches affected, the adequacy of collateral blood flow, and whether the lesion involves the dominant hemisphere. Acute, complete occlusion of the MCA near its origin (Fig. 9-35) causes contralateral hemiplegia, hemianesthesia, and hemianopsia. Global aphasia is present if the lesion is in the domi-

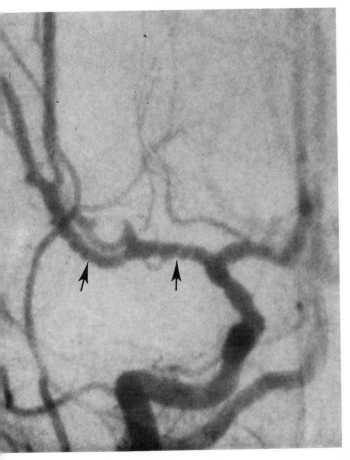

Fig. 9-40. Right common carotid angiogram (arterial phase, AP view). This is a case of fibromuscular dysplasia involving the MCA **(arrows).** This "string of beads" appearance was also present in the cervical ICA. *(From Osborn AG, Anderson RE: Angiographic spectrum of cephalocervical fibromuscular dysplasia. Stroke 8:617–626, 1977.)*

nant hemisphere. Profound coma and death often result. If only the lenticulostriate arteries are involved, the clinical findings may vary from a moderate degree of hemiplegia of equal severity in both extremities to severe hemiplegia, particularly affecting the lower extremity.[59]

Most cases of MCA occlusion involve individual branches rather than the entire MCA distribution (Fig. 9-43). Occlusion of the dominant orbitofrontal artery produces expressive aphasia while involvement of precentral artery (supplying Broca's area) results in paresis of the opposite side of the face and tongue plus motor aphasia (if the lesion is in the dominant hemisphere). Obliteration of the central or rolandic artery results in contralateral paresis and hypoesthesia of the face and tongue. Anterior parietal branch occlusion causes contralateral astereognosis. Posterior parietal and angular artery lesions cause contralateral hemanopia and mild sensory defects (including visual verbal aphasia and agraphia if on the dominant side). Posterior temporal artery occlusion causes hemianopia (due to involvement of the visual radiation) and auditory receptive aphasia (if on the dominant side). Wernicke's aphasia occurs if the superior temporal gyrus is involved.[59]

NON-ATHEROMATOUS ARTERIOPATHIES

Atherosclerosis is the most common cause of intracranial arterial stenosis and predominantly involves the circle of Willis or initial segments of the major cerebral vessels. However, a variety of non-atheromatous processes can produce intracranial occlusive vascular disease.

Arteritis

Single or multiple peripheral segmental stenoses, often alternating with areas of fusiform dilatation, have been identified in a variety of arteritides such as giant cell arteritis, fibromuscular dysplasia, and angiitis secondary to drug abuse (Figs. 9-39, 9-40).[7, 8, 45, 53]

Miscellaneous Arteriopathies

The differential diagnosis of peripheral arteritic changes is extensive. In addition to arteritis, vascular spasm secondary to subarachnoid hemorrhage, trauma, emboli, atheromata (Fig. 9-41A) focal or infiltrating tumors such as lymphoma (Fig. 9-41B), pyogenic meningoencephalitis (see Fig. 5-19), fibromuscular dysplasia, neurocutaneous syndromes (*i.e.,* von Recklinghausen's disease or encephalotrigeminal angiomatosis), and postirradiation vasculopathy may all cause localized stenosis and dilatation of the arterial lumen with or without tapered occlusions.[3A, 6, 23, 28, 29, 31, 37, 45, 55] The pyogenic meningitides such as tuberculous meningitis predominantly affect the circle of Willis, while peripheral vascular disease with relative sparing of the basilar vessels is more characteristic of arteritis. The clinical history is often helpful in distinguishing hemorrhage, radiation therapy, and drug abuse. Stenosis or arterial wall irregularities associated with intracranial neoplasms are usually confined to a single artery or group of arteries in or adjacent to the mass. Non-contiguous vessels may be involved if the lesion is diffuse or infiltrating.[23]

Fig. 9-41. Left carotid angiogram (**A**, arterial phase, lateral view). Diffuse atherosclerotic changes are present in the supraclinoid ICA as well as branches of the ACA and MCA (**arrows**). Left common carotid angiogram (**B**, arterial phase, lateral view) of a temporal lobe glioma. Note elevation and encasement of MCA branches by the tumor (**arrows**).

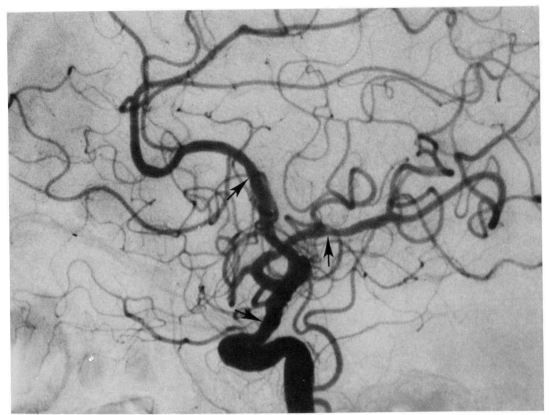

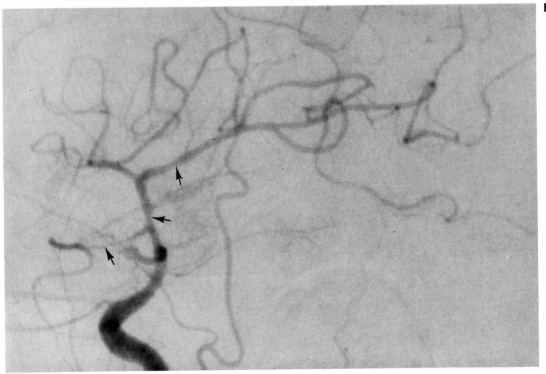

A

B

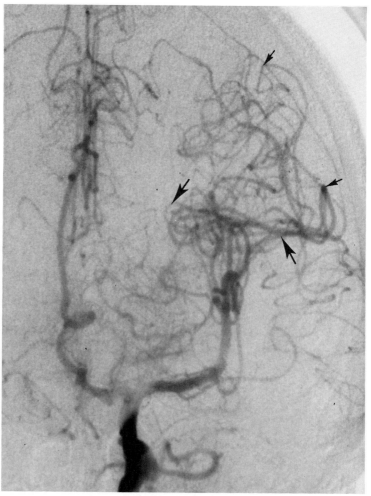

A

B

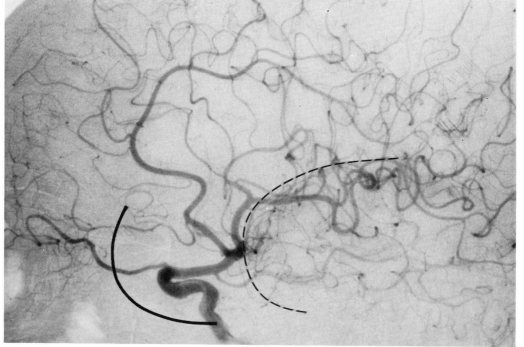

Fig. 9-42A. Left internal carotid angiogram (arterial phase, AP view) of a large middle cranial fossa arachnoid cyst. The extra-axial cyst has displaced the Sylvian point medially and stretched the temporal MCA branches posterosuperiorly **(large arrows)**. Note the relatively minor left to right shift of the ACA. A small subdural hematoma is associated with the cyst and has displaced the cortical MCA branches away from the calvarium **(small arrows)**.

Fig. 9-42B. Same patient as 9-42**A** (lateral view). A large avascular space is seen in the anterior middle cranial fossa. An attenuated temporal lobe is present **(dotted lines)**. The temporal lobe in the middle cranial fossa normally extends to the greater sphenoid wing **(solid curved line)**.

MISCELLANEOUS LESIONS AFFECTING THE MIDDLE CEREBRAL ARTERY

Arachnoid Cysts

Cerebral arachnoid cysts are uncommon, comprising approximately one percent of all intracranial space-occupying lesions. The middle cranial fossa is the most common location followed by the cerebral convexities, posterior fossa, suprasellar cistern and collicular region.[32] Arachnoid cysts are often congenital although they may be associated with unhealed skull fractures or meningeal inflammation.[24, 32]

Angiographically, uncomplicated middle cranial fossa arachnoid cysts are associated with displacement of MCA branches in the face of minimal or no ACA shift (Fig. 9-42). The temporal lobe is attenuated and foreshortened. Symptomatic arachnoid cysts are frequently associated with subdural hematoma.[51]

Extra-axial Fluid Collections

Extra-axial fluid collections can be subarachnoid, subdural, or epidural. They can be acute or chronic and usually occur secondary to effusions, hemorrhage, or inflammatory disease. While CT scans have largely replaced angiography in the evaluation of extra-cerebral collections, angiography remains a useful diagnostic modality in the evaluation of iso-attenuating extra-axial fluid.[4, 36, 41]

Subdural Hematomas over the cerebral hemispheres displace the MCA cortical branches away from the calvarium. While an acute subdural hematoma classically tends to appear as an avascular crescentic extra-axial space at angiography (Fig. 9-43) and chronic lesions are more often biconvex or lentiform (Fig. 9-44), shape alone is an unreliable indicator of temporal relationship. Some subdural hematomas, particularly those with an irregular contour that cannot be classified as either crescentic or lentiform, have a "transitional" shape defying accurate temporal classification.[11] It is safe to diagnose the subdural hematoma as chronic only if the extra-axial collection is truly lentiform.[6A]

Large subtemporal subdural hematomas may elevate the MCA genu and displace the Sylvian triangle superiorly. On the lateral view, the temporal cortical arteries may be displaced away from the middle cranial fossa floor. Submentovertex views may demonstrate an extracerebral space that is not readily apparent on routine projections.[13]

Subdural Empyemas are collections of purulent fluid located between the dura mater and the arachnoid. Arteriography may demonstrate an extra-axial fluid collection. Diffuse irregularities or multifocal constrictions of the arterial walls may be present in cortical branches adjacent to the empyema.[17,46A]

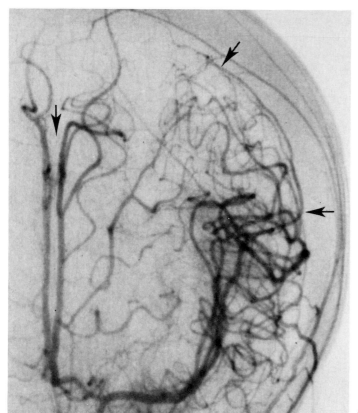

A

B

Fig. 9-43. Left common carotid angiograms (AP view). This case illustrates an abused two-year-old with an acute subdural hematoma. Arterial **(A)** and late capillary-early venous **(B)** phases. A large crescentic extra-axial fluid collection extends over the cerebral hemispheres and into the interhemispheric fissure **(arrows).**

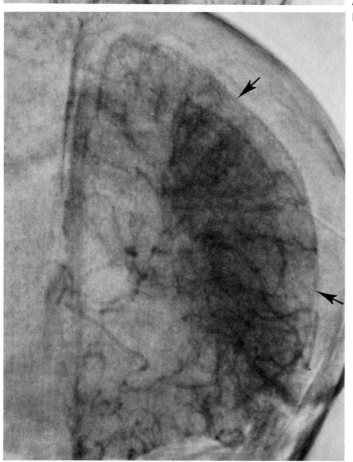

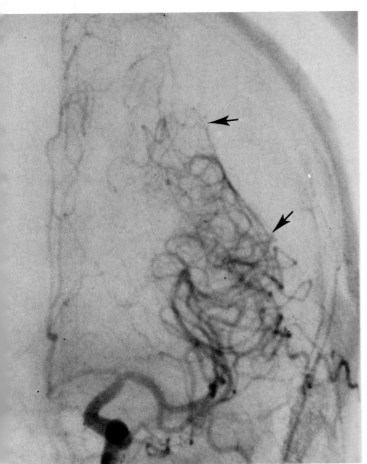

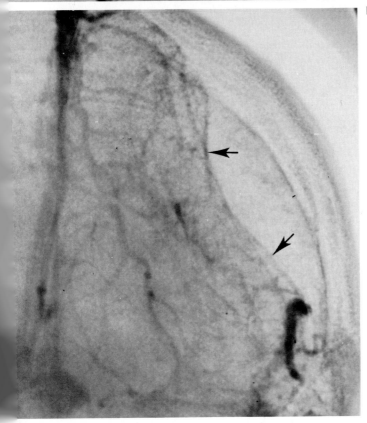

Fig. 9-44. Left common carotid angiogram (AP view). Arterial **(A)** and early venous **(B)** phases. A large chronic subdural hematoma displaces the cortical arteries and veins away from the calvarium **(arrows).** Note the biconvex or lentiform shape of the extracerebral fluid collection.

A

B

REFERENCES

1. **Blatt ES, McLaurin RL:** The arteriographic pattern accompanying centrosylvian mass lesions. Am J Roentgenol 101:52–60, 1967
2. **Bradac GB:** Early filling of veins in the parietal region. Neuroradiology 13:41–43, 1977
3. **Bradac GB, Simon RS, Fiegler W:** The early filling of a vein in the carotid angiogram. Neuroradiology 129:409–417, 1978
3A. **Brant-Zawadzki M, Anderson M, DeArmond SJ et al:** Radiation-induced large intracranial vessel occlusive vasculopathy. Am J Roentgenol 134:51–55, 1980
4. **Cornell SH, Chiu LC, Christie JH:** Diagnosis of extra-cerebral fluid collections by computed tomography. Am J Roentgenol 131:107–110, 1978
5. **Davis JM, Davis KR, Kleinman GN et al:** Computed tomography of herpes simplex encephalitis, with clinicopathological correlation. Radiology 129:409–417, 1978
6. **Enzmann D, Scott WR:** Intracranial involvement of giant-cell arteritis. Neurology 27:794–797, 1977
6A. **Ericson K, Bergstrand G, Levander B:** Angiographic findings in subdural hematoma correlated with CT attenuation valves. J Comp Asst Tomogr 3:789–794, 1979
7. **Faer MJ, Mead JH, Lynch RD:** Cerebral granulomatous angiitis: case report and literature review. Am J Roentgenol 129:458–467, 1977
8. **Ferris EJ, Levine HL:** Cerebral arteritis: classification. Radiology 109:327–341, 1973
9. **Ferris EJ, Rudikoff JC, Shapiro JH:** Cerebral angiography of bacterial infection. Radiology 90:727–734, 1968
10. **Gammill SL, Shipkey FH, Himmelfarb EH et al:** Roentgenography-pathology correlative study of neovascularity. Am J Roentgenol 126:376–385, 1976
11. **Gilday DL, Wortzman, G, Reid M:** Subdural hematoma: is it or is it not acute? Radiology 110:141–145, 1974
12. **Gillilan LA:** Potential collateral circulation to the human cerebral cortex. Neurology 24:941–948, 1974
13. **Glickman MG, McNamara TO, Margolis MT:** Arteriographic diagnosis of subtemporal subdural hematoma. Radiology 109:607–615, 1973
14. **Hacker H:** Abnormal middle cerebral artery. In Newton TH, Potts DG (eds): Radiology of the Skull and Brain, Vol 2, pp. 1479–1526. St. Louis, CV Mosby, 1974
15. **Ito J, Maeda H, Inoue K et al:** Fenestration of the middle cerebral artery. Neuroradiology 13:37–39, 1977
16. **Ito J, Sato T, Arai H et al:** The accessory middle cerebral artery and duplication of the middle cerebral artery. Jpn J Clin Radiol 20:449–457, 1975
17. **Kaufman DM, Leeds NE:** Focal angiographic abnormalities with subdural empyema. Neuroradiology 11:169–173, 1976
18. **Kaufman SL, White RI Jr, Harrington DP et al:** Protean manifestations of mycotic aneurysms. Am J Roentgenol 131:1019–1025, 1978
19. **Kier EL:** Development of cerebral vessels. In Newton TH, Potts DG (eds): Radiology of the Skull and Brain, Vol 2, pp 1089–1130. St. Louis, CV Mosby, 1974
20. **Kilgore BB, Fields WS:** Arterial occlusive disease in adults. In Newton TH, Potts DG (eds): Radiology of the Skull and Brain, Vol. 2, pp 2310–2343. St. Louis, CV Mosby, 1974
21. **Krayenbuhl HA, Yasargil MG:** Cerebral Angiography, 2nd ed. Philadelphia, JB Lippincott, 1968
22. **Kricheff II, Taveras JM:** The angiographic localization of suprasylvian space-occupying lesions. Am J Roentgenol 82:602–614, 1964
22A. **Latchaw RE, Ausman JI, Lee MC:** Superficial temporal-middle cerebral artery bypass. J Neurosurg 51:455–465, 1979
23. **Launay M, Fredy D, Merland JJ et al:** Narrowing and occlusion of arteries by intracranial tumors. Neuroradiology 14:177–179, 1977
24. **Lee BCP:** Intracranial cysts. Radiology 130:667–674, 1979
25. **Lee SH, Goldberg HI:** Hypervascular pattern associated with idiopathic focal status epilepticus. Radiology 125:159–163, 1977
26. **Lee SH, Goldberg HI:** The normal angiographic sylvian point on the lateral cerebral angiogram. Neuroradiology 17:101–103, 1979
27. **Leeds NE, Goldberg HI:** Abnormal vascular patterns in benign intracranial lesions of the brain. Am J Roentgenol 118:576–586, 1973
28. **Leeds NE, Rosenblatt R:** Arterial wall irregularities in intracranial neoplasms. Radiology 103:121–124, 1972
29. **Leeds NE, Rosenblatt R, Zimmerman HM:** Focal angiographic changes of cerebral lymphoma with pathologic correlation. Radiology 99:595–599, 1971
30. **Lehrer HZ:** Temporal arterial geodesics. II. Effects of masses deep to the temporal lobe. Acta Radiol [Diagn] (Stockh) 7:124–128, 1968
31. **Lemahieu SF, Marchau MMB:** Intracranial fibromuscular dysplasia and stroke in children. Neuroradiology 18:99–102, 1979
32. **Leo JS, Pinto RS, Hulvat GF et al:** Computed tomography of arachnoid cysts. Radiology 130:674–680, 1979
33. **Lukin RR, Chambers AA, McLaurin R et al:**

Thrombosed giant middle cerebral aneurysms. Neuroradiology 10:125–129, 1975

34. **Michotey P, Moscow NP, Salamon G:** Anatomy of the cortical branches of the middle cerebral artery. In Newton TH, Potts DG (eds): Radiology of the Skull and Brain, Vol 2, pp 1471–1478. St. Louis, CV Mosby, 1974

35. **Mishkin MM, Schreiber MN:** Colleratal circulation. In Newton TH, Potts DG (eds): Radiology of the Skull and Brain, Vol 2, pp 2344–2374. St. Louis, CV Mosby, 1974

36. **Moller A, Ericson K:** Computed tomography of isoattenuating subdural hematomas. Radiology 130:149–152, 1979

37. **Mori K, Takeuchi J, Ishikawa M et al:** Occlusive arteriopathy and brain tumor. J Neurosurg 49:22–35, 1978

38. **Nielsen H, Halaburt H:** Cerebral abscess with special reference to the angiographic changes. Neuroradiology 12:73–78, 1976

39. **Norton GA, Kishore PRS, Lin J:** CT contrast enhancement in cerebral infarction. Am J Roentgenol 131:881–885, 1978

40. **Olmsted WW, McGee TP:** The pathogenesis of peripheral aneurysm of the central nervous system: A subject review from the AFIP. Radiology 123:661–666, 1977

41. **Osborn AG:** Computed tomography in neurological diagnosis. Annu Rev Med 30:189–198, 1979

41A. **Parkinson D, West M:** Traumatic intracranial aneurysms. J Neurosurg 52:11–20, 1980

42. **Pinto RS, Kricheff II, Butler AR et al:** Correlation of computed tomographic, angiographic and neuropathological changes in giant cerebral aneurysms. Radiology 132:85–92, 1979

43. **Radcliffe WB, Guinto FC Jr, Adcock DF et al:** Early localization of herpes simplex encephalitis by radionuclide imaging and carotid arteriography. Radiology 105:603–605, 1972

43A. **Rao VRK, Pillai SM, Shenoy KT et al:** Hypervascular cavernous angioma at angiography. Neuroradiology 18:211–214, 1979

43B. **Rhoton AL Jr, Saeki N, Perlmutter D et al:** Microsurgical anatomy of common aneurysm sites. Clin Neurosurg 26:248–306, 1979

44. **Ring BA:** The middle cerebral artery. In Newton TH, Potts DG (eds): Radiology of the Skull and Brain, Vol. 2, pp 1442–1478. St. Louis, CV Mosby, 1974

45. **Rumbaugh CL, Bergeron RT, Fang HCH et al:** Cerebral angiographic changes in the drug abuse patient. Radiology 101:335–344, 1971

46. **Russell DS, Rubinstein LJ:** Pathology of Tumors of the Nervous System, 4th ed. Baltimore, Williams & Wilkins, 1977

46A. **Sadhu VK, Handel SS, Pinto RS et al:** Neuroradiologic diagnosis of subdural empyema and CT limitations. Am J Neuroradiol 1:39–44, 1980

47. **Sarwan M, Batnitzky S, Schechter MM:** Tumorous aneurysms. Neuroradiology 12:79–97, 1976

48. **Scatliff JH, Guinto FC, Radcliffe WB:** Vascular patterns in cerebral neoplasms and their differential diagnosis. Semin Roentgenol 6:59–69, 1971

48A. **Schubiger O, Valavanis A, Hayek J:** Computed tomography in cerebral aneurysms with special emphasis on giant intracranial aneurysms. J Comp Asst Tomogr 4:24–32, 1980

49. **Segall HD, Rumbaugh CL, Bergeron RT et al:** Brain and meningeal infections in children: radiological considerations. Neuroradiology 6:8–16, 1973

50. **Serrats AA, Vlahovitch B, Parker SA:** The arteriographic pattern of the insula: its normal appearance and variations in cases of tumor of the cerebral hemispheres. J Neurol Neurosurg Psychiatry 31:379–390, 1968

51. **Smith RA, Smith WA:** Arachnoid cysts of the middle cranial fossa. Surg Neurol 5:246–252, 1979

52. **Sole-Llenas J, Mercader JM, Pons-Tortella E:** Morphological aspects of the vessels of brain tumors. Neuroradiology 13:51–54, 1977

53. **Sole-Llenas J, Pons-Torella E:** Cerebral angiitis. Neuroradiology 15:1–11, 1978

54. **Stephens RB, Stilwell DL:** Arteries and Veins of the Human Body, pp. 33–70. Springfield, IL, CC Thomas, 1969

55. **Suwanwela C, Suwanwela N:** Intracranial arterial narrowing and spasm in acute head injury. J Neurosurg 36:314–323, 1972

56. **Taveras J, Poser C:** Roentgenologic aspects of cerebral angiography in children. Am J Roentgenol 82:371–390, 1959

57. **Taveras JM, Gilson JM, Davis DO et al:** Angiography in cerebral infarction. Radiology 93:549–558, 1969

58. **Teal JS, Rumbaugh CL, Bergeron RT et al:** Anomalies of the middle cerebral artery: accessory artery, duplication, and early bifurcation. Am J Roentgenol 118:567–575, 1973

59. **Tichy F:** Syndromes of cerebral arteries. Arch Pathol 48:475–488, 1949

60. **Waddington MM:** Atlas of Cerebral Angiography with Anatomic Correlation. Boston, Little, Brown, 1974

61. **Wickbom I:** Tumor circulation. In Newton TH, Potts DG (eds): Radiology of the Skull and Brain, Vol 2, pp 2257–2285. Springfield, IL, CV Mosby, 1974

62. **Wood JH, Doppman JL, Lightfoote WE II et al:** Role of vascular proliferation on angiographic appearance and encapsulation of experimental traumatic and metastatic brain abscesses. J Neurosurg 48:264–273, 1978

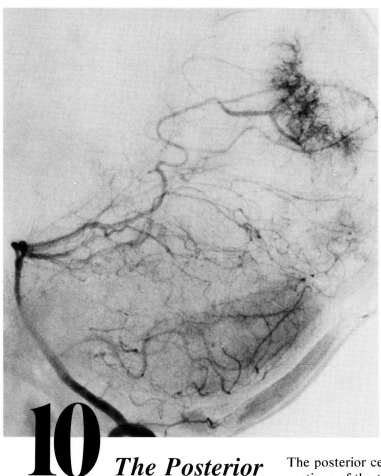

10 *The Posterior Cerebral Artery*

The posterior cerebral artery (PCA) supplies portions of the temporal, parietal, and occipital lobes as well as the thalamus, midbrain, and other deep structures such as the choroid plexus and ependyma of the third and lateral ventricles. More than any other intracranial vessel the PCA subserves the function of vision including ocular reflexes, eye movements, the transmission and integration of visual information and memory, and perception.[11]

NORMAL GROSS ANATOMY

P1 Segment

The posterior cerebral artery originates from the terminal basilar artery bifurcation ventral to the midbrain. The P1 segment, also termed the *peduncular* or *precommunicating portion,* lies within the interpeduncular cistern and ex-

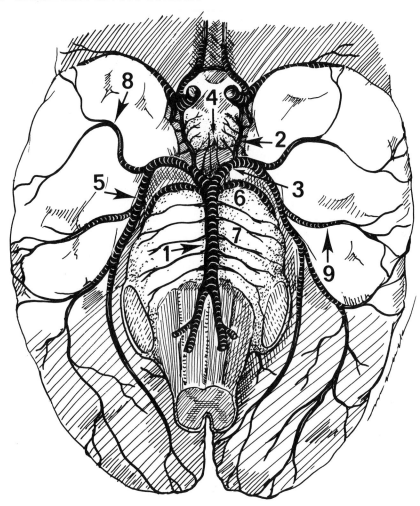

Fig. 10-1. Anatomic drawing of the posterior cerebral artery and adjacent structures (anteroinferior view). **1.** Basilar artery. **2.** Posterior communicating artery. **3.** P1 (peduncular) segment of the PCA. **4.** Thalamoperforating arteries. **5.** P2 (ambient) segment of the PCA. **6.** Superior cerebellar arteries. **7.** Pontine branches of the basilar artery. **8.** Anterior temporal artery. **9.** Posterior temporal artery.

tends from the PCA origin to its junction with the posterior communicating artery (PCoA). As it curves posterolaterally around the midbrain above the third nerve, the P1 segment gives rise to a number of perforating branches that supply the brainstem and thalamus (Figs. 10-1, 10-2).

Thalamoperforating Arteries. These are a group of vessels that arise from the PCoA and P1 segment and enter the brain by passing through the posterior perforating substance just behind the mammillary bodies (Figs. 10-1, arrow 4, and 10-2, arrows 1 and 2).[23] They course superiorly in the interpeduncular fossa, then pass between the cerebral peduncles to supply the thalamus, hypothalamus, subthala-

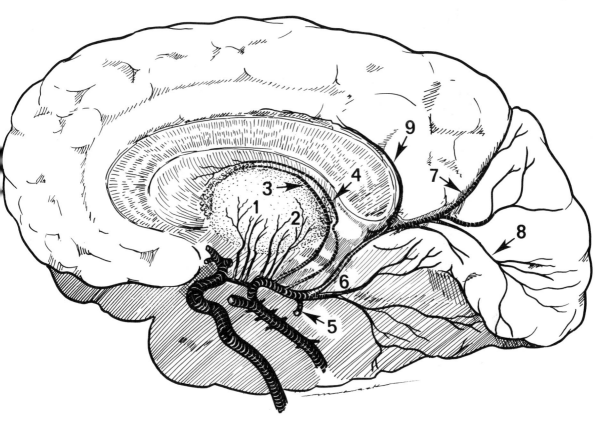

Fig. 10-2. Anatomic drawing of the posterior cerebral arteries and their branches (inferomedial view). Portions of the temporal and occipital lobe have been removed to demonstrate the cortical PCA branches. **1.** Anterior thalamoperforating arteries. **2.** Posterior thalamoperforating and thalamogeniculate arteries. **3.** Medial posterior choroidal artery. **4.** Lateral posterior choroidal artery. **5.** Anterior temporal artery (cut off). **6.** Posterior temporal artery. **7.** Parieto-occipital artery. **8.** Calcarine artery. **9.** Splenial arteries.

mus, nuclei of CNs III and IV, the oculomotor nerve, posterior portion of the internal capsule, and other important structures.[29] The thalamoperforating arteries arising from the PCoA are designated as **anterior thalamoperforating arteries** (ATPAs) while those originating from the precommunicating PCA are termed the **posterior thalamoperforating arteries** (PTPAs).[4]

Meningeal Branches. An inconstant meningeal branch arises from the peduncular PCA segment and courses around the midbrain to the tentorial apex. An anterior branch pierces the tentorium and extends anterosuperiorly along the falx cerebri. A posterior ramus courses superiorly along the falx. This PCA meningeal branch has been termed the artery of Davidoff and Schechter. It has only been identified in abnormal angiographic studies when vascular lesions have induced hypertrophy of this vessel.[28]

P2 Segment

The P2 portion, also termed the *ambient segment,* includes that segment of the PCA extending from the PCoA to about the posterior aspect of the midbrain. The P2 segment sweeps around the cerebral peduncle above the level of the tentorium (Fig. 10-1, arrow 5). It courses posteriorly within the ambient cistern parallel to the optic tract and basal vein and between the midbrain and hippocampal gyrus.[16] The P2 segment has central (brain stem) branches, ventricular branches, and cortical branches.

Brain Stem Branches. One to seven **thalamo-geniculate arteries** arise directly from P2 to supply part of the thalamus, posterior limb of the internal capsule, geniculate bodies, and optic tract (Fig. 10-2, arrow 2). Peduncular **perforating branches** also arise from P2 to supply the corticospinal and corticobulbar pathways as well as other segmental structures.[29]

Ventricular and Choroid Plexus Branches. The **medial posterior choroidal artery** (MPChA) usually arises as a single vessel from the P2 segment (Figs. 10-2, arrow 4, and 10-3, arrow 9). Occasionally it may be multiple or may arise from the precommunicating PCA. After coursing around the brainstem, the MPChA turns superomedially to reach the roof of the third ventricle.[21] It then courses anteriorly toward the foramen of Monro, supplying the thalamus, pineal body, and choroid plexus of the third and lateral ventricles.[22, 26] The MPChA has a reciprocal relationship with both the anterior and lateral posterior choroidal arteries since they share portions of the same vascular territory (see Chapter 7).[2B]

One to nine **lateral posterior choroidal arteries** (LPChAs) arise either directly from P2 or from various cortical PCA branches. They pass laterally through the choroidal fissure to the choroid plexus of the temporal horn and atrium. Together with the choroid plexus the LPChAs curve around the pulvinar of the thalamus within the atrium and body of the lateral ventricle (Figs. 10-2, arrow 3, and 10-3,

arrow 10). Branches of the LPChA also supply the cerebral peduncle, posterior commissure, lateral geniculate body and parts of the thalamus, fornix, and caudate nucleus.[26] Rich anastomoses between all the choroidal arteries are present on the surfaces of the choroid plexus, geniculate bodies, and temporal lobe.[2B]

Cortical Branches. The PCA has four main cortical branches: the inferior temporal group of arteries, and the parieto-occipital, calcarine, and splenial branches.[15, 29] The inferior temporal arteries arise from the P2 segment while the latter three vessels originate more distally.

The **inferior temporal arteries** include hippocampal as well as anterior, middle, posterior, and common temporal arteries. These vessels arise from the PCA near the origin of the LPChAs (Fig. 10-1, arrows 8 and 9, and Fig. 10-2, arrows 5 and 6) and supply the inferior parts of the temporal lobe (Fig. 10-2). On occasion, the posterior temporal artery can extend to the occipital pole and supply the macular area of the striate cortex.[15]

P3 Segment

The P3 segment courses posteriorly in the quadrigeminal cistern from the pulvinar to the anterior limit of the calcarine fissure. However, the PCA often divides into its major terminal branches before reaching the calcarine fissure itself.[29]

Cortical Branches. The **parieto-occipital artery** is one of the two major terminal PCA branches. It usually arises within the ambient cistern as a single trunk and courses posteriorly in the parieto-occipital sulcus (Fig. 10-2, arrow 7). It vascularizes part of the cuneus and precuneus, superior occipital gyrus, and, occasionally, the precentral and superior parietal lobule. Accessory blood supply to the visual cortex is present in 35% of anatomic specimens.[15]

The **calcarine artery,** the other terminal branch, usually arises at the distal bifurcation of the main PCA (Fig. 10-2, arrow 8). It courses posteriorly deep within the calcarine

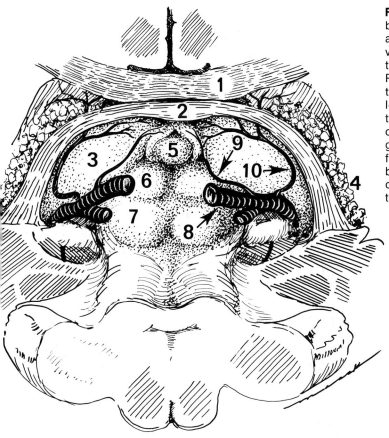

Fig. 10-3. Anatomic drawing of brainstem, quadrigeminal plate, and corpus callosum (posterior view). The relationship between the choroidal branches of the PCA and their adjacent structures is depicted. **1.** Corpus callosum. **2.** Fornix. **3.** Pulvinar of the thalamus. **4.** Choroid plexus of the lateral ventricle. **5.** Pineal gland. **6.** Superior colliculi. **7.** Inferior colliculi. **8.** Posterior cerebral artery. **9.** Medial posterior choroidal artery. **10.** Lateral posterior choroidal artery.

sulcus to supply the visual cortex, inferior cuneus, and part of the lingual gyrus.[26]

The **splenial arteries** are small rami arising either directly from the PCA or from the parieto-occipital artery (Fig. 10-2, arrow 9). Sometimes termed the "posterior pericallosal artery," they ramify over the splenium of the corpus callosum and may anastomose with the pericallosal branches of the ACA.[15]

The cortical distribution of the major PCA branches is depicted in Figure 10-4, A-C.

NORMAL ANGIOGRAPHIC ANATOMY

P1 Segment

The P1 segment is best seen at vertebral angiography in the AP Towne or submentovertex projection. The proximal portions of the PCA have a variable configuration so considerable side-to-side asymmetry is common (Figs. 10-5, 10-6). The maximum normal difference in height of the two proximal PCA segments is about 8 mm.[16]

P2 Segment

The P2 segment lies within the ambient cistern. Coursing posteriorly around the midbrain, it is well visualized in both frontal and lateral views. As with the P1 portion, the ambient segment varies in appearance. It usually follows a relatively straight or inferiorly convex course (Figs. 10-5, 10-6). Posterior to the midbrain, the two PCAs approach each other at a variable distance within the quadrigeminal cistern, then continue posterosuperiorly to terminate in their cortical branches.

(Text continued on p. 303)

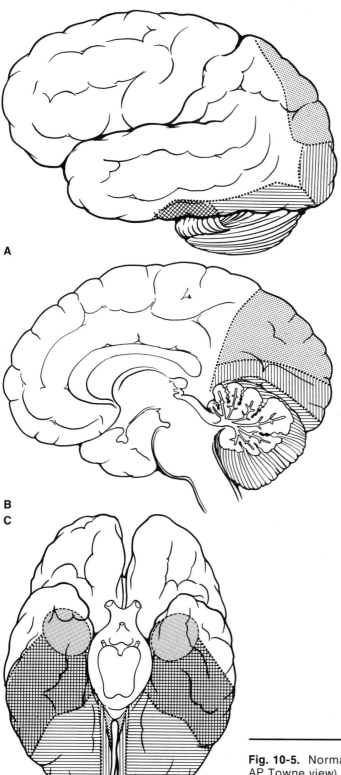

Fig. 10-4. Sketches depicting the most common vascular distribution of the PCA cortical branches. Lateral view **(A),** medial view **(B),** and base view **(C).** Parieto-occipital artery, **dotted area;** Calcarine artery, **vertical stripes;** Anterior temporal artery, **cross-hatched area;** Posterior temporal artery, **horizontal stripes;** Hippocampal artery, **gray area.** *(Adapted from Zeal AA, Rhoton AL Jr: Microsurgical anatomy of the posterior cerebral artery. J Neurosurg 48:534–559, 1978.)*

Fig. 10-5. Normal vertebral angiogram (arterial phase, AP Towne view). Note the variable configuration of the P1 and P2 PCA segments.

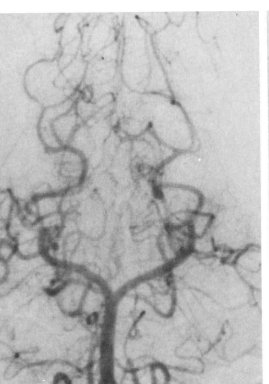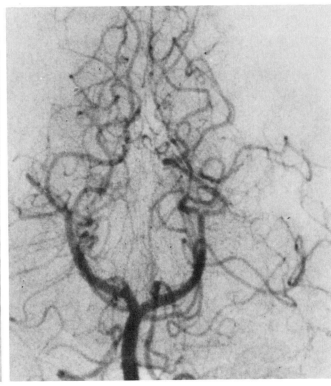

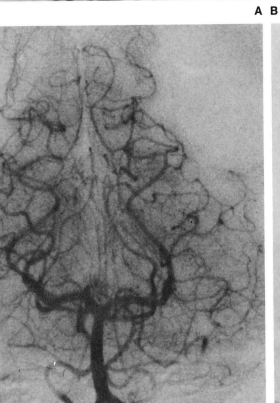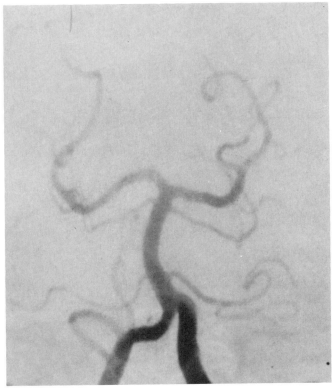

A B

C D

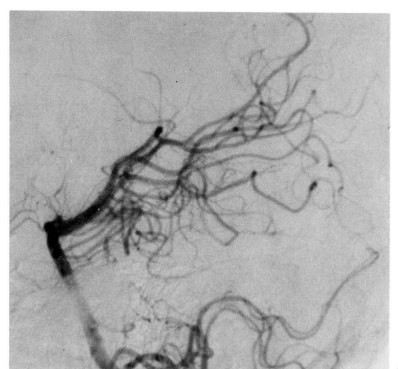

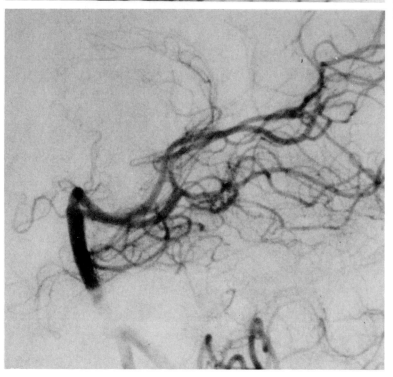

A

B

Fig. 10-6. Normal vertebral angiograms (arterial phase, lateral view). Note the various normal P1 and P2 configurations.

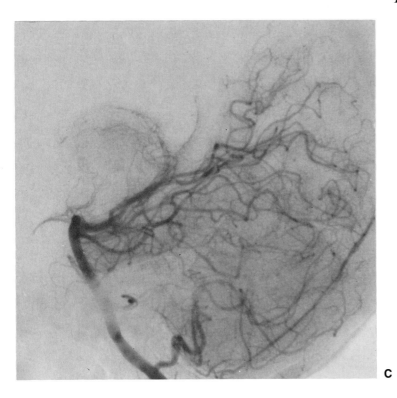

c

Thalamoperforating Arteries. Arising at a slight angle from the PCoA, the anterior group of thalamoperforating arteries is best seen in the lateral projection when there is retrograde filling of the PCoAs (Fig. 10-7C, arrow 2, also see Fig. 6-6). Initially, the ATPAs loop posteriorly, then follow a somewhat undulating superiorly-directed course adjacent to the hypothalamus and walls of the third ventricle. The PTPAs are also well seen in the lateral view as they arise from the P1 segment. Initially, they follow a very sinuous course in the interpeduncular cistern, then often assume a characteristically straight appearance as they traverse the midbrain (Fig. 10-7C, arrow 1). Both groups of thalamoperforating vessels are poorly seen in the frontal projection (Fig. 10-7A, arrow 1).[4, 9] The thalamogeniculate arteries are rarely identifiable on normal vertebral angiograms.

Posterior Choroidal Arteries. The MPChA is identified in the lateral projection as it curves posterosuperiorly around the pineal gland. Its configuration resembles the number 3 (Fig. 10-7C, arrow 3). The MPChA courses forward in the roof of the third ventricle and usually ends in a characteristic tight hairpin turn as its terminal branches ascend through the foramen of Monro.[3, 22] The LPChAs originate from the PCA in the ambient cistern, initially coursing laterally to enter the choroidal fissure. They then turn superiorly, following an anteriorly concave course around the pulvinar of the thalamus (as seen on the lateral view) where they course several millimeters above the MPChA (Fig. 10-7C, arrow 4). The LPChAs demarcate the choroidal fissure and temporal horn.[24]

During the late arterial or early capillary phase of angiography, a definite vascular blush of the choroid plexus is often identified (Fig. 10-7A, D). The two sides should be symmetrical as seen in the AP projection.

(Text continued on p. 306)

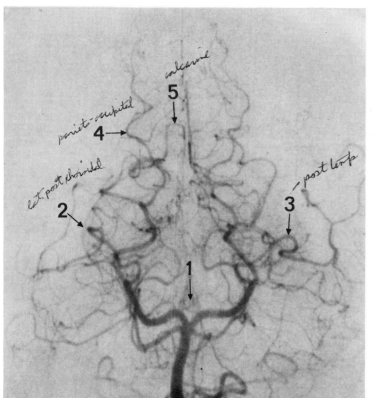

Fig. 10-7A. Normal AP vertebral angiogram, arterial phase
1. Thalamoperforating arteries. **2.** Lateral posterior choroidal artery.
3. Posterior temporal artery.
4. Parieto-occipital artery. **5.** Calcarine artery.

A
B

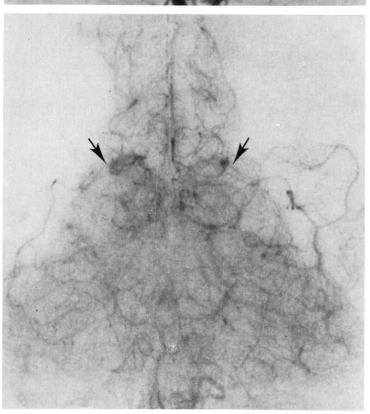

Fig. 10-7B. Normal AP vertebral angiogram (capillary phase). Same patient as 10-7A. Note the symmetry of the choroidal plexus blush **(arrows).**

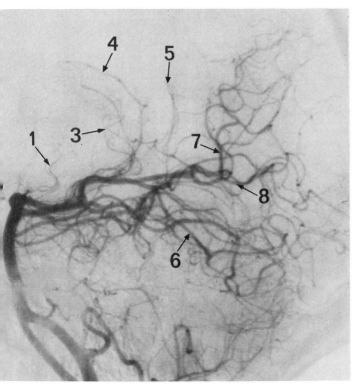

C

D

Fig. 10-7C. Normal lateral vertebral angiogram (arterial phase). Same patient as 10-7A. **1.** Posterior thalamoperforating arteries. **2.** Anterior thalamoperforating arteries. **3.** Medial posterior choroidal arteries. **4.** Lateral posterior choroidal artery. **5.** Splenial (posterior pericallosal) arteries. **6.** Posterior temporal artery. **7.** Parieto-occipital artery. **8.** Calcarine artery. **9.** Anterior temporal artery.

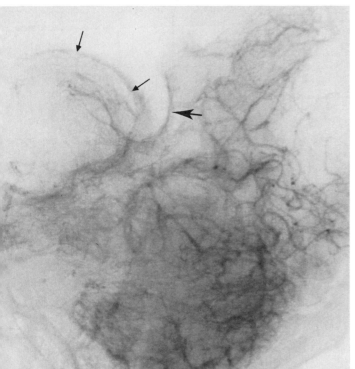

Fig. 10-7D. Normal lateral vertebral angiogram (capillary phase). Same patient as 10-7C. Note the distinct choroid blush **(small arrows).** The splenium of the corpus callosum is also well seen **(large arrow).**

Cortical PCA Branches

The **hippocampal** and **anterior temporal arteries** are frequently the first and second cortical branches to arise from the PCA. The hippocampal arteries are usually too small to be visualized at angiography. The anterior and posterior temporal arteries are often seen in the lateral projection (Fig. 10-7C). The **posterior temporal artery** is also easily identified on the AP view (Fig. 10-7A, arrow 3) although the anterior temporal branch is frequently obscured by overlapping branches from the superior cerebellar artery.[16]

The **parieto-occipital artery** courses posterosuperiorly and is seen in the lateral view as the uppermost of the three posterior cortical PCA branches (Fig. 10-7C, arrow 7). In the frontal projection, the proximal parieto-occipital artery is also the most medial of these vessels as it initially hugs the inner surface of the parieto-occipital lobe. Its distal branches then extend superiorly and laterally as the artery courses deep into the parieto-occipital fissure (Fig. 10-7, arrow 4).[15]

The **calcarine artery** is easily identified in the lateral view by its relatively straight course between the parieto-occipital branches above and the posterior temporal branches below (Fig. 10-7C, arrow 8). In the AP projection, the calcarine artery initially lies lateral to the parieto-occipital artery, then crosses medially as it follows its winding posterior course deep within the calcarine fissure (Fig. 10-7A, arrow 5).[16]

The **posterior pericallosal artery** and splenial branches of the PCA arise within the quadrigeminal cistern. Best seen in the lateral view of vertebral angiograms, these vessels first course anteriorly for a short distance, then bend backwards on themselves to sweep around the splenium of the corpus callosum in a smooth anteriorly concave curve. They then run anteriorly and slightly superiorly in the pericallosal cistern where they eventually anastomose with the pericallosal branch of the ACA (Fig. 10-7C, arrow 5). Capillary phase films of vertebral angiograms often outline the splenium of the corpus callosum (Fig. 10-7D).

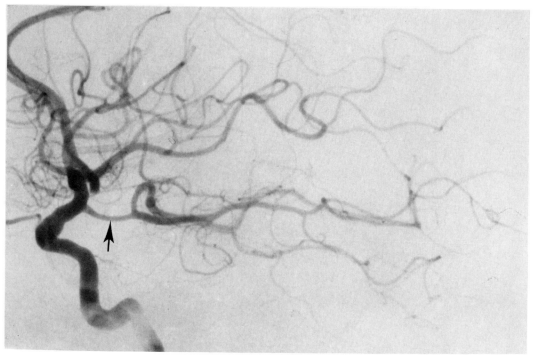

A

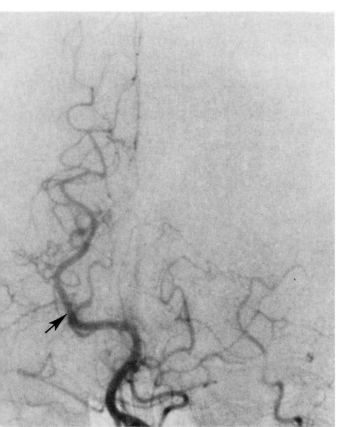

Fig. 10-8. Fetal origin of the posterior cerebral artery from the ICA. Fetal origin of the PCA **(A)** is indicated **(arrow)** on this selective left internal carotid angiogram (lateral view). AP vertebral angiogram **(B)** does not opacify the left PCA. The right PCA is indicated **(arrow)**. AP left internal carotid angiogram **(C)** also opacifies the left PCA **(arrow)**.

B
C

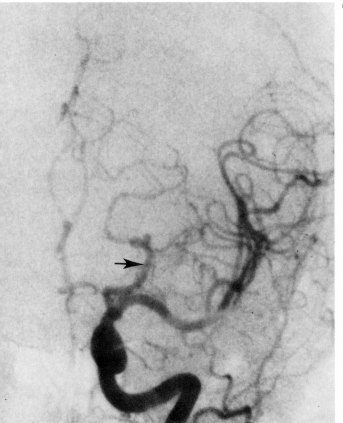

NORMAL VARIATIONS AND ANOMALIES

Anomalies of the posterior circle of Willis are common, occurring in nearly half of all anatomic specimens. These consist of either a hypoplastic PCoA or a "fetal" arrangement in which the communicating artery provides the major blood supply to the PCA (Fig. 10-8A). In such cases, the P1 segment is smaller than the PCoA or is hypoplastic. Complete absence of either segment is rare. Fetal origin of the PCA from the internal carotid circulation is seen in approximately 20% of anatomic dissections.[23] In such instances vertebral angiograms fail to visualize the PCA. It is identified with an ipsilateral carotid study (Fig. 10-8B, C).

In some types of persistent carotid-basilar anastomoses, the PCAs may be supplied via a proatlantal intersegmental artery, persistent trigeminal artery, or other anomalous vessel (see Chapter 6).

VASCULAR LESIONS INVOLVING THE PCA AND ITS BRANCHES

Stenosis and Occlusions

Occlusive vascular disease limited to the PCA is an uncommon occurrence in individuals of any age group and is usually seen as part of a more generalized process.[1, 8] Progressive atheromatous disease is the most common cause of PCA stenosis although embolic and traumatic occlusions have been reported. Hippocampal or combined uncal and hippocampal descending transtentorial herniation may also occlude the PCA as it is compressed against the posterior margin of the tentorium (see below). Rarely, some forms of collagen vascular disease or fibromuscular dysplasia can affect the PCA.

Angiographic Findings. Most angiographically identifiable PCA stenoses and occlusions occur in the P2 or ambient segment (Fig. 10-9), although occlusions proximal to the PCoA have been reported. Occlusions occurring at the origin of the PCA are rare.[2] Failure to visualize an entire PCA at vertebral angiography is usually due to the fetal-type origin of the PCA from the ICA (Fig. 10-8B, C) (see above).

Stenoses appear as smooth or irregular foci with vascular tapering (Fig. 10-9). Most occlusions are unilateral and are usually identified by an abrupt termination or discontinuity in the opacified PCA. Occlusions distal to the P2 segment are usually not identified at angiography. However, retrograde filling of the occluded PCA and its branches via leptomeningeal collaterals from the MCA is often seen in such cases.

Clinical Manifestations. The clinical manifestations and actual extent of the infarcted area vary widely in PCA occlusions depending on the site of obstruction and the adequacy of collateral flow.[16] For example, the rare PCA occlusion at its origin may be asymptomatic if collateral flow from the circle of Willis is sufficient. Infarction of the area supplied by the thalamogeniculate arteries results in the thalamic syndrome of Dejerine and Roussy (*i.e.*, contralateral loss of superficial and deep sensation), extreme hypersensitivity to touch, pain, and temperature ("thalamic pain"), contralateral hemiplegia, and often a homonymous hemianopsia.[29] Cerebellar ataxia with or without choreoathetoid movements may be present.[16]

Posterior temporal artery occlusions result in a mild but transient dysphasia. Since the calcarine artery supplies the visual cortex, the hallmark of its occlusion is a contralateral homonymous visual field defect usually occurring with macular sparing. PCA occlusions may result initially in cortical blindness followed by crossed homonymous hemianopsia with sparing of macular vision.[10]

Occlusion of various PCA branches may also produce somesthetic disturbances due to involvement of afferent pathways in the medial lemniscus or thalamus, motor weakness due to corticospinal tract involvement, memory deficits, autonomic imbalance secondary to disturbances of the sympathetic and para-

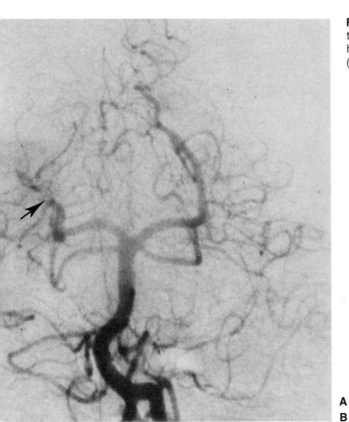

Fig. 10-9. AP **(A)** and lateral **(B)** vertebral angiograms in a patient with a high grade stenosis of the ambient (P2) segment of the PCA **(arrows).**

A
B

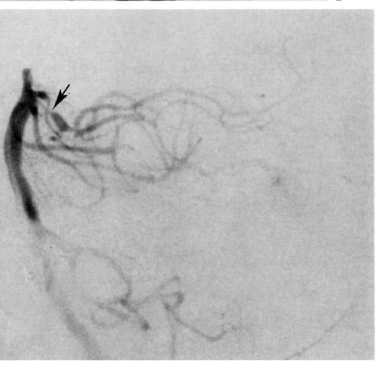

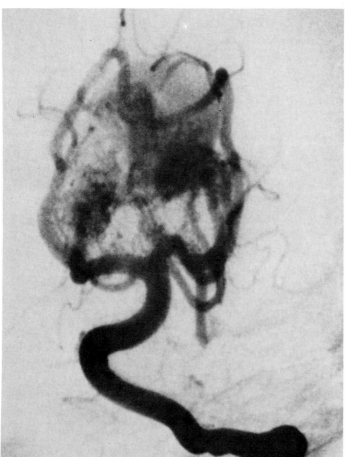

Fig. 10-10. Left vertebral angiogram (arterial phase). This shows a three-year-old child with a diencephalic arteriovenous malformation and aneurysmal dilatation of the vein of Galen (same patient as Figure 11-46). AP **(A)** and lateral **(B)** views show marked enlargement of the PCAs and their choroidal branches.

A
B

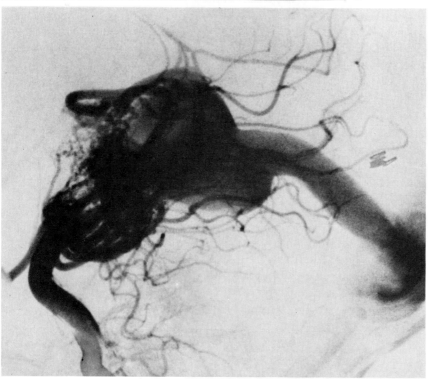

sympathetic pathways in the diencephalon, alterations of consciousness due to ischemia of the midbrain reticular activating system, abnormal movements, and endocrine disturbances due to involvement of the hypothalamic-pituitary axis.[29]

Aneurysms

While aneurysms of the terminal basilar artery are relatively common, congenital saccular aneurysms of the PCA itself are rare. When present, they are usually located at or adjacent to the basilar artery bifurcation. Distal cortical branch aneurysms are usually idiopathic or mycotic and result from deposition of infected emboli in these branches.[16] Trauma and tumor embolus (from chorococarcinoma or cardiac myxoma) are rare causes of peripheral aneurysms.[19, 21A] Fusiform aneurysms are most often located in the basilar artery and proximal PCA. They are usually secondary to atheromatous disease (see Fig. 6-17).

Arteriovenous Malformations

Branches of the PCA supply arteriovenous malformations (AVMs) involving the thala-mus, midbrain, or occipital lobes and may contribute to similar lesions elsewhere. An unusual type of thalamic vascular malformation is associated with aneurysmal dilatation of the vein of Galen. This congenital arteriovenous fistula is usually between diencephalic vessels that are embryologically choroidal and drain into the great cerebral vein.[18, 25A] The anterior and posterior choroidal arteries are usually markedly enlarged (Fig. 10-10).

Malformations primarily involving the occipital lobe often present with headache and visual symptoms. The parieto-occipital, calcarine, and temporal branches of the PCA as well as the angular branch of the MCA are the most common contributing vessels. Dural supply to these malformations via the ECA is frequent.[2A, 27]

Vascular Tumors

The medial and lateral posterior choroidal arteries are often involved in supplying primary vascular neoplasms of the thalamus, pineal gland, and midbrain (Fig. 10-11). They are also frequently enlarged and distorted with intraventricular tumors such as meningiomas. Enlargement of a choroidal artery (with or

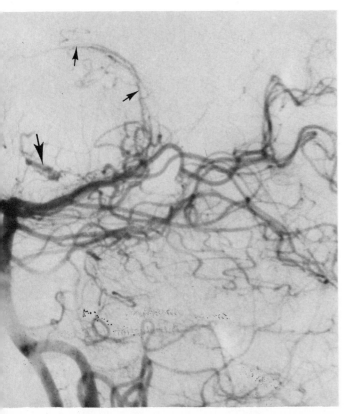

Fig. 10-11. Left vertebral angiogram (arterial phase, lateral view) of pinealoma. The thalamoperforating and choroidal arteries are prominent and supply the vascular neoplasm **(large arrow)**. Note posterosuperior displacement and bowing of the posterior choroidal arteries **(small arrows)**.

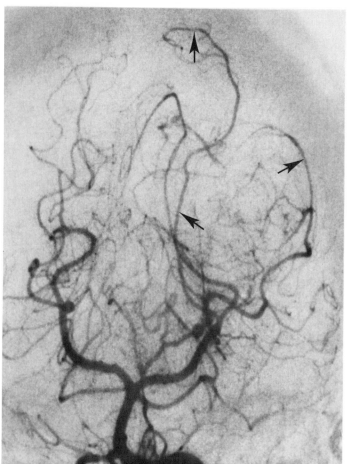

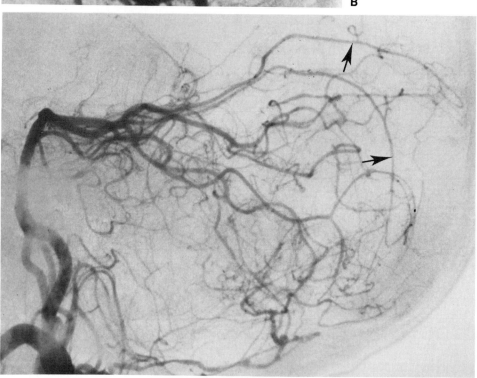

Fig. 10-12. AP **(A)** and lateral **(B)** vertebral angiograms in a patient with a huge transtentorial meningioma. Note stretching and draping of the parieto-occipital branches around the lesion **(arrows).**

A
B

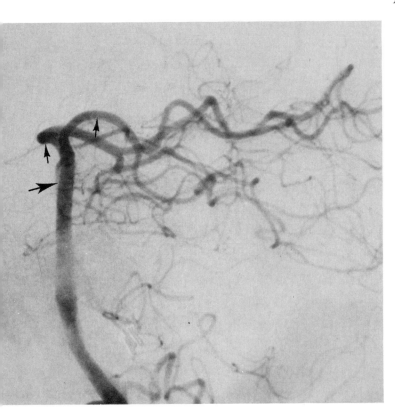

Fig. 10-13. Left vertebral angiogram (arterial phase, lateral view) of a large anterior tentorial meningioma. The PCAs are elevated **(small arrows)** and the basilar artery is displaced posteriorly by the mass **(large arrow).**

without neovascularity or vascular blush) is characteristic but not pathognomonic of intraventricular meningioma. Other intraventricular lesions (*i.e.,* choroid plexus papilloma, ependymoma, glioma, and vascular metastases or malformations) may also produce enlargement of these vessels. Association vascular displacements are due to the neoplasm itself or secondary to ventricular entrapment and hydrocephalus.[13]

Occipital lobe neoplasms are primarily supplied by cortical PCA branches. As with parenchymal vascular tumors elsewhere, angiographic findings vary from a faint diffuse vascular blush to marked neovascularity with tortuous, bizarre-appearing vessels, accumulation of contrast in irregular vascular channels, and arteriovenous shunting. Meningiomas arising from the tentorium or posterior falx often displace adjacent cortical PCA branches as well as receive significant vascular contribution from these vessels (Fig. 10-12).

DISPLACEMENTS OF THE POSTERIOR CEREBRAL ARTERY AND ITS BRANCHES

P1 Segment

Distortions of the P1 or peduncular segment are best appreciated in the AP view. Posteromedial or superior displacement is most commonly due to an extra-axial lesion such as a tentorial meningioma or clivus chordoma (Fig. 10-13). Sufficiently large sellar or suprasellar mass lesions may displace the distal basilar artery and proximal PCA posteriorly (Fig. 10-14). A midbrain glioma is rarely primarily exophytic, angiographically mimicking the findings of an extra-axial mass (Fig. 10-15). Intrinsic midbrain neoplasms or other mass lesions producing anterior displacement of the brainstem may also be associated with anterolateral PCA displacement.[17]

(Text continued on p. 317)

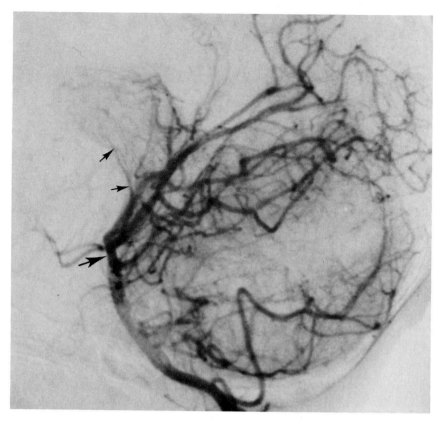

Fig. 10-14. Left vertebral angiogram (arterial phase, lateral view) of a large craniopharyngioma. The large suprasellar mass has displaced the posterior thalamoperforating arteries superiorly **(small arrows).** The distal basilar artery is also displaced posteriorly **(large arrow).**

Fig. 10-15. Left vertebral angiogram (arterial phase). This shows a four-year-old child with a huge exophytic brainstem glioma. The basilar artery is displaced posteriorly and the PCAs are elevated. Note encasement of these arteries **(arrows).** AP **(A)** and lateral **(B)** views are shown. This intra-axial lesion angiographically mimics an extra-axial tumor. *(Case courtesy of R. Jaffe, M.D.)*

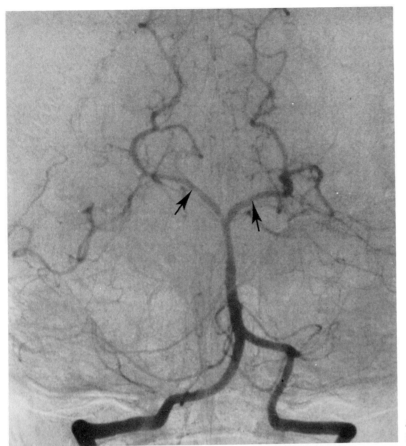

A
B

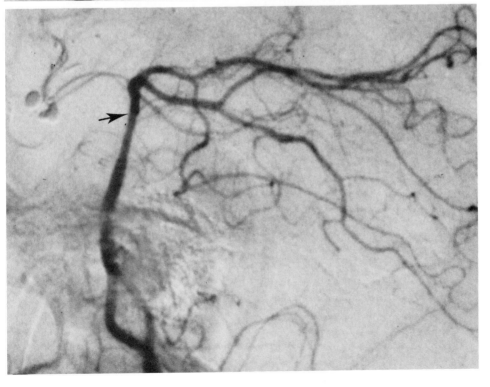

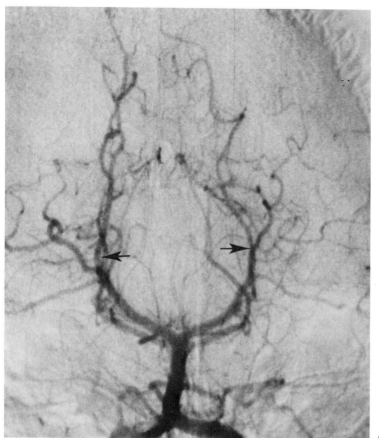

A

B

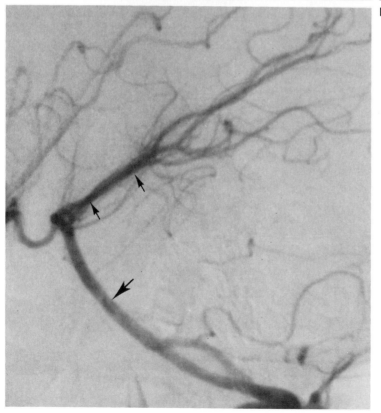

Fig. 10-16. Left vertebral angiogram (arterial phase). This shows a three-year-old with a midbrain glioma. In the AP view **(A),** note the outward bowing of the PCAs by the mass **(arrows).** In the lateral view **(B),** the PCAs appear stretched as they pass around the enlarged midbrain **(small arrow).** Note anterior displacement of the basilar artery **(large arrow).**

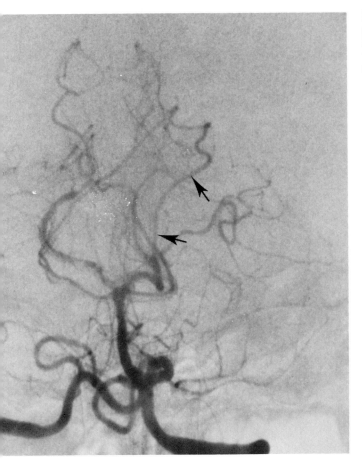

Fig. 10-17. Left vertebral angiogram (arterial phase, AP view) of a large tumor of the middle and posterior left temporal lobe. The P2 segment of the PCA is displaced medially **(arrows).**

P2 Segment

Distortions of the PCA within the ambient cistern can be recognized in both the AP and lateral projections. Unusually large brainstem masses cause lateral displacement and loss of the normal undulations of the PCA as it curves around the brainstem (Fig. 10-16). Large extra-axial masses in the quadrigeminal plate cistern and inferior herniation of a massively enlarged suprapineal recess can also produce this appearance.

Medial displacement of the P2 segment can be caused by masses in or adjacent to the tentorium, large mid or posterior temporal tumors, and descending herniation of the hippocampal gyrus (Fig. 10-17). Marked inferior dislocation of the PCA through the tentorial incisura may occur with severe descending herniations (Fig. 10-18). Cortical PCA branches (which must remain in the supratentorial compartment) appear draped or kinked as they cross the tentorial edge. The compression of these branches against the tentorium can become so severe that it can cause actual occlusion. In anterior (uncal) descending herniation, the PCoA and proximal PCA are usually displaced medially by the uncus. The PCoA may appear compressed inferiorly and kinked over the posterior clinoid process (see Fig. 8-45B).[12]

Superior displacement of the P2 segment is uncommon but can be identified in upward herniation of the cerebellar vermis through the tentorial incisura (Fig. 10-19). Occasionally, tentorial meningiomas or large infiltrative posterior temporal neoplasms may produce a similar appearance.

(Text continued on p. 320)

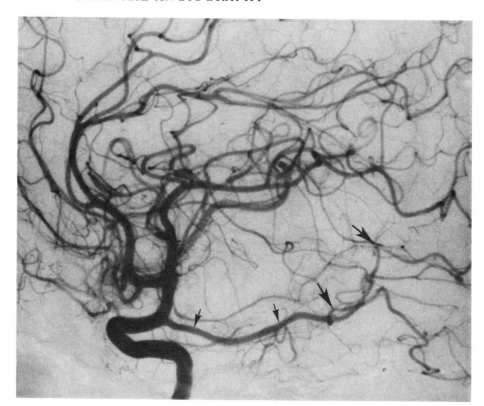

Fig. 10-18

Fig. 10-19

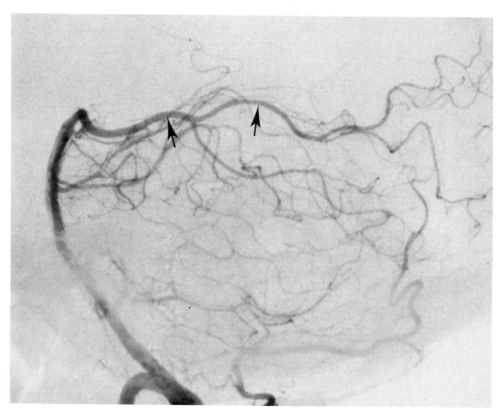

◀ **Fig. 10-18.** Left carotid angiogram (arterial phase, lateral view) of a large temporal lobe neoplasm that has caused descending transtentorial herniation. The PCA has a fetal origin from the ICA. Note inferior displacement of the proximal PCA **(small arrows).** Sharp angulation of the PCA branches is present where they are draped against the tentorium **(large arrows).**

Fig. 10-20. Left vertebral angiogram (arterial phase, lateral view) in a patient with enlarged third and lateral ventricles. Note the stretching and elongation of the thalamoperforating arteries **(arrows).**

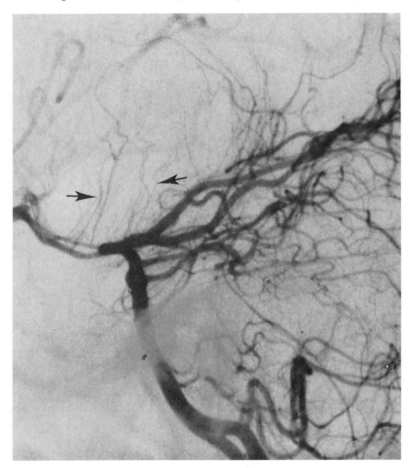

◀ **Fig. 10-19.** Left vertebral angiogram (arterial phase, lateral view). A large superior vermian tumor extends through the tentorial incisura, elevating the PCA **(arrows).**

Thalamoperforating Arteries

Mild non-tumoral third ventricular dilatation produces stretching and straightening of the paraventricular portions of the anterior thalamoperforating arteries (ATPAs). With moderate third ventricular enlargement, these vessels also appear somewhat elongated (Fig. 10-20). Severe enlargement of the lateral ventricles may also produce anteroinferior displacement of both the anterior and posterior thalamoperforating groups.[5] With third ventricular dilatation secondary to cerebral atrophy, the thalamoperforating vessels may appear elongated but retain their slightly undulating course and do not appear stretched.

Large mass lesions within the suprasellar or interpeduncular cisterns stretch and bow the thalamoperforating arteries posteriorly and superiorly (Fig. 10-14). Not infrequently the vertebral angiogram may be more striking than changes apparent on the carotid study (see Figs. 6-21B, C, 6-22). Mesencephalic tu-mors may bow the thalamoperforating arteries anteriorly (Fig. 10-21). Thalamic lesions displace the thalamoperforating arteries laterally (Fig. 10-23C).

Pinealomas and other mass lesions in the quadrigeminal plate area may produce both the characteristic angiographic changes associated with obstructive hydrocephalus as well as compress the thalamoperforating vessels anteroinferiorly.[7]

Choroidal Arteries

The distance between the MPChA and LPChA as seen on the lateral view tends to diminish with severe hydrocephalus as the markedly enlarged lateral ventricles cause downward displacement of both distal posterior choroidal arteries (Fig. 10-22).[21]

Fig. 10-21. Left vertebral angiogram (arterial phase, lateral view). A glioma involving the cerebral peduncles displaces the thalamoperforating vessels anteriorly **(arrows)**.

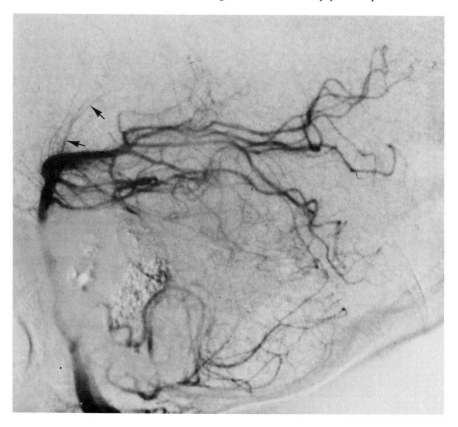

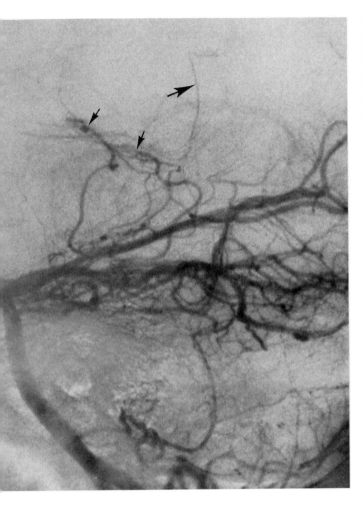

Fig. 10-22. Left vertebral angiogram (arterial phase, lateral view) of severe obstructive hydrocephalus secondary to aqueductal stenosis. Note anteroinferior displacement of the posterior choroidal arteries **(small arrows)** while the splenial vessels are bowed posterosuperiorly **(large arrow)** by the massive ventricular enlargement.

Thalamic tumors produce posterosuperior displacement of the LPChA and, to a lesser degree, the MPChA (Fig. 10-23). The normal arc of the LPChA as it passes around the pulvinar appears widened and accentuated.[14]

Lesions above the choroidal arteries, such as those located in or adjacent to the quadrigeminal plate cistern, tend to depress these vessels (Figs. 10-24, 10-25) while most pinealomas and posterior third ventricular tumors elevate them (Fig. 10-11).[21] Some authors feel that pinealoma is unlikely if anterior displacement of the MPChA is present.[25]

Posterior Pericallosal Artery

The posterior pericallosal artery is displaced posterosuperiorly in lesions of the corpus callosum splenium. The distance between the posterior choroidal and splenial vessels may also be increased (although arterial changes are actually present in relatively few cases.) These findings can also be associated with severe hydrocephalus since marked dilatation of the lateral ventricles can elevate the corpus callosum and displace the splenium posterosuperiorly (Figs. 10-22, 10-25).[20]

Cortical Branches

As with mass lesions elsewhere, those located in PCA territory may produce focal strengthening and bowing of its cortical branches (Fig. 10-12). Extra-axial lesions such as meningioma or subdural hematoma may displace some of the distal cortical branches away from the calvarium.

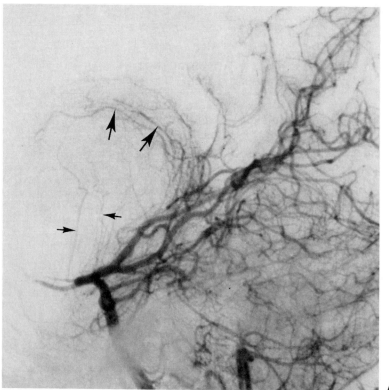

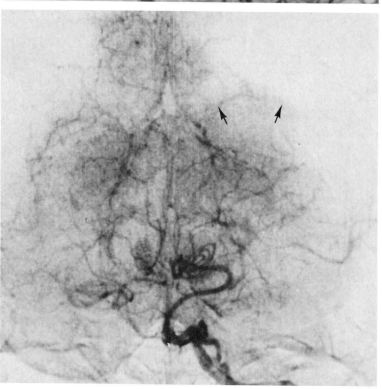

Fig. 10-23. Left vertebral angiogram in two patients with left thalamic gliomas. In the first patient, **(A,** arterial phase lateral view) both the medial and lateral posterior choroidal arteries are displaced posterosuperiorly and the distance between them diminished **(large arrows).** Note the stretching and elongation of the thalamoperforating vessels secondary to the tumor **(small arrows).** In the capillary phase (**B,** AP view), the left choroid plexus blush is elevated **(arrows)** compared to the normal right side. (Same patient as 10-29A.) In the second patient, (**C,** arterial phase, AP view), the thalamoperforating arteries are displaced from left to right **(arrows)** by the tumor in the pulvinar.

A

B

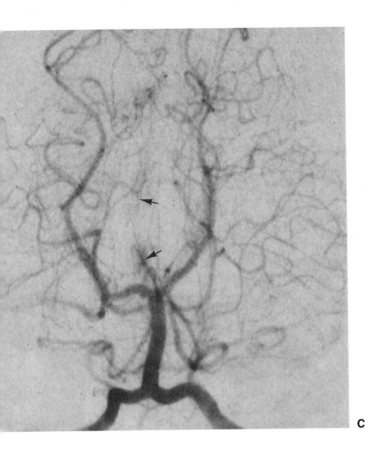

C

Fig. 10-24. Left vertebral angiogram (arterial phase, lateral view) of a large quadrigeminal plate tumor depressing the posterior choroidal arteries (**arrows**).

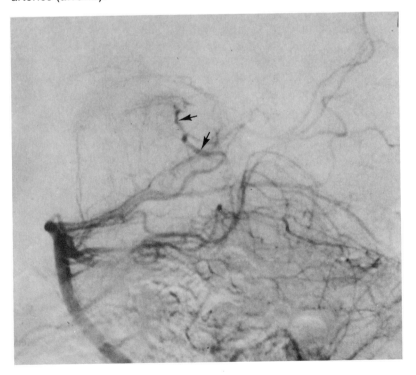

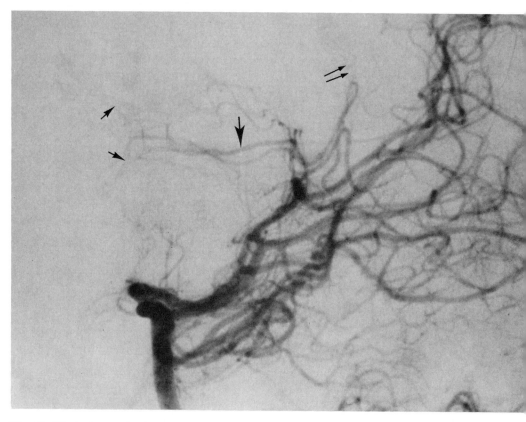

Fig. 10-25. Left vertebral angiogram (arterial phase, lateral view) of an ependymoma adjacent to the foramen of Monro (same patient as Figure 11-39). The distal portions of the PTPAs are draped around the lesion **(small black arrows)** while the more proximal segments are depressed by massively enlarged lateral ventricles **(large black arrow).** The splenial (posterior pericallosal) arteries are also displaced posterosuperiorly **(small double arrows).**

REFERENCES

1. **Billewicz O, Babin E, Massot R et al:** Thrombosis of the posterior cerebral artery. Neuroradiology 1:99–100, 1970
2. **Einsiedel-Lechtape H, Lechtape-Gruter R, Hennemann U:** The angiographic diagnosis of occlusions of the posterior cerebral artery. Neuroradiology 4:47–57, 1977
2A. **Faria MA, Fleischer AS:** Dual cerebral and meningeal supply to giant arteriovenous malformations of the posterior cerebral hemisphere. J Neurosurg 52:153–161, 1980
2B. **Fujii K, Lenkey C, Rhoton AL Jr:** Microsurgical anatomy of the choroidal arteries: Lateral and third ventricles. J Neurosurg 52:165–188, 1980
3. **Galloway JR, Greitz T:** The medial and lateral choroid arteries. An anatomic and roentgenographic study. Acta Radiol [Diagn] (Stockh) 53:353–366, 1960
4. **George AE, Raybaud CH, Salamon G et al:** Anatomy of the thalamoperforating arteries with special emphasis on arteriography of the third ventricle. Part I. Am J Roentgenol 124:220–230. 1975
5. **George AE, Salamon G, Krichell II:** Pathologic anatomy of the thalamoperforating arteries in lesions of the third ventricle. Part II. Am J Roentgenol 124:231–240, 1975
6. **Goto K, Tagawa K, Uemura K et al:** Posterior cerebral artery occlusion: clinical, computed tomographic, and angiographic corelation. Radiology 132: 357–368, 1979

7. **Greitz T:** Tumors of the quadrigeminal plate and adjacent structures. Acta Radiol [Diagn] (Stockh) 12:513–538, 1972

8. **Hahn FJY, Rice AC, Christie JH:** Occlusion of the posterior cerebral artery: scintiscan and angiographic findings. Radiology 112:131–133, 1974

9. **Hara K, Fujino Y:** The thalamoperforate artery. Acta Radiol [Diagn] (Stockh) 5:192–200, 1966

10. **Haymaker W:** Bing's Local Diagnosis in Neurological Diseases. St. Louis, CV Mosby, 1956

11. **Hoyt WF, Newton TH, Margolis MT:** The posterior cerebral artery: embryology and developmental anomalies. In Newton TH, Potts DG (eds): Radiology of the Skull and Brain, Vol 2, pp 1540–1550. St. Louis, CV Mosby, 1974

12. **Komaki S, Handel S:** Molding of the posterior communicating artery in downward transtentorial herniation. Radiology 113:107–110, 1974

13. **Mani RL, Hedgcock MW, Mass SI et al:** Radiographic diagnosis of meningioma of the lateral ventricle. J Neurosurg 49:249–255, 1978

14. **Margolis MT, Hoffman HB, Newton TH:** Choroidal arteries in the diagnosis of thalamic tumors. J Neurosurg 36:287–298, 1972

15. **Margolis MT, Newton TH, Hoyt WF:** Cortical branches of the posterior cerebral artery. Anatomic-radiologic correlation. Neuroradiology 2:127–135, 1971

16. **Margolis MT, Newton TH, Hoyt WF:** The posterior cerebral artery: gross and roentgenographic anatomy. In Newton TH, Potts DG (eds): Radiology of the Skull and Brain, Vol 2, pp 1551–1578. St. Louis, CV Mosby, 1974

17. **Newton TH, Hoyt WF, Margolis MT:** The posterior cerebral artery. III. Pathology. In Newton TH, Potts DG (eds): Radiology of the Skull and Brain, Vol 2, pp 1580–1627. St. Louis, CV Mosby, 1974

18. **O'Brien MS, Schechter MM:** Arteriovenous malformations involving the galenic system. Am J Roentgenol 110:50–55, 1970

19. **Olmstead WW, McGee TP:** The pathogenesis of peripheral aneurysms of the central nervous system: a subject review from the AFIP. Radiology 123:661–666, 1977

20. **Osborn AG, Poole GJ:** Angiographic signs of corpus callosal tumors: a reappraisal. Radiology 115:97–105, 1975

21. **Pachtman H, Hilal SK, Wood EH:** The posterior choroidal arteries. Radiology 112:343–352, 1974

21A. **Parkinson D, West M:** Traumatic intracranial aneurysms. J Neurosurg 52:11–20, 1980

22. **Rothman SLG, Allen WE III, Simeone JF:** The medial posterior choroidal artery as an indicator of masses at the foramen of Monro. Neuroradiology 11:123–129, 1976

23. **Saeki N, Rhoton AL Jr:** Microsurgical anatomy of the upper basilar artery and the posterior circle of Willis. J Neurosurg 46:563–578, 1977

24. **Salamon G, Lecaque GL, Strother CM:** An angiographic study of the temporal horn. Radiology 128:387–392, 1978

25. **Sones PJ Jr, Hoffman JC Jr:** Angiography of tumors involving the posterior third ventricle. Am J Roentgenol 124:241–249, 1975

25A. **Spallone A:** Computed tomography in aneurysms of the vein of Galen. J Comp Asst Tomogr 3:779–782, 1979

26. **Stevens RB, Stilwell DL:** Arteries and Veins of the Human Brain, pp 96–99. Springfield IL, CC Thomas, 1969

27. **Troost BT, Newton TH:** Roentgen analysis of arteriovenous malformations of the occipital lobe. Am J Roentgenol 122:538–544, 1974

28. **Weinstein MA, Duchesneau PM, Dohn DF:** Angiographic identification of the meningeal branch of the posterior cerebral artery. Am J Roentgenol 128:326–327, 1977

29. **Zeal AA, Rhoton AL Jr:** Microsurgical anatomy of the posterior cerebral artery. J Neurosurg 48:534–559, 1978

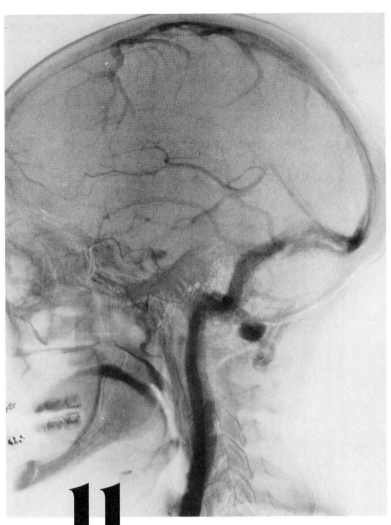

11 *Veins of the Head and Neck*

The extracranial veins, cortical veins, deep cerebral venous system, and dural sinuses may participate either directly or indirectly in a variety of pathological processes affecting the brain. Familiarity with normal anatomy, common variations, and anomalies is thus a prerequisite for correct interpretation of the complete cerebral angiographic series. A study of the cerebral venous system begins with an anatomic-radiographic consideration of the veins of the face and neck, the superficial and deep cerebral venous system, and the dural sinuses. Common pathologic processes affecting these structures will be discussed in this chapter. Venous drainage of the posterior fossa is considered in Chapter 12.

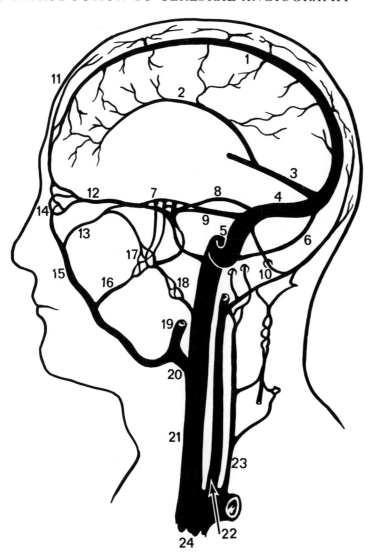

Fig. 11-1. Anatomic drawing depicting the craniofacial venous plexuses. *(Modified from Gray H., Anatomy of the Human Body. M. Goss (ed), Lea and Febiger, 1966)* **1.** Superior sagittal sinus. **2.** Inferior sagittal sinus. **3.** Straight sinus. **4.** Transverse sinus. **5.** Sigmoid sinus. **6.** Occipital sinus. **7.** Cavernous sinus. **8.** Superior petrosal sinus. **9.** Inferior petrosal sinus. **10.** Emissary veins. **11.** Frontal scalp veins. **12.** Superior ophthalmic vein. **13.** Inferior ophthalmic vein. **14.** Angular vein. **15.** Anterior facial vein. **16.** Deep facial vein. **17.** Pterygoid venous plexus. **18.** Pharyngeal venous plexus. **19.** Posterior facial vein. **20.** Common facial vein. **21.** Internal jugular vein. **22.** External jugular vein. **23.** Vertebral vein. **24.** Subclavian vein.

NORMAL GROSS ANATOMY

Scalp and Emissary Veins

Veins of the scalp are connected via emissary veins to the cranial dural venous sinuses. Parietal emissary veins pass through channels in the parietal bones and are located anterior to the lambda on each side of the sagittal suture. Mastoid emissary veins receive the occipital and posterior auricular veins, then pass through the mastoid foramina to drain into the sigmoid sinus. Other scalp veins communicate with the ophthalmic veins (Fig. 11.1, number 10).[17]

Facial Veins

The superficial and deep facial veins are major tributaries of the internal and external jugular veins. The **anterior facial vein** (a continuation of the angular vein) descends obliquely across the face, communicating with the ophthalmic veins and cavernous sinus. It receives tributaries from the anterior scalp, orbit, and nose (Fig. 11-1, number 15). The **deep facial vein** connects the anterior facial vein with the pterygoid venous plexus (Fig. 11-1, number 16). The **pterygoid plexus** lies between the temporalis and lateral pterygoid muscles. It receives tributaries that generally correspond to branches of the maxillary artery. The pterygoid plexus communicates freely with the facial veins. It also anastomoses with the cavernous sinus, ophthalmic veins, and maxillary (retromandibular) vein (Fig. 11-1, number 17).

The **posterior facial vein** (also called the **retromandibular vein**) is formed by the superficial temporal and maxillary veins (Fig. 11-1, number 19). The posterior and anterior facial veins unite to form the **common facial vein.** After receiving lingual, submental, and thyroid tributaries, the common facial vein joins the internal jugular vein at the level of the hyoid bone (Fig. 11-1, number 20).

Veins of the Neck

The **external jugular vein** is formed by segments of the retromandibular and posterior auricular veins. It receives tributaries from the scalp and deep facial structures. The external jugular vein varies considerably in size, coursing inferiorly and obliquely across the sternomastoid muscle to terminate in the subclavian vein (Fig. 11-1, number 22).

The **internal jugular vein** (IJV) begins within the pars vascularis of the jugular fossa as the caudad continuation of the sigmoid sinus. The slight dilatation present at the origin of each internal jugular vein is termed the jugular bulb. The IJV courses inferiorly, lateral to the internal and common carotid arteries. Posterior to the medial ends of the clavicles, the IJVs unite with their respective subclavian veins to form the right and left innominate veins. Tributaries of the IJV include the inferior petrosal sinus (which drains into the jugular bulb), the common facial vein, and lingual, pharyngeal, and thyroid veins (Fig. 11-1, number 21)[17, 38]

The **vertebral vein** is formed in the suboccipital triangle by numerous small tributaries from the cranial vertebral venous plexuses and cervical musculature (Fig. 11-1, number 23). It descends with the vertebral artery through the foramina transversaria, emerges from this bony canal at the C6 or C7 level, and terminates in the brachiocephalic vein. Via the mastoid emissary veins, the vertebral veins also anastomose with the transverse sinus (see below) and external jugular system.[8]

Venous Drainage of the Brain and Meninges

The veins of the human brain are usually divided into four groups: diploic veins, meningeal veins, dural sinuses, and cerebral veins. The latter are further subdivided into superficial, or cortical, and deep cerebral veins.

Diploic Veins. Diploic veins are small, irregularly shaped endothelial-lined channels that run between the two tables of the skull and drain the diploë. They communicate directly with the extracranial venous system as well as with the meningeal veins and dural sinuses. These diploic veins are rarely visualized on normal carotid angiograms. However,

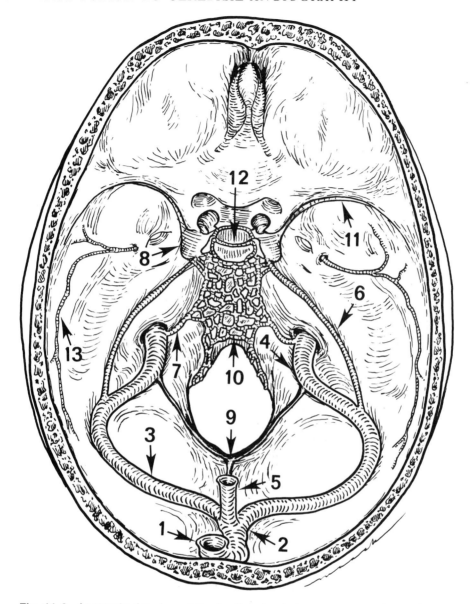

Fig. 11-2. Anatomic drawing of the basilar dural sinuses as seen from above. **1.** Superior sagittal sinus. **2.** Torcular Herophili. **3.** Transverse sinus. **4.** Sigmoid sinus. **5.** Straight sinus. **6.** Superior petrosal sinus. **7.** Inferior petrosal sinus. **8.** Cavernous sinus. **9.** Occipital sinus. **10.** Clival venous plexus. **11.** Sphenoparietal sinus. **12.** Intercavernous sinus. **13.** Middle meningeal sinus.

they may become enlarged with chronic increased intracranial pressure or arteriovenous malformations.[18, 45]

Meningeal Veins. The meningeal veins are epidural vessels contained within the dura. They lie in a shallow groove on the inner table of the calvarium. They usually accompany the meningeal arteries, providing venous drainage for the falx cerebri, the tentorium, and the cranial dura mater. The meningeal veins either empty into the dural sinuses or pass extracranially and drain into the pterygoid or vertebral plexuses (Fig. 11-2, arrow 13).

Dural Sinuses. The cranial dural sinuses are trabeculated, endothelial-lined channels whose walls are formed by the two layers of dura mater. These channels collect blood from the cerebral veins, meninges, and calvarium, forming the major drainage pathway for the cranial cavity and its contents. The dural sinuses also communicate with the meningeal and diploic veins. Via a network of emissary veins that pass both directly through the cranial vault and basilar foramina, the dural sinuses also communicate with the extracranial venous system.[8] These intercommunications can become an important pathway for collateral venous drainage in case of cerebral venous occlusion (see below).

The major dural sinuses include the superior and inferior sagittal sinuses, the cavernous and intercavernous sinuses, the superior and inferior petrosal sinuses, the occipital sinus, and the straight, transverse, and sigmoid sinuses.

The **superior sagittal (longitudinal) sinus** (SSS) originates near the crista galli where it communicates with facial and nasal veins. It arcs posteriorly, lying in the midline along the upper margin of the falx cerebri and its junction with the dural lining of the calvarium (Fig. 11-1, number 1; and 11-3, arrow 4). Throughout most of its course, the SSS is midline. However, it often deviates slightly to the right as it descends along the occipital bone where it usually terminates by becoming the right transverse sinus. It may also join the torcular

Herophili (confluens sinuum) at the internal occipital protuberance. Venous lakes are contained within the dura mater adjacent to the SSS; they communicate freely with this structure. Arachnoid (Pacchionian) granulations project into the floor and walls of these venous lacunae and into the superior sagittal and other dural sinuses.[18, 43]

In addition to the SSS, the **torcular Herophili** also receives the occipital and straight sinuses as well as some tentorial and cerebellar veins (Figs. 11-2, arrow 2; and 11-3, arrow 7). It usually has two major components—the right and left transverse sinuses—which are united by variable cross channels. The right transverse sinus is usually the larger of the two. Tributaries of the torcular are highly variable. Fifty-seven percent of all anatomic specimens have freely communicating superior sagittal, straight, occipital and transverse sinuses. The remainder have various anomalous venous patterns.[26]

The **inferior sagittal (longitudinal) sinus** (ISS) is a channel that courses posteriorly in the inferior free edge of the falx cerebri (Fig. 11-3, arrow 5). Tributaries from the falx, the corpus callosum, cingulum, and medial hemispheres unite at the junction of the anterior and middle thirds of the falx to form the ISS.[33]

The **straight sinus** (SS) is formed by the confluence of the great cerebral vein (vein of Galen) and the inferior sagittal sinus (Figs. 11-1, number 3; and 11-3, arrow 6). The straight sinus runs posteroinferiorly in the confluence of the falx cerebri and tentorial leaves. It terminates at the internal occipital protuberance, usually by becoming the left transverse sinus. Venous patterns at the junction of the ISS and vein of Galen are quite variable. In approximately 85% of anatomic specimens the straight sinus is represented by a single midline tentorial channel. Duplication of the ISS is seen in 7 to 15% of cases.[10, 16]

The **occipital sinus,** usually the smallest of the major dural sinuses, begins at the margins of the foramen magnum and passes superiorly into the confluens sinuum (Figs. 11-1, number 6; and 11-2, arrow 9). The occipital sinus communicates with the internal jugular vein or

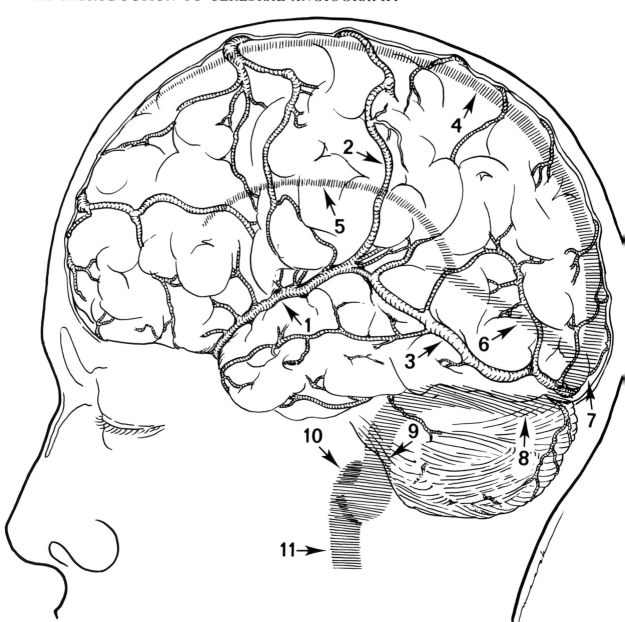

Fig. 11-3. Anatomic drawing of the superficial cerebral veins (the major dural sinuses are shown in the shaded areas). **1.** Superficial middle cerebral vein. **2.** Vein of Trolard. **3.** Vein of Labbé. **4.** Superior sagittal sinus. **5.** Inferior sagittal sinus. **6.** Straight sinus. **7.** Torcular Herophili. **8.** Transverse sinus. **9.** Sigmoid sinus. **10.** Jugular bulb. **11.** Internal jugular vein.

vertebral venous plexus through venous plexuses that accompany the hypoglossal nerves. In approximately two percent of anatomic specimens, the occipital sinus forms a major draining channel for the SS or SSS.[27]

The **transverse sinuses** originate at the torcular Herophili and course anterolaterally between the attachments of the tentorial leaves to the calvarium (Figs. 11-1, number 4; and 11-2, arrow 3). The transverse sinuses then turn downward and medially at the posterior edges of the petrous temporal bones to become the sigmoid sinuses. Along their course the transverse sinuses receive venous blood from the superior sagittal and straight sinuses as well as the cerebellum and inferolateral surfaces of the temporal and occipital lobes. In about 25% of all cases the transverse sinuses are unequal in size, with the right sinus usually larger than the left. In five to six percent of anatomic specimens, a narrowed or atretic segment can be identified in one of the transverse sinuses.[26]

The **sigmoid sinuses** represent the anteroinferior continuation of the transverse sinuses. The sigmoid sinuses pass inferiorly and medially in a gentle S-shaped curve towards the jugular foramen. There they terminate by becoming the paired internal jugular veins (Figs. 11-1, number 5; and 11-2, arrow 4).

The **superior petrosal sinus,** a channel extending from the cavernous sinus to the sigmoid sinus, runs along the dorsal ridge of the petrous temporal bone at the dural attachment of the tentorium cerebelli (Figs. 11-1, number 8; and 11-2, arrow 6). Its tributaries include veins from the pons, upper medulla, cerebellum, and inner ear.

The **inferior petrosal sinus** also originates from the cavernous sinus (Figs. 11-1, number 9; and 11-2, arrow 7). Passing posterolaterally along the petro-occipital suture, it courses between the ninth and tenth cranial nerves to drain into the jugular bulb. The paired inferior petrosal sinuses are interconnected with the basilar venous plexus of the clivus and the intercavernous sinus. In turn, the clival or basilar venous plexus communicates with the cavernous, superior petrosal, and occipital sinuses as well as the inferior vertebral veins.

The **sphenoparietal sinus** (SPS) is the anteroinferior continuation of the meningeal sinus. It follows the curve of the greater sphenoid wing to reach the cavernous sinus (Fig. 11-2, arrow 11). In addition to receiving the meningeal sinus and meningeal veins it also frequently drains the superficial middle cerebral vein. The SPS often anastomoses with the basal vein of Rosenthal.[45]

The **cavernous sinuses** are irregularly shaped, paired venous spaces lying on either side of the body of the sphenoid bone (Figs. 11-1, number 7; and 11-2, arrow 8). The tributaries and interconnections of the cavernous sinuses are complex. Anteriorly they receive the superior and inferior ophthalmic veins and the SPS. Laterally they communicate with the pterygoid plexus through the foramen ovale. Medially each cavernous sinus communicates with its counterpart on the opposite side via intercavernous sinuses that surround the hypophysis. Posteriorly the cavernous sinuses communicate with the transverse sinus. They also drain into the internal jugular veins via the inferior petrosal veins. Unlike most dural sinuses, the cavernous sinuses are heavily trabeculated and compartmentalized. They transmit the ICA, the oculomotor, trochlear, and abducens nerves, and the ophthalmic and maxillary divisions of the trigeminal nerve (see Chapter 5).[8, 17, 38, 45]

Superficial Cerebral Veins. The superficial cerebral veins lie along the surface sulci. They drain the cortex and some of the white matter of the brain (Fig. 11-3). These veins are highly variable both in number and configuration. In general, the superficial veins are arranged in a wheel or spoke-like pattern. They radiate outward toward the calvarium with the stem of the Sylvian fissure representing the hub.[12] The superficial veins drain into the dural sinuses (see below). Abundant anastomoses between the superficial and deep groups of draining veins are present but are normally quite inconspicuous.

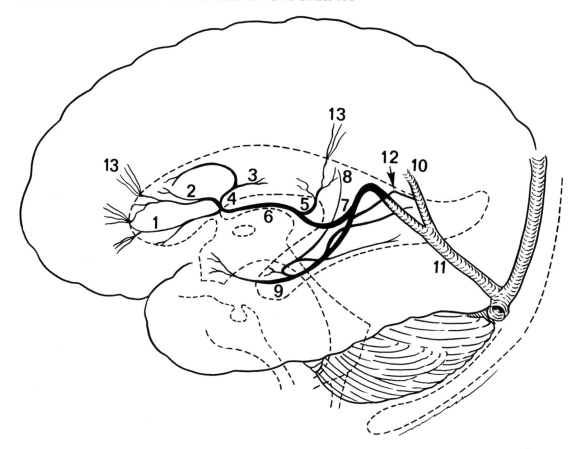

Three large superficial cerebral veins can often be identified: the Sylvian or superficial middle cerebral vein, the vein of Trolard, and the vein of Labbé. The **superficial middle cerebral vein** runs along the surface of the Sylvian fissure (Figs. 11-3, arrow 1). It is the most variable of all the superficial veins.[51] The superficial middle cerebral vein drains the opercular areas adjacent to the Sylvian fissure, curves anteriorly around the tip of the temporal lobe, then empties into the cavernous or sphenoparietal sinus. It anastomoses with the deep cerebral venous system (via uncal, insular, and basal veins) and with other superficial veins and dural sinuses. It also communicates with the facial veins and pterygoid plexus.[14]

Rather large, but inconstant end-to-end anastomoses between the superficial middle cerebral vein and superior sagittal sinus or transverse sinus may be present. These variable channels are called the anastomotic **veins of Trolard and Labbé**, respectively. The anastomotic vein of Trolard courses over the mid-

Fig. 11-4. Anatomic drawing of the subependymal veins of the lateral ventricle (lateral view). *(Adapted from Wolf BS, Huang YP: Am J Roentgenol 91:406–426, 1964)* **1.** Septal vein. **2.** Anterior caudate veins. **3.** Terminal vein. **4.** Thalamostriate vein. **5.** Direct lateral vein. **6.** Internal cerebral vein. **7.** Vein of Galen. **8.** Inferior ventricular vein. **9.** Basal vein of Rosenthal. **10.** Inferior sagittal sinus. **11.** Straight sinus. **12.** Medial atrial vein. **13.** Medullary veins.

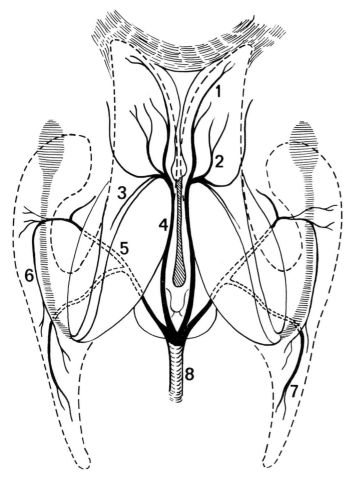

Fig. 11-5. Anatomic drawing of subependymal veins as seen from above. Most of the medial draining group is shown. *(Adapted from Wolf BS, Huang YP: Am J Roentgenol 91:406–426, 1964)* **1.** Septal vein. **2.** Anterior caudate vein. **3.** Terminal vein. **4.** Internal cerebral vein. **5.** Basal vein of Rosenthal. **6.** Inferior ventricular vein. **7.** Lateral atrial vein. **8.** Vein of Galen.

hemispheric convexity joining the posterior aspect of the Sylvian vein with the SSS (Fig. 11-3, arrow 2).[25] In 70% of anatomic specimens, the vein of Labbé arises as a posterior continuation of the superficial middle cerebral vein that crosses the posterior temporal lobe diagonally and joins the transverse sinus (Fig. 11-3, arrow 3). These anastomotic veins cross the subdural space to enter the dural sinuses.

Deep Cerebral Veins. A single, but nevertheless, important exception to the generalization that the brain is drained radially in a centrifugal fashion is that the deep cerebral white matter and basal ganglia drain centrally via medullary veins into the subependymal veins of the lateral ventricles.[45]

A number of small, deep **medullary veins** originate 1 to 2 cm below the cortical gray matter. They pass through the deep cerebral white matter in a perpendicular direction, draining into subependymal veins that course along the walls of the lateral ventricles. The medullary veins are distributed radially along the anterior and superior surface of the frontal horn, the superolateral angle of the body of the lateral ventricle, and the posterior and superolateral surface of the atrium (Fig. 11-4, number 13). The occipital and temporal lobes have fewer deep medullary veins.[21, 22]

After receiving the medullary veins the subependymal veins aggregate into larger tributaries that drain into the internal cerebral vein and great cerebral vein (vein of Galen). The subependymal veins are conveniently divided into medial and lateral draining groups. Of all the **lateral subependymal veins** the *thalamostriate vein* is usually the largest (Fig. 11-4,

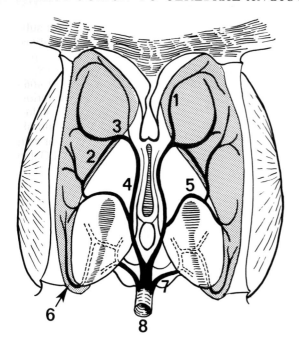

Fig. 11-6. Anatomic drawing of the subependymal veins as seen from above. The lateral draining group and their relationships to caudate nuclei and thalami are shown. The caudate nuclei are dotted. *(Modified from Wolf BS, Huang YP: Am J Roentgenol 9:406–426, 1964)* **1.** Anterior caudate vein. **2.** Terminal vein. **3.** Thalamostriate vein. **4.** Internal cerebral vein. **5.** Direct lateral vein. **6.** Inferior ventricular vein. **7.** Basal vein of Rosenthal. **8.** Vein of Galen.

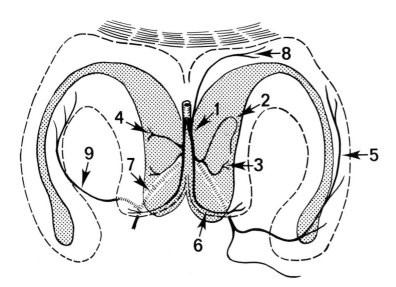

Fig. 11-7. Anatomic drawing of the subependymal veins as seen from in front, slightly above. The lateral ventricles are indicated **(dotted lines).** The caudate nuclei are shaded. *(Modified from Wolf BS, Huang YP: Am J Roentgenol 9:406–426, 1964)* **1.** Internal cerebral vein. **2.** Thalamostriate vein. **3.** Anterior caudate vein. **4.** Direct lateral vein. **5.** Inferior ventricular vein. **6.** Septal vein. **7.** Basal vein of Rosenthal. **8.** Medial atrial vein. **9.** Lateral atrial vein.

number 4). This vessel is formed by the union of the *terminal vein*, a vessel that runs beneath the stria terminalis between the thalamus and body of the caudate nucleus (Fig. 11-4, number 3) and the *anterior caudate veins* that drain the head of the caudate nucleus (Fig. 11-4, number 2). The thalamostriate vein curves anteroinferiorly over the thalamus to enter the internal cerebral vein behind the foramen of Monro.[4, 44, 50]

The *direct lateral vein* is another member of the lateral subependymal group. It lies posterior to the thalamostriate vein. The direct lateral vein begins in the superolateral corner of the ventricle and courses medially over the thalamus to reach the internal cerebral vein (Figs. 11-4, number 5; 11-6, number 5; and 11-7, number 4).

The most important of the **medial subependymal veins** is the *septal vein*. This vessel receives intramedullary tributaries that reach the anterior wall of the lateral ventricle just in front of the head of the caudate nucleus. The septal vein initially passes medially along the flared rostral portion of the frontal horns, then courses posteromedially along the septum pellucidum (Figs. 11-5, number 1; and 11-7, number 6). It has a slight, laterally convex curve as it passes around the pillars of the fornix to enter the internal cerebral vein behind the foramen of Monro.[53] This forms the so-called "true venous angle" (*i.e.*, on cerebral angiography it indicates the position of the intraventricular foramen). Occasionally, the septal vein follows an anomalous course, running more posterior before entering the internal cerebral vein. This forms the so-called "false venous angle" (*i.e.*, it does not demarcate the foramen of Monro).

Other subependymal veins assist in draining the deep cerebral white matter and gray nuclei. Both lateral and medial *atrial veins* as well as inferior *ventricular veins* may drain the ventricular walls (Figs. 11-5 thru 11-7).

A number of **thalamic veins** can sometimes be identified. The *superior thalamic vein*, the largest and most constant of these vessels, follows a course roughly parallel to the internal cerebral vein. It terminates in the basal vein of Rosenthal or the posterior aspect of the internal cerebral vein.[50] The thalamic veins are discussed in further detail in Chapter 12 since they are usually identified on posterior fossa angiograms.

The **basal vein of Rosenthal** (BVR) usually arises in the Sylvian fissure (Figs. 11-5, number 5; 11-6, number 7; 11-7, number 7). Formed from the confluence of the anterior and deep middle cerebral veins, it also receives the tributaries from the insula and the cerebral peduncles.[49] Also joining the BVR are veins of the temporal horn and medial temporal lobe as well as inferior striate veins that drain the inferior aspects of the basal ganglia. After receiving these tributaries, the basal vein courses posteriorly around the cerebral peduncle and across the colliculi to the vein of Galen. Midway in its course, the BVR may also receive the lateral mesencephalic vein, a collateral channel joining the BVR with the superior petrosal sinus.[44]

The internal cerebral veins (ICV) are paired structures that originate behind the foramen of Monro. They are formed by the union of the septal and thalamostriate veins (Figs. 11-5, number 4; 11-6, number 4; 11-7, number 1). Just after its origin, the ICV enters the subarachnoid space of the transverse cerebral fissure. Running posteriorly near the midline in the velum interpositum, the ICV follows a somewhat sinusoidal course that is at first concave inferiorly, than convex. As it passes posteriorly, the ICV receives a number of small subependymal tributaries.

Under or just behind the splenium of the corpus callosum the paired ICVs unite with the basal veins to form the great cerebral vein or **vein of Galen** (VG). The vein of Galen is a short, U-shaped structure that curves posterosuperiorly around the splenium. It terminates near the apex of the tentorial incisura where it joins the inferior sagittal sinus to form the straight sinus (Figs. 11-5, number 8; and 11-6, number 8). The vein of Galen also receives occipital, posterior pericallosal, mesencephalic, and superior cerebellar tributaries.[23, 45]

338

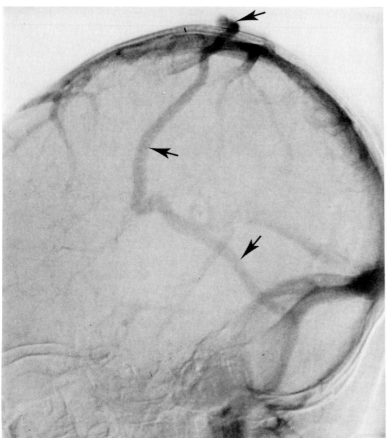

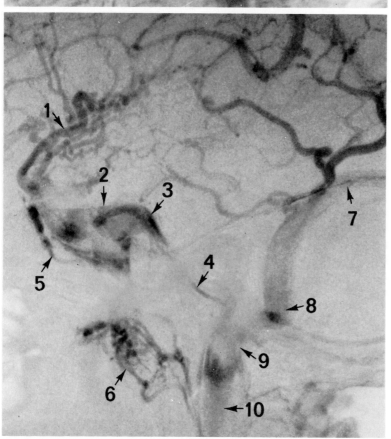

Fig. 11-8. Normal left carotid angiogram (**A,** late venous phase, lateral view). A prominent scalp vein is indicated **(arrows).** Normal left internal carotid angiogram (**B,** venous phase, lateral view). **1.** Multiple superficial middle cerebral veins. **2.** Cavernous sinus. **3.** Clival venous plexus. **4.** Inferior petrosal sinus. **5.** Sphenoparietal sinus. **6.** Pterygoid venous plexus. **7.** Transverse sinus. **8.** Sigmoid sinus. **9.** Jugular bulb. **10.** Internal jugular vein.

A

B

NORMAL ANGIOGRAPHIC ANATOMY

Scalp Veins

While scalp veins may be visualized with selective external carotid angiography they are only occasionally seen in normal internal or common carotid studies (Fig. 11-8A). Filling of scalp veins at carotid angiography has been identified with a variety of lesions such as arteriovenous malformations or neoplasms involving the scalp, sinus pericranii, increased intracranial pressure, and dural sinus occlusion or thrombosis.[46]

Veins of the Face and Neck

A number of the facial veins and their tributaries can be seen on the late venous phase films of normal cerebral angiograms. The pterygoid plexus and anterior facial vein are often identified as are the petrosal and cavernous sinuses (Fig. 11-8B). The pterygoid plexus is seen as a network of vessels that lies over the infratemporal fossa and pterygoid muscles, posterior to the pterygopalatine fossa. The pharyngeal veins are less commonly seen and lie posterior and slightly inferior to the pterygoid plexus. The anterior facial vein is frequently identified on common carotid studies. Orbital and ophthalmic veins are also seen on selective internal carotid angiograms.[37A]

Diploic and Meningeal Veins

Diploic and meningeal veins are rarely seen in normal carotid angiograms. Very prominent diploic veins may develop in the presence of an arteriovenous malformation that involves the scalp or dura.[18] Occasionally, meningeal veins are seen with vascular malformations. The middle meningeal veins are sometimes visualized with a traumatic arteriovenous fistula or epidural hematoma (see Fig. 3-23).

Dural Venous Sinuses

Many of the dural sinuses are clearly delineated on the venous phase of cerebral angiograms. On the lateral view, the **superior sagittal sinus** appears as a curvilinear structure hugging the inner table of the skull. Usually the SSS originates near the crista galli and gradually increases in size as it extends posteriorly along the inner table of the skull to the torcular Herophili (Fig. 11-9, arrow 1). Occa-

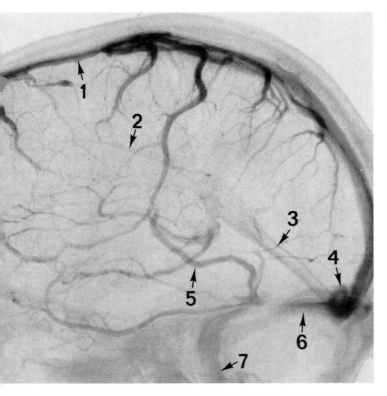

Fig. 11-9. Normal left internal carotid angiogram (venous phase, lateral view). **1.** Superior sagittal sinus. **2.** Inferior sagittal sinus. **3.** Straight sinus. **4.** Torcular Herophili. **5.** Vein of Labbé. **6.** Transverse sinus. **7.** Sigmoid sinus.

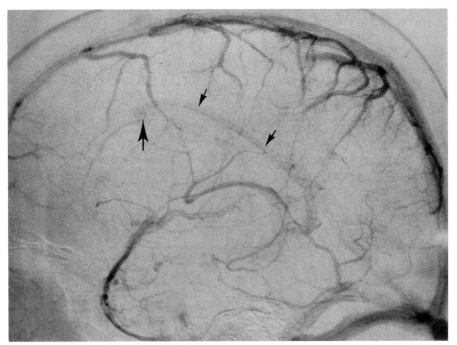

Fig. 11-10. Left internal carotid angiogram (venous phase, lateral view) of a pituitary adenoma. The normal inferior sagittal sinus is particularly well seen **(small arrows).** Note the characteristic anterior "hook" **(large arrow)** where a large vein draining the medial frontal lobe joins the ISS.

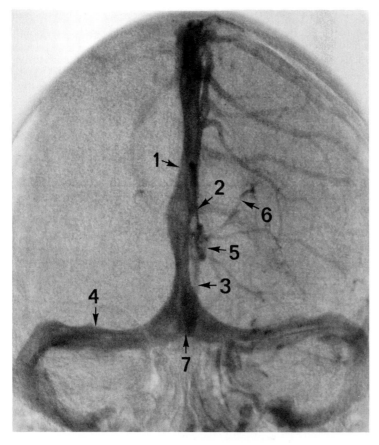

Fig. 11-11. Left internal carotid angiogram (venous phase, AP view). The superior sagittal sinus drains equally into the transverse sinuses. **1.** Superior sagittal sinus. **2.** Inferior sagittal sinus. **3.** Straight sinus. **4.** Transverse sinus. **5.** Internal cerebral vein. **6.** Thalamostriate vein. **7.** Torcular Herophili.

sionally, the SSS is absent anteriorly and is formed more posteriorly by the union of several large superior cerebral veins (Fig. 3-30).[24] This anatomic variation should not be mistaken for SSS displacement due to an extra-axial fluid collection.

The **inferior sagittal sinus** lies within the inferior free edge of the falx cerebri and is best seen on lateral views (Fig. 11-9). The degree of opacification of the ISS and its tributaries varies. A "button-hook" shaped acute bend is often present at the anterior margin of the ISS where it is formed by a tuft of tributaries from the falx, corpus callosum, and cingulate gyrus (Fig. 11-10).[33] Near its origin, the ISS is closer to the inner table of the skull. As it arcs posteriorly, the ISS follows an increasingly more inferior course toward its union with the internal cerebral veins. It usually overlies the SSS on AP views (Fig. 11-11, arrow 2).

Formed by the confluence of the ISS and vein of Galen, the **straight sinus** extends posteroinferiorly toward the internal occipital protuberance and is almost always well delineated on lateral cerebral angiograms (Fig. 11-9, arrow 3). On anteroposterior views this vessel is usually superimposed on other prominent midline venous structures and hence may be difficult to identify (Fig. 11-11, arrow 3).

As one of the smallest major dural sinuses, the **occipital sinus** is rarely well defined on normal carotid angiograms. The occipital sinus extends posterosuperiorly from the jugular vein or vertebral venous plexus to the torcular Herophili (Fig. 11-12, arrow 3).

The **torcular Herophili** and the **transverse sinuses** are easily identified. On the AP view, the torcular and transverse sinuses usually form an inverted "T" with the superior sagittal sinus (Fig. 11-11). Venous drainage into the transverse sinuses is often quite asymmetric (Fig. 11-12). From their origin at the torcular Herophili, the transverse sinuses usually slope downward slightly toward their anteroinferior continuations, the sigmoid sinuses. On lateral cerebral angiograms, the **sigmoid sinuses** have an anteriorly convex curve as they course inferomedially toward the jugular foramen where they terminate by becoming the internal jugular veins (Fig. 11-8, arrow 8; and 11-9, arrow 7).

Near its origin each **internal jugular vein** has a prominent enlargement, the jugular bulb, that is easily identified on the late venous phase of both AP and lateral angiograms (Fig. 11-8, arrow 9). After they exit from the skull base, the IJVs can be seen for some distance as they course inferiorly within the cervical neurovascular bundle (Fig. 11-8, arrow 10).

The various dural sinuses at the skull base (the **superior** and **inferior petrosal sinuses, cavernous sinus,** and **clival venous plexuses**) are inconstantly visualized at carotid angiography. Obscured by the dense bone of the skull base, they are best delineated with careful subtraction prints (Fig. 11-8).

Superficial Cerebral Veins

On lateral venous phase angiograms, the **superficial cortical veins** resemble the spokes of a wheel radiating from the hub (represented by the Sylvian fissure)[12] Six to eight major superficial vessels of roughly similar caliber are usually identified. The anastomotic **vein of Trolard** may be single or double; it courses superiorly from the Sylvian fissure to the SSS (Fig. 11-13, arrow 1). The inferior anastomotic *vein of Labbé* connects the Sylvian region with the transverse sinus (Figs. 11-13 and 11-14).

The **superficial middle cerebral vein** generally follows the course of the Sylvian fissure, curving anteroinferiorly to enter the sphenoparietal sinus or pterygoid plexus (Fig. 11-8).

Deep Cerebral Veins

While early reports indicated that radiographic visualization of the deep **medullary veins** indicated the presence of significant pathology, more recent studies demonstrate that these vessels are normally seen with selective magnification subtraction angiograms.[21] They are best identified on the lateral view where they are seen as small, fine vessels of uniform caliber that course perpendicular to the ventricular ependyma. They are most often identified adjacent to the frontal horn, body, and atrium of the lateral ventricle (Fig. 11-15).

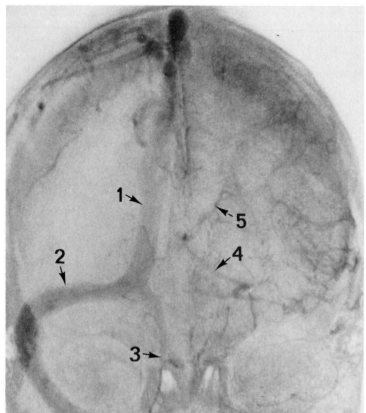

Fig. 11-12. Left internal carotid angiogram (venous phase, AP view). Note absence of the left transverse sinus. The superior sagittal sinus **(arrow 1)** ends in the right transverse sinus **(arrow 2).** The occipital sinus **(arrow 3),** left basal vein of Rosenthal **(arrow 4)** and thalamostriate vein **(arrow 5)** are well seen.

Fig. 11-13. Left internal carotid angiogram (venous phase, lateral view). **1.** Vein of Trolard. **2.** Vein of Galen. **3.** Internal cerebral vein. **4.** Basal vein of Rosenthal.

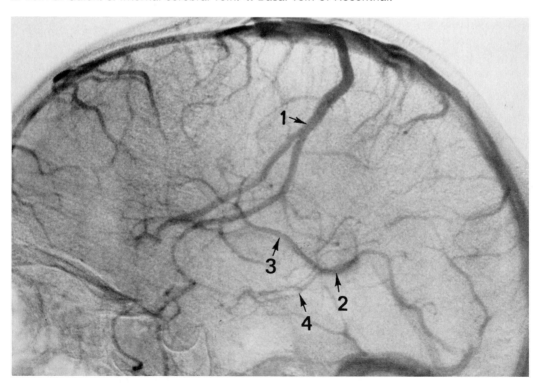

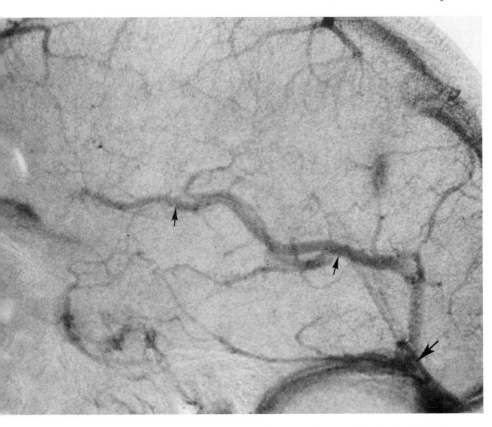

Fig. 11-14. Left internal carotid angiogram (venous phase, lateral view). A large anastomotic vein of Labbé **(small arrows)** drains into the transverse sinus **(large arrow).**

The **deep middle cerebral** vein is formed by the union of several insular veins that drain anteroinferiorly to form a common stem near the anterior aspect of the island of Reil (Fig. 11-16). The deep middle cerebral vein courses medially within the Sylvian fissure (Fig. 11-17, arrow 2). It unites with anterior cerebral and inferior striate veins to form the **basal vein of Rosenthal** (BVR). The radiographic appearance of the BVR is quite characteristic (Fig. 11-17, arrows 3 and 4). In the AP view it resembles the leg of a frog lying on its back with its toes pointing anterolaterally. The "ankle" corresponds to the medial aspect of the uncus, the knee to the most lateral aspect of the BVR as it courses around the cerebral peduncles.[23] On lateral views, the BVR follows an anteriorly concave curve as it runs posterosuperiorly in the ambient cistern to join the internal cerebral vein (Fig. 11-13, arrow 4). The posterior segment of the BVR may be hypoplastic. In such instances it may drain anteriorly into the basilar plexus, via a lateral mesencephalic vein to the superior petrosal sinus, or posteriorly via the transverse sinus.[2]

The **vein of Galen** forms an arc under the splenium of the corpus callosum, curving posterosuperiorly towards the tentorial apex. It is well seen on the lateral view (Fig. 11-13, arrow 2) but is often obscured by the overlying SSS on AP projections.[48]

Subependymal Veins

The various subependymal veins are well seen on both AP and lateral venous phase angiograms. They outline the margins of the lateral

(Text continued on p. 346)

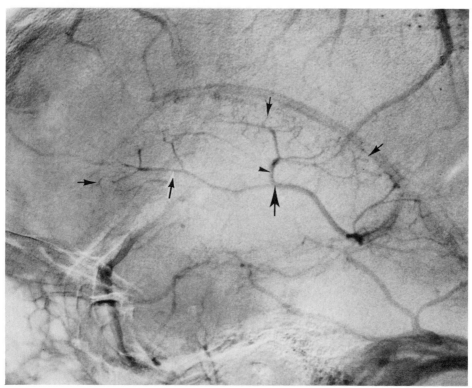

Fig. 11-15. Left internal carotid angiogram (venous phase, lateral view). Numerous tiny medullary veins **(small arrows)** drain into the subependymal veins. A "false" venous angle, **(large arrow)** is formed by the junction of the septal **(outlined arrow)** and direct lateral **(arrowhead)** veins. Note the prominent inferior sagittal sinus.

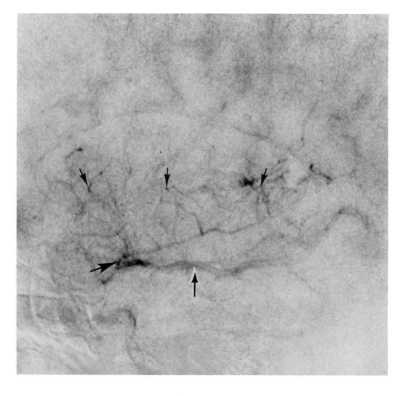

Fig. 11-16. Left internal carotid angiogram (late capillary phase, lateral view). Multiple insular veins **(small arrows)** unite to form a common trunk **(large arrow)** that extends medially under the anterior pole of the insula and then backward into the basal vein of Rosenthal **(outlined arrow).**

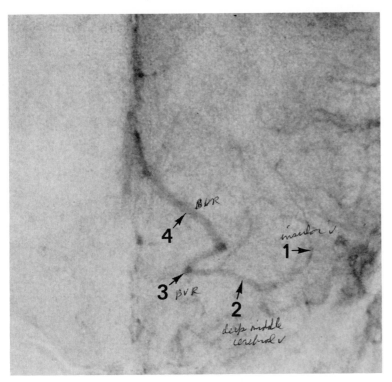

Fig. 11-17. Left internal carotid angiogram (early venous phase, AP view). The basal vein of Rosenthal is particulary well seen.
1. Insular vein. **2.** Deep middle cerebral vein.
3. Basal vein of Rosenthal medial to the uncus.
4. Peduncular segment of the basal vein.

see p 343 for description

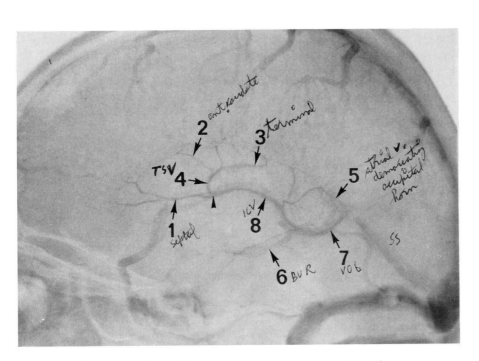

Fig. 11-18. Left internal carotid angiogram (venous phase, lateral view). The arrowhead indicates a true venous angle and demarcates the foramen of Monro. **1.** Septal vein. **2.** Anterior caudate veins. **3.** Terminal vein. **4.** Thalamostriate vein. **5.** Atrial vein (demarcating the occipital horn). **6.** Basal vein of Rosenthal. **7.** Vein of Galen. **8.** Internal cerebral vein.

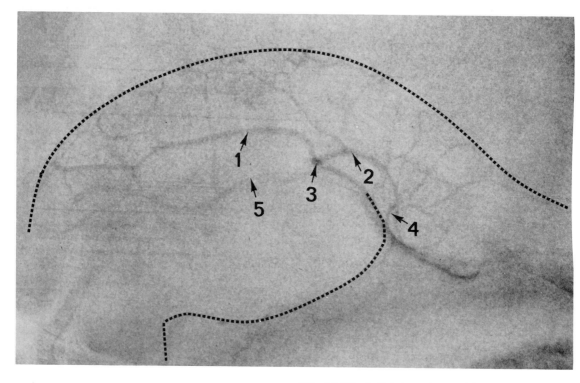

ventricles (Figs. 11-18, 11-19). The **septal vein** follows a straight or gently undulating posterior course as seen on the lateral view (Fig. 11-18, arrow 1). On AP projections, the anterior tributaries of the septal vein course medially along the anterior wall of the frontal horn (Fig. 11-20, arrow 1). When they reach the septum they form an obtuse angle with the main septal vein. This distinct angulation is termed the "septal point" and should lie between 1 to 1.5 mm from the midline (Fig. 11-20, large black arrow).[44, 53] The septal and caudate veins usually unite to form the *thalamostriate vein* (TSV). In the lateral view, the TSV receives the terminal vein and curves anteriorly along the stria terminalis (Fig. 11-18, arrow 4). The TSV and terminal vein thus demarcate the superior margin of the thalamus and inferomedial border of the caudate nucleus. On the AP view, the TSV has a characteristic double curve that resembles an antler (Fig. 11-20, arrow 4).[18] The superolateral aspect of the TSV represents the lateral margin of the lateral ventricle. Numerous other subependymal veins (*i.e.*, the direct lateral, atrial

Fig. 11-19. Left internal carotid angiogram (late venous phase, lateral view). The superficial veins have emptied; the subependymal veins form a partial outline of the lateral ventricle **(dotted line)**. Multiple anomalous veins are present. An anomalous septal vein **(arrow 1)** and lateral atrial vein **(arrow 2)** unite to form a common atrial vein **(arrow 3)**. Medial atrial veins **(arrow 4)** are also present. The internal cerebral vein **(arrow 5)** is also indicated.

Fig. 11-20. AP venous phase angiograms **(A, B). 1.** Septal vein (large arrow on septal point). **2.** Internal cerebral vein. **3.** Direct lateral vein. **4.** Thalamostriate vein. **5.** Atrial vein.

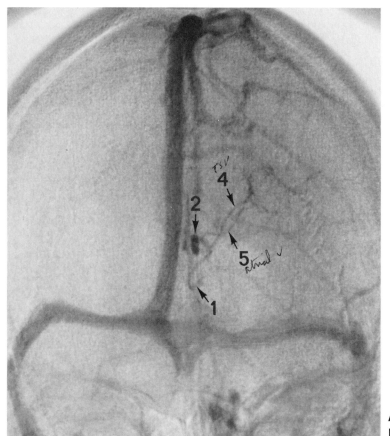

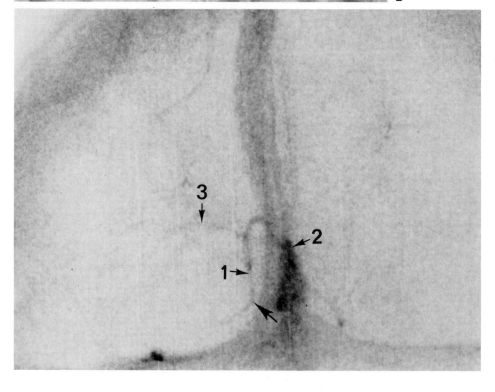

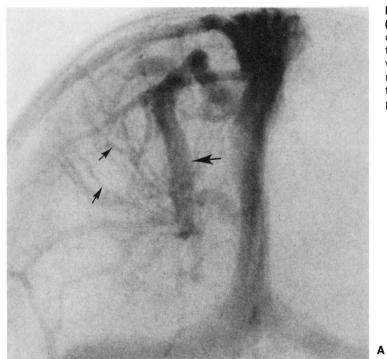

Fig. 11-21. AP **(A)** and lateral **(B)** venous phase angiograms of a venous angioma. Note tuft of enlarged medullary veins **(small arrows).** The arterial phase was normal. No arteriovenous shunting was present.

A

B

and inferior ventricular veins) can also be identified on normal carotid angiograms (Figs. 11-18 to 11-20).

The **internal cerebral vein** extends from the foramen of Monro to the vein of Galen (Figs. 11-18, arrow 8; and 11-19, arrow 5). Since the curved anterior and posterior segments of the ICV are superimposed on the AP view, the ICV appears as an elliptical area of increased density in this projection (Fig. 11-20, arrow 2).[18] Because the ICVs are paired structures, the most medial aspect of each vessel should lie within 2 mm of the midline as seen on AP venous phase angiograms.

CONGENITAL ANOMALIES AND MALFORMATIONS

Venous Angiomas

Intracranial venous angioma is a relatively common incidental finding at autopsy although it is an uncommon angiographic diagnosis.[41] The lesion has a characteristic "caput medusae," wedge-shaped appearance with its base at the meninges and its apex directed toward the ventricles.[13] Prominent medullary veins drain into a markedly enlarged transcortical cerebral vein (Fig. 11-21). The arterial phase is usually normal and no arteriovenous shunting is seen.[3, 15, 30, 39, 47] In the more common arteriovenous malformation, grossly enlarged arteries and multiple dilated draining veins with marked arteriovenous shunting are present (see below).

Sturge-Weber Syndome

Sturge-Weber syndrome (encephalofacial angiomatosis) is a regional angiomatous phacoma characterized by a hemifacial angioma confined to the trigeminal nerve distribution. There is a related angiomatosis of the ipsilateral cerebral leptomeninges that may also involve the ocular choroid.[19] The lesion primarily affects the occipital pole but may extend to involve the parietal and temporal lobes. Calcification appears after one to two years of age and is located in the second and third cortical layers. It occurs in a typical serpiginous configuration.[46A]

The angiographic findings are characteristic (Fig. 11-22). No arterial abnormalities are seen although a diffuse capillary blush may be present. There is a distinct paucity of superficial cortical veins beneath the area of leptomeningeal angiomatosis. Enlarged medullary veins and dilated, tortuous, deep cerebral veins provide collateral venous drainage.[6]

Maldevelopments and Congenital Anomalies of the Dural Sinuses

Malposition of the attached falx and superior sagittal sinus is associated with severe developmental anomalies such as hydranencephaly, cerebral hypoplasia, or absent corpus callosum with interhemispheric cyst.[35]

Chiari II Malformations are characterized by an abnormally low, elongated fourth ventricle, cerebellar hypoplasia, elongation of the inferior vermis, and an abnormal tentorium cerebelli (see Chapter 12). The quadrigeminal plate is often fused into a tectal spur, while the cerebellum grows upward through a malformed tentorial incisura.[33A–C] The slope of the tentorium in the midline is steeper than normal while its posterolateral attachments are unusually low.[54] The transverse sinuses and torcular Herophili are frequently located only a few millimeters above the foramen magnum (Fig. 11-23); the straight sinus appears more vertical and is often shorter than normal due to the broad tentorial hiatus and small posterior fossa.[19] An inferiorly positioned torcular with low transverse sinuses has also been identified with aqueduct stenosis and large congenital supratentorial cysts.[52]

Dandy-Walker Malformation is characterized by absence of the caudal vermian lobules and a markedly dilated fourth ventricle that probably represents a developmental anomaly of the posterior medullary velum.[29] Venous phase angiograms disclose an elevated, flattened vein of Galen with a high torcular positioned

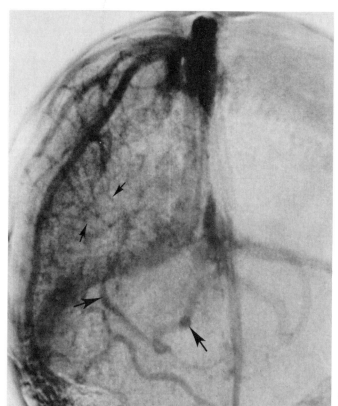

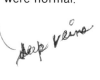

Fig- 11-22. AP **(A)** and lateral **(B)** venous phase angiograms of Sturge-Weber syndrome. Note the paucity of superficial cortical veins in the parietal-occipital area. Prominent medullary veins **(small arrows)** drain into markedly enlarged, tortuous subependymal veins **(large arrows).** The arterial and capillary phases were normal.

deep veins

A
B

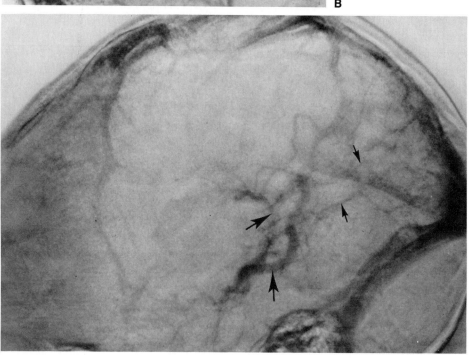

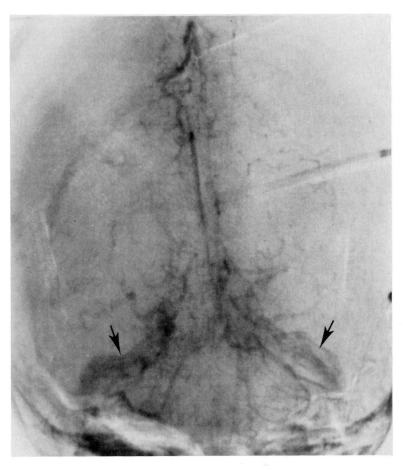

Fig. 11-23. AP venous phase angiogram of a Chiari II malformation. Note the abnormally low position of the transverse sinuses **(arrows).**

above the lambda. The transverse sinuses cross the lambdoid suture and angle steeply down to the sigmoid sinus.[19] High transverse sinuses and an elevated torcular Herophili can also be seen with **posterior fossa arachnoid cyst** although they are not positioned above the level of the lambda (Fig. 11-24). A normally formed, but displaced cerebellum and fourth ventricle are present in this developmental anomaly.[19]

High jugular bulb can occur secondary to congenital or acquired dehiscence of the bony plate that normally separates the jugular vein from the middle ear structures. This anomaly should not be mistaken for a vascular tumor of the middle ear.[31, 45A]

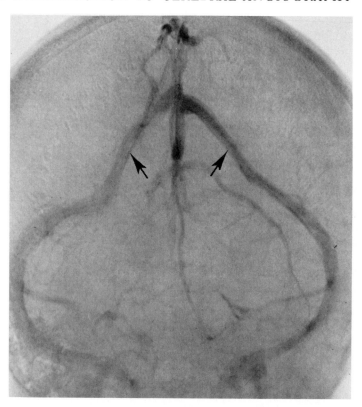

Fig. 11-24. AP venous phase angiogram of a huge congenital posterior fossa arachnoid cyst. Note marked elevation of the transverse sinuses **(arrows).**

ABNORMALITIES OF THE CEREBRAL VENOUS SYSTEM

Displacement or Occlusion of Dural Sinuses

Compression of the SSS by trauma or neonatal calvarial molding has been reported (Fig. 11-31).[34] Extradural masses such as neoplasm or epidural hematoma can displace the dural sinuses away from the calvarium (Figs. 11-25, 11-26). Tumors such as meningiomas may also compress or occlude the dural sinuses.

The transverse and sigmoid sinuses may become occluded secondary to mastoid inflammatory disease (Fig. 11-27). Venous sinus thrombosis can also be associated with trauma, dehydration, or hypercoagulable states although it may occur in the absence of any predisposing condition.[42] While intracranial circulation time may be prolonged, characteristic angiographic findings include delayed venous emptying, occluded or absent dural sinuses (Fig. 11-28), increased trans-medullary drainage into the deep cerebral venous systems, and marked tortuousity and irregularity of the cortical veins (Fig. 11-29). The cavernous sinus may become compressed or occluded by pituitary or skull base tumors as well as by primary venous thrombosis.[9]

Displacement of Superficial Cortical Veins

Epidural or subdural masses or fluid collections may displace the superficial cerebral veins from the calvarial vault (Fig. 11-30). Elongation and stretching of the bridging cortical veins may be striking (Fig. 11-31).[20] Focal intraparenchymal lesions may also cause localized deformation or displacement of the superficial cerebral veins (Fig. 11-32).

Displacement of Subependymal Veins

The subependymal veins are invaluable in the angiographic localization of deep median and

(Text continued on p. 359)

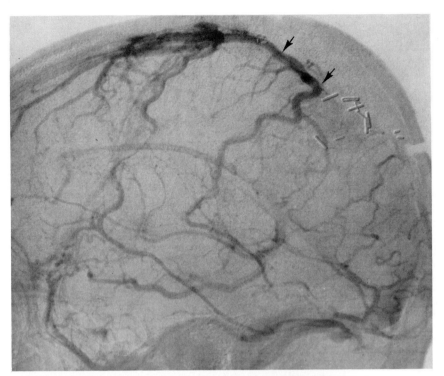

A

B

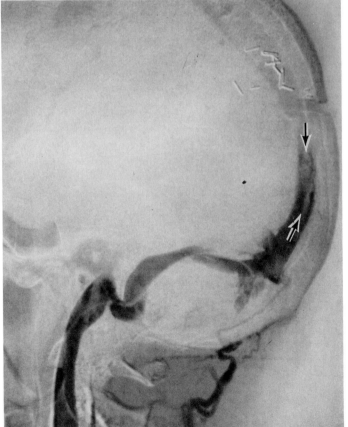

Fig. 11-25. Left internal carotid angiogram (**A,** venous phase, lateral view) of a recurrent parasagittal meningioma. The superior sagittal sinus is displaced away from the inner table of the skull **(arrows)** and occluded near the previous operative site. Left internal jugular venogram **(B).** Same patient as Figure 11-25A. The SSS is occluded; note the negative filling defect caused by tumor growing within the sinus **(arrows).**

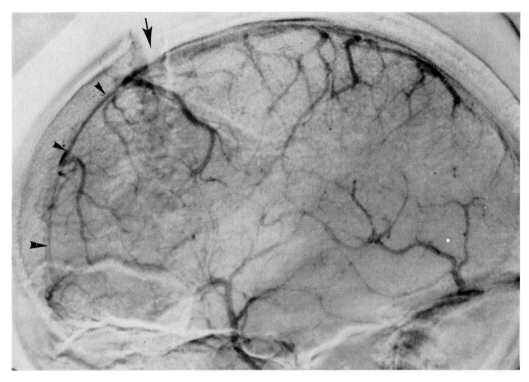

Fig. 11-26. Left common carotid angiogram (venous phase, lateral view) of traumatic diastasis of the coronal suture **(large arrow).** An epidural hematoma displaces the anterior SSS away from the calvarium **(arrowheads).**

Fig. 11-27. AP **(A)** and lateral **(B)** venous phase films in a four-year-old child with acute mastoiditis. The right transverse sinus is occluded **(outlined arrows).** Note marked collateral drainage via the superficial middle cerebral and ophthalmic veins, occipital, superior petrosal, and cavernous sinuses **(black arrows).**

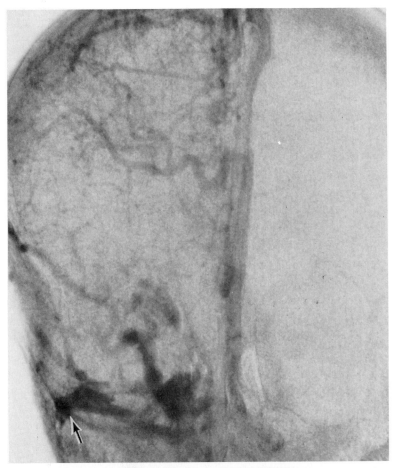

A
B

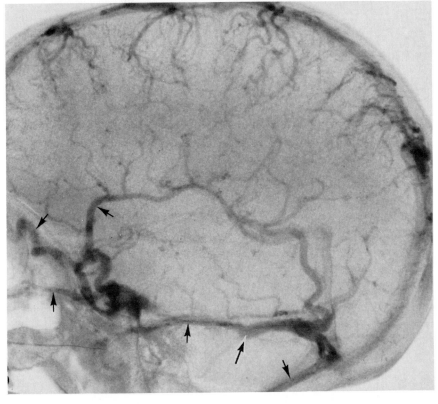

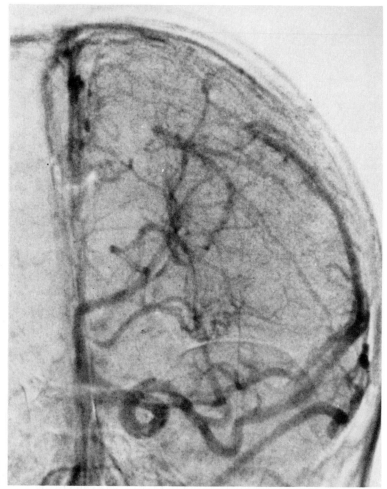

A

B

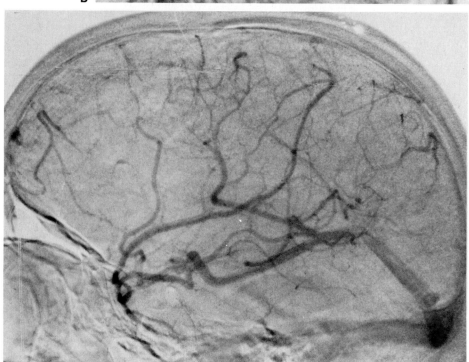

◀ **Fig. 11-28.** AP **(A)** and lateral **(B)** venous phase angiograms in a patient with thrombosis of the anterior segment of the superior sagittal sinus. Note the prominent subependymal and cortical veins providing collateral drainage to the superficial middle cerebral veins and posterior dural sinuses.

Fig. 11-29. Left internal carotid angiogram (venous phase, lateral view). This 34-year-old post-partum female had SSS thrombosis. Multiple cortical veins are also occluded as indicated by the paucity of superficial veins in the frontal and anterior parietal areas.

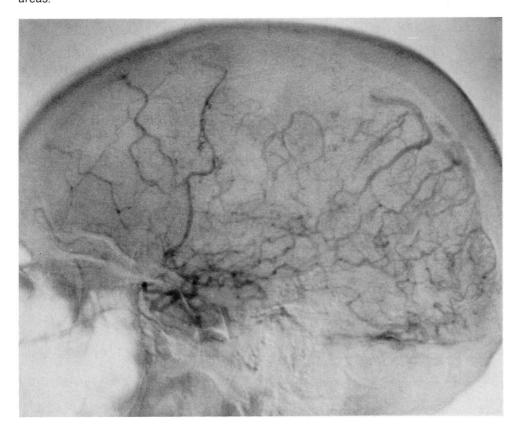

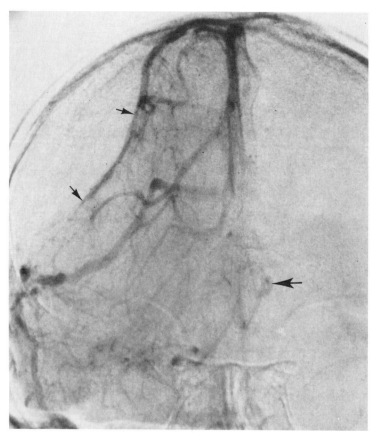

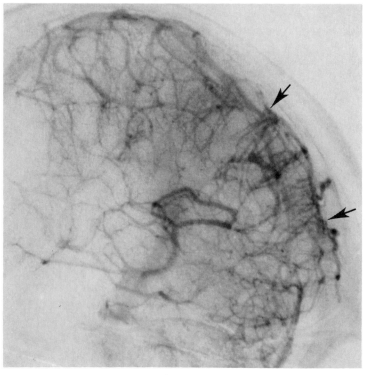

Fig. 11-30. Right common carotid angiogram (**A,** venous phase, AP view) of a large chronic subdural hematoma that displaces the cortical veins away from the inner table of the calvarium **(small arrows).** Note displacement of the thalamostriate and internal cerebral veins across the midline **(large arrows).** Left internal carotid angiogram (**B,** early venous phase, oblique view). An acute subdural hematoma, represented by a small crescentic extra-axial fluid collection, has displaced the cortical veins away from the inner table of the skull **(arrows).** Routine AP and lateral views failed to demonstrate the lesion.

A
B

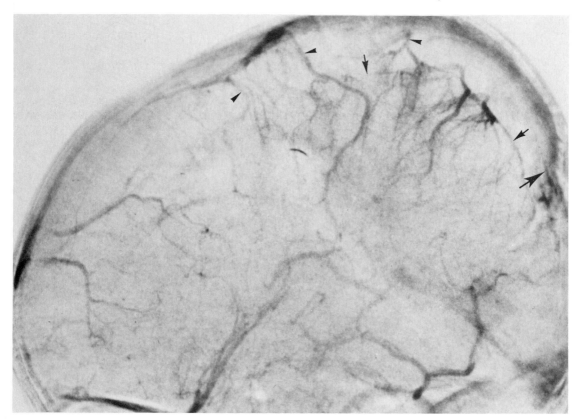

Fig. 11-31. Left common carotid angiogram (venous phase, arterial view). This shows a two-year-old child with a depressed occipital skull fracture compressing the superior sagittal sinus **(large arrow).** A large subdural hematoma has displaced the brain and accompanying cortical veins away from the calvarium **(small arrows).** Note stretching of the cortical veins **(arrowheads)** as they must bridge the subdural space to reach the SSS.

paramedian pathologic processes since there is a paucity of arterial markers in these areas.[40]

Subfalcine herniation of the lateral ventricles also shifts the subependymal veins across the midline. Displaced thalamostriate and internal cerebral veins are easily identified on AP venous phase angiograms (Fig. 11-30A). If a mass effect is sufficiently large the TSV and anterior aspect of the ICV will be significantly displaced. However, the posterior portion of the ICV is tethered in the midline by the vein of Galen which is anchored within the rigid falcotentorial junction. As the ICV returns to the midline, it may form an "alpha" configuration with the anteriorly herniated TSV (Fig. 11-33).

On lateral views, the subependymal veins may be displaced along their anteroposterior axis (Figs. 11-34, 11-35). Closure (Fig. 11-36) or widening of the venous angle formed by the TSV can sometimes be identified with large frontal or thalamic masses respectively.

(Text continued on p. 363)

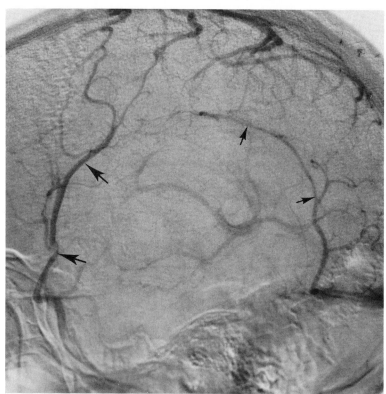

Fig. 11-32. Left internal carotid angiogram (venous phase, lateral view) of a huge cystic ganglioglioma of the temporal lobe. The superficial middle cerebral vein is displaced anterosuperiorly **(large black arrows).** The vein of Labbé is displaced posterosuperiorly **(small black arrows).**

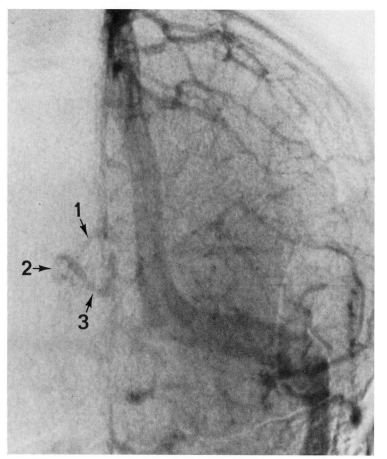

Fig. 11-33. Left internal carotid angiogram (venous phase, AP view) of a large left hemisphere mass. The thalamostriate vein **(arrow 1)** and anterior aspect of the internal cerebral vein **(arrow 2)** are displaced across the midline. Posteriorly, the ICV returns to the midline **(arrow 3)** where it is tethered by the vein of Galen. Note the "alpha" configuration of the displaced TSV and ICV.

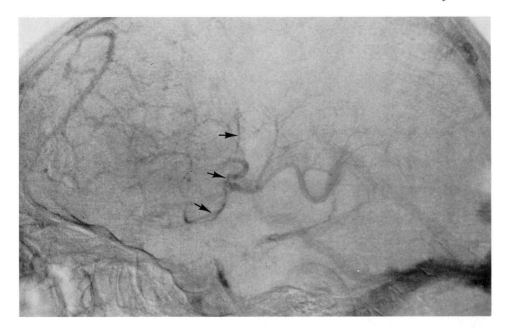

Fig. 11-34. Left internal carotid angiogram (venous phase, lateral view). A huge vascular tumor in the frontal lobe has displaced the lateral ventricle and its accompanying subependymal veins posteriorly **(arrows)**. Note the compression and buckling of the internal cerebral vein.

Fig. 11-35. Left internal carotid angiogram (venous phase, lateral view) of a large parietal-occipital meningioma. Note the prominent medullary veins **(arrowheads)**. Compression of the SSS was present. The subependymal veins are displaced anteriorly **(large arrows)**.

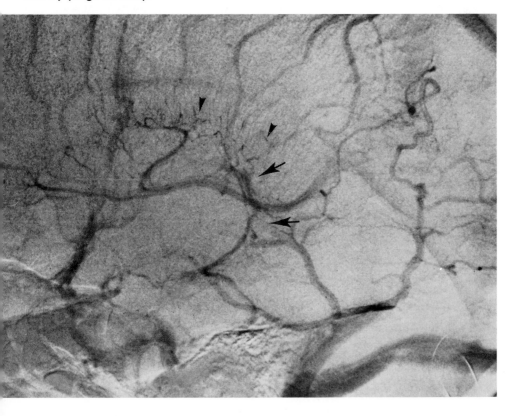

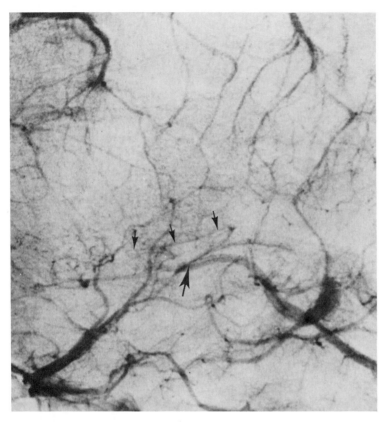

Fig. 11-36. Left internal carotid angiogram (venous phase, lateral view). A large frontal mass has depressed the roof of the lateral ventricle **(small arrows)** and compressed the venous angle at the foramen of Monro **(large arrow).**

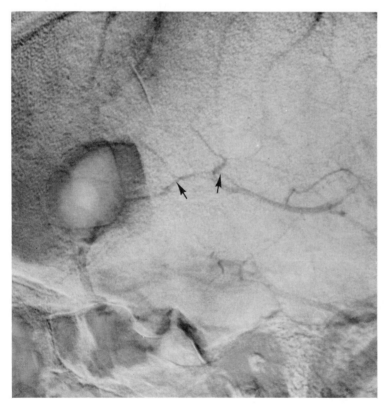

Fig. 11-37. Left internal carotid angiogram (venous phase, lateral view). A colloid cyst displaces the posterior segment of the septal vein superolaterally **(arrows).**

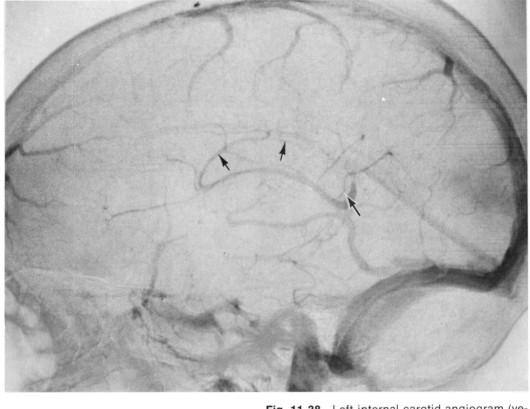

Fig. 11-38. Left internal carotid angiogram (venous phase, lateral view). A large avascular thalamic tumor elevates the terminal and thalamostriate veins **(small arrows)**. Note the broadened arc of the lateral atrial vein **(outlined arrow)** as it crosses over the enlarged thalamus. The venous angle is slightly increased.

Focal deformation of individual subependymal veins may be produced by masses in specifiic locations. For example, colloid cysts or mass lesions adjacent to the foramen of Monro characteristically displace the posterior aspect of septal vein superolaterally (Fig. 11-37). Thalamic masses often elevate the thalamostriate and terminal or direct lateral veins (Fig. 11-38).[40]

An intraventricular or intracerebral tumor with ventricular extension may distort the subependymal veins (Fig. 11-39). Some vascular intraventricular neoplasms (*i.e.*, choroid plexus papilloma or meningioma) may also be associated with a vascular blush and enlargement of the choroidal arteries and subependymal veins (Fig. 11-40).[32] Abnormal subependymal veins may occasionally be the only angiographic sign of a tumor originating within or invading the ventricular system.[1]

Since the subependymal veins outline the lateral ventricles, ventricular size can be determined by careful analysis of venous phase angiograms. In hydrocephalus, the thalamostriate and lateral atrial veins appear bowed outwardly on the AP projection (Fig. 11-41A). On capillary or early venous phase films, the enlarged lateral ventricle may appear as an avascular space (Fig. 11-41C). Lateral films usually disclose flattening and depression of the internal cerebral vein and basal vein of Rosenthal. The elongated, stretched subependymal veins outline the ventricular roof (Fig. 11-41B).

Absence of Cortical Veins

Diminution in the number of superficial cerebral veins occurs with Sturge-Weber syndrome (see above). Absence of cortical draining veins can sometimes be identified in areas of cortical ischemia or infarction (Fig. 11-42). Sufficiently large intracranial masses may compress adjacent superficial veins, producing a relatively avascular area on venous phase angiograms (Fig. 11-43).

Absence of Deep Cerebral Veins

The subependymal and deep cerebral veins show considerable normal variation. Deficiency of entire segments of the deep system is unusual, but has been reported in association with holoprosencephaly and other severe cerebral malformations.[37]

Enlargement of the Cortical Veins and Dural Sinuses

While mild to moderate enlargement of the cortical veins can occur in the presence of vascular neoplasms, marked engorgement of these vessels and the dural sinuses is seen primarily with venous angiomas and arteriovenous malformations (Fig. 11-44).

Angiomas involving the transverse sinus may produce massive enlargement of these structures. They are often associated with venous sinus thrombosis and retrograde filling of other dural sinuses (Fig. 11-45).[28]

Aneurysmal dilatation of the vein of Galen accompanies AVMs of the diencephalic vessels. Occasionally, branches of the posterior cerebral artery may communicate directly with the vein of Galen. The massively enlarged vein of Galen may produce obstructive hydrocephalus by compromising the cerebral aqueduct (Fig. 11-46).[28, 36, 42A] Secondary dilatation of the torcular Herophili may also accompany this condition.[47A]

Enlargement of the Deep Cerebral Veins

The deep medullary veins can be visualized with careful magnification-subtraction prints of normal selective angiographic studies. These vessels may enlarge as well as increase in number with a variety of pathologic processes (Fig. 11-47, small arrows). Malignant gliomas, arteriovenous malformations, vascular metastases, cortical vein or dural sinus thrombosis, Sturge-Weber syndrome, and encephalitis have all been reported in association with abnormally prominent medullary veins.[5] Enlarged subependymal veins may also be present (Fig. 11-47, large arrow).

Fig. 11-39. Left internal carotid angiogram (venous phase, lateral view) of a large lobulated ependymoma adjacent to the foramen of Monro. The septal vein is deformed and bowed superiorly **(arrows).**

Fig. 11-40. Left internal carotid angiogram (venous phase, lateral view) of an intraventricular meningioma confined to the temporal horn. Note the vascular blush **(arrows).**

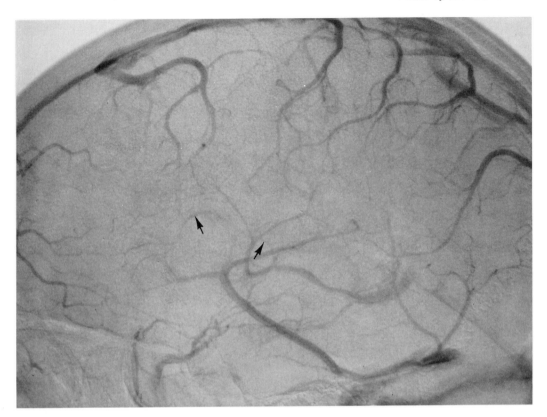

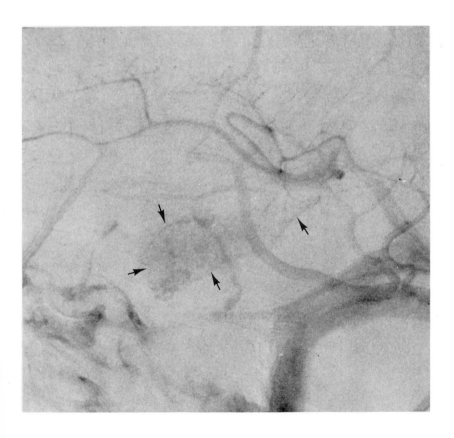

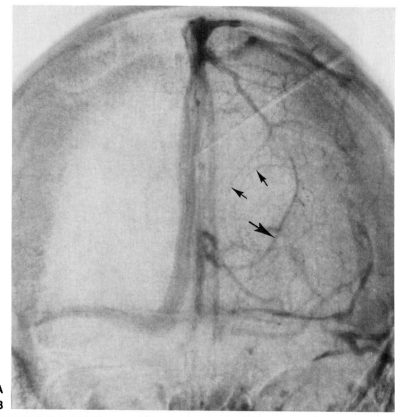

A
B

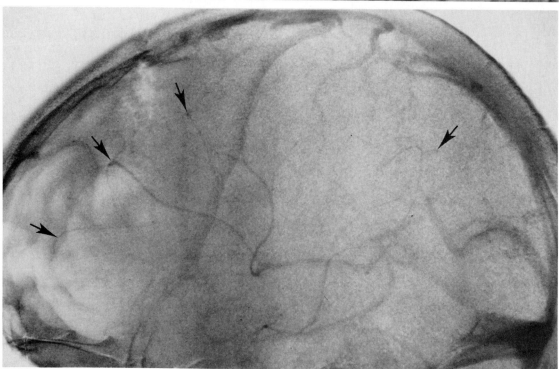

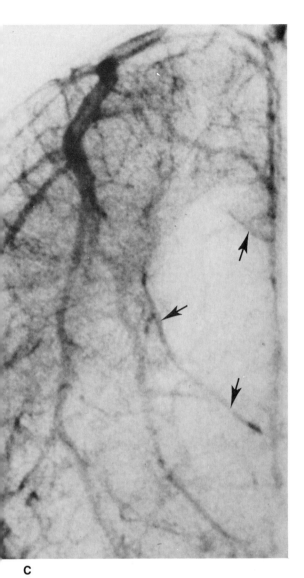

C

Fig. 11-41. Three patients with hydrocephalus. AP venous phase study **(A)** in a patient with aqueductal stenosis. The thalamostriate vein is bowed laterally **(large arrows)**. Note the enlarged occipital horn as indicated by the stretched, draped atrial veins **(small arrows)**. Lateral view **(B)** in another case of aqueduct stenosis. The stretched subependymal veins indicate the extent of the massive ventricular enlargement **(arrows)**. Late capillary-early venous phase **(C,** AP view) showing moderately severe ventricular enlargement. The cerebrospinal fluid-filled lateral ventricle is clearly outlined **(arrows)**.

Early Draining Veins

Early filling of a vein has been defined as the filling of a vein within the first three seconds after the beginning of intracerebral contrast circulation or as an abnormal sequence of venous filling.[7] The thalamostriate and internal cerebral veins are normally the first of the deep veins to fill following injection of contrast into the carotid artery. These veins are also opacified earlier than any other group (deep or superficial) except the posterior frontal and Sylvian (insular) veins. The basal vein usually appears next, followed by the septal vein which is often the last subependymal vein to become opacified. The dural sinuses fill relatively late with the ISS usually the last to appear. The superficial cortical veins are normally opacified before any of the dural sinuses with the exception of the vein of Trolard (which fills after the SS and SSS). The posterior frontal veins are the first of the superficial group to fill and are followed by the middle cerebral and parietal groups. The vein of Labbé, the occipital vein, and vein of Trolard are usually the last to become opacified.[11]

Arteriovenus shunting with early appearance of contrast in adjacent draining veins is not pathognomonic of any particular lesion (see Chapter 9). Early draining veins may be seen with primary and metastatic vascular neoplasms, angiomas and arteriovenous malformations, inflammatory disease (*i.e.*, encephalitis or cerebritis), trauma, toxic encephalopathy, cerebral ischemia with "luxury perfusion", and elipeptogenic foci (see Figs. 9-22 to 9-32 and 11-48 to 11-53).

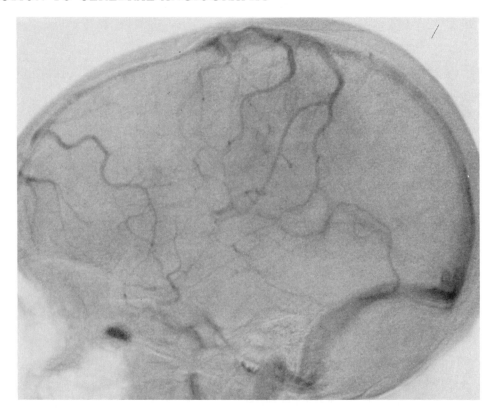

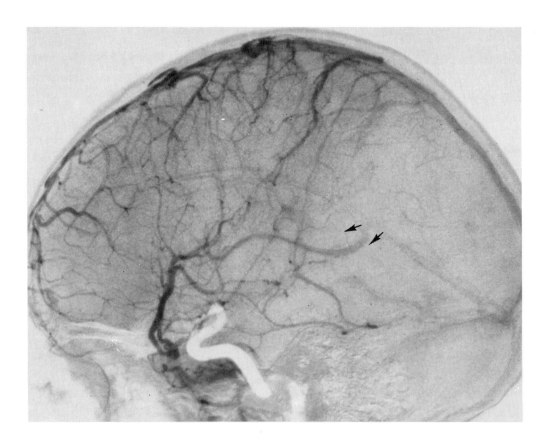

Fig. 11-42. Left internal carotid angiogram (venous phase, lateral view). Multiple ischemic infarcts are present. Note the paucity of cortical veins draining the devascularized areas.

Fig. 11-43. Left internal carotid angiogram (venous phase, lateral view) of a huge avascular tumor involving the parietal and occipital lobes. Note the virtual absence of draining veins in this area. The occipital horn of the lateral ventricle is displaced anteroinferiorly as indicated by the acute inferior angulation of the atrial veins **(arrows).**

Fig. 11-44. Left internal carotid angiogram (early venous phase, lateral view) of a large arteriovenous malformation involving the frontal and temporal lobes. Note massive enlargement of the superficial cerebral veins as well as the basal vein of Rosenthal and vein of Galen.

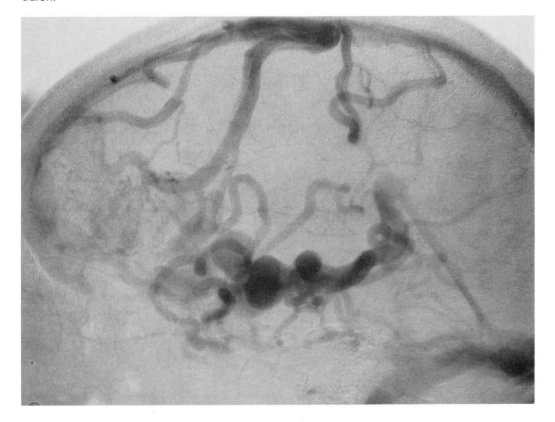

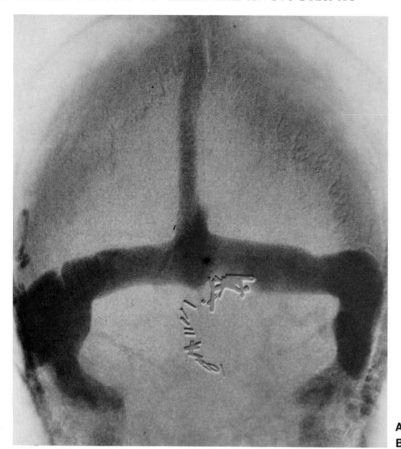

Fig. 11-45. AP **(A)** and lateral **(B)** left vertebral angiograms (venous phase) of a massive posterior fossa dural AVM. Note the huge transverse sinuses. The superior sagittal sinus, not ordinarily opacified during vertebral angiography, has been filled in retrograde fashion as a consequence of the increased venous pressure in the transverse sinuses.

A
B

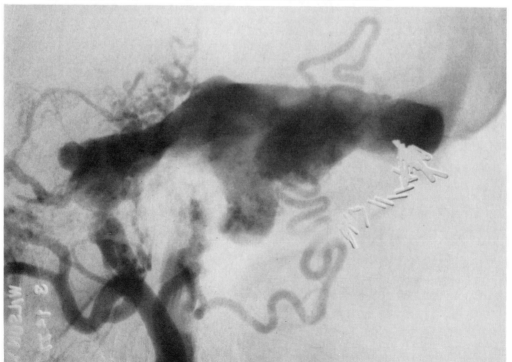

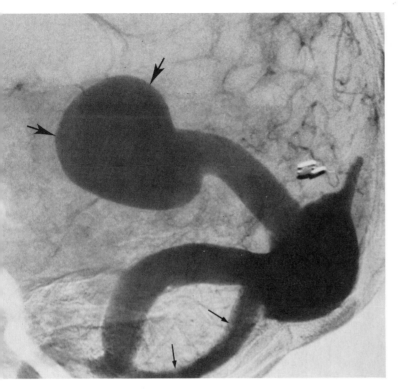

Fig. 11-46. Selective left vertebral angiogram (late arterial phase, lateral view). This was seen in a three-year-old child with aneurysmal dilatation of the vein of Galen **(large arrows).** Severe obstructive hydrocephalus was present. Note enlargement of all the draining sinuses including the torcular Herophili and occipital sinus **(small arrows).**

Fig. 11-47. Left internal carotid angiogram (early venous phase, lateral view) of a corpus callosum glioma. A vascular blush and multiple enlarged medullary veins **(small arrows)** are present. The anterior caudate and thalamostriate veins are also enlarged **(large arrow).**

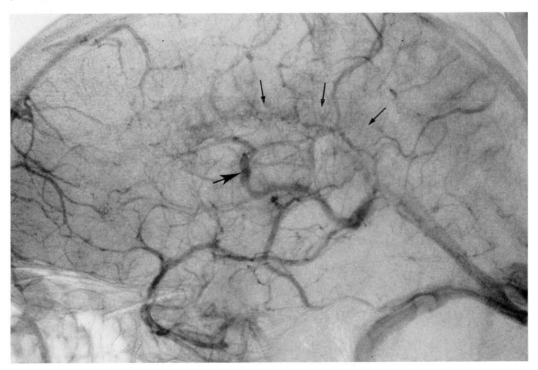

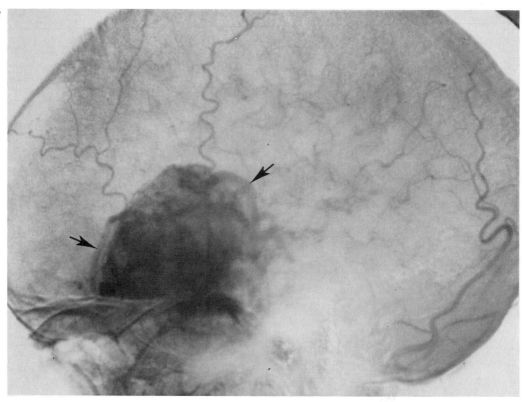

Fig. 11-48. Left common carotid angiogram (capillary phase, lateral view). A large meningioma with early draining veins **(arrows)** is present. *(Case courtesy of B. McIff, M.D.)*

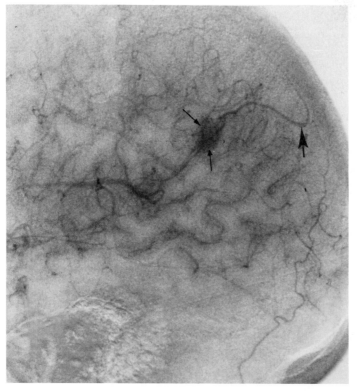

Fig. 11-49. Left common carotid angiogram (late arterial phase, lateral view) of a solitary metastasis **(small arrows)** from carcinoma of the lung. Note early opacification of the adjacent cortical vein **(large arrow).**

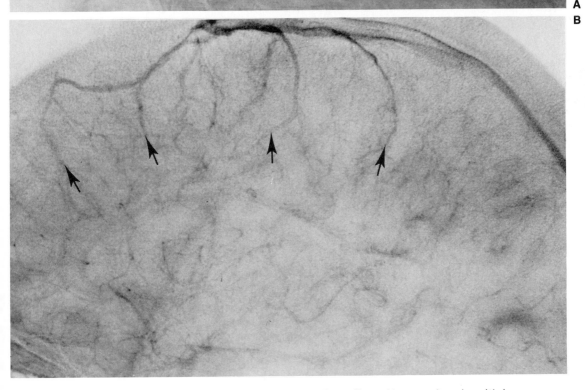

Fig. 11-50. Two patients with capillary angiomas. Note the solitary **(A, arrow)** and multiple **(B, arrows)** early draining veins.

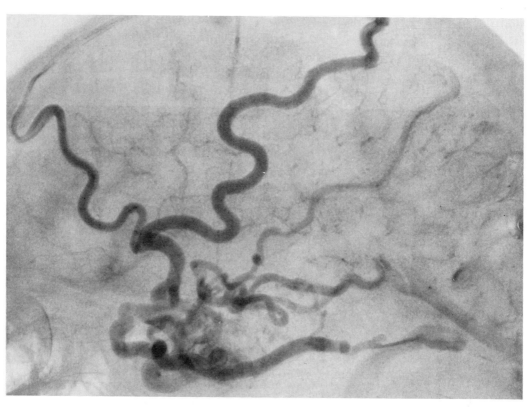

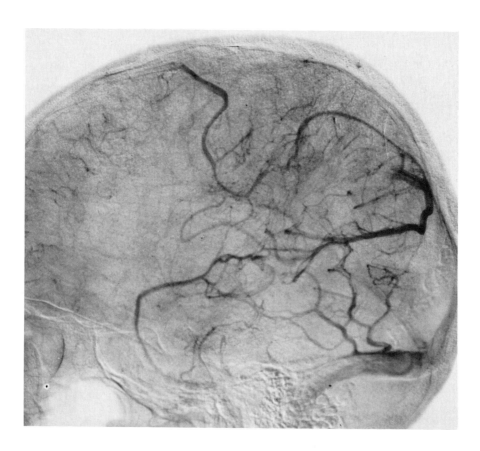

Fig. 11-51. Left internal carotid angiogram (capillary phase, lateral view) of a large temporal lobe AVM. Note early opacification of multiple enlarged cortical veins.

Fig. 11-52. Left internal carotid angiogram (late arterial phase, lateral view) of herpes encephalitis. Multiple early draining veins are present (same patient as Figure 9-25)

Fig. 11-53. Left common carotid angiogram (late arterial phase, lateral view) of a cerebral infarction. A prominent early draining vein is present **(arrow).**

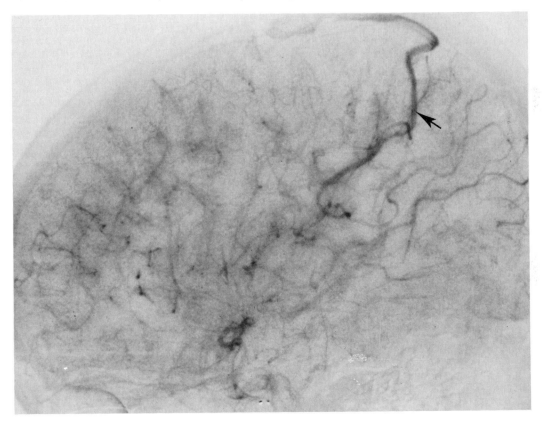

REFERENCES

1. **Azar-Kia B, Sarwar M, Schechter MM, Batnitzky S:** Subependymal veins and ventricular tumors. Radiology 113:81–88, 1974
2. **Babin E, Megret M:** Variations in the drainage of the basal vein. Neuroradiology 6:154–161, 1973
3. **Bartlett JE, Kishore PRS:** Intracranial cavernous angioma. Am J Roentgenol 120:635–656, 1977
4. **Belloni G, di Rocco C:** A practical approach to the phlebographic study of the lateral cerebral ventricles. Neuroradiology 10:111–119, 1975
5. **Bentson JR, Hasso AN:** Transient enlargement of deep medullary veins in encephalitis. Neuroradiology 9:217–222, 1975
6. **Bentson JR, Wilson GH, Newton TH:** Cerebral venous drainage pattern of the Sturge-Weber syndrome. Radiology 101:111–118, 1971
7. **Bradac GB, Simon RS, Fiegler W:** The early filling of a vein in the carotid angiogram. Neuroradiology 9:13–19, 1975
8. **Braun JP, Tournade A:** Venous drainage in the craniocervical region. Neuroradiology 13:155–158, 1977
9. **Brismar G, Brismar J:** Thrombosis of the intraorbital veins and cavernous sinus. Acta Radiol [Diagn] (Stockh) 18:145–153, 1977
10. **Browder J, Kaplan HA, Krieger AJ:** Anatomic features of the straight sinus and its tributaries. J Neurosurg 44:55–61, 1976
11. **Bub B, Ferris EJ, Levy PS, Navani S:** The cerebral venogram: a statistical analysis of the sequence of venous filling in cerebral angiograms. Radiology 91:1112–1118, 1968
12. **DiChiro G:** Angiographic patterns of cerebral convexity veins and superficial dural sinuses. Am J Roentgenol 87:308–321, 1962
13. **Fierstein SB, Pribram HW, Hieshima G:** Angiography and computed tomography in the evaluation of cerebral venous malformations. Neuroradiology 17:137–148, 1979
14. **Galligioni F, Bernardi R, Pellone M, Iraei G:** The superficial sylvian vein in normal and pathologic cerebral angiography. Am J Roentgenol 107:565–579, 1969
15. **Golden JB, Kramer RA:** The angiographically occult cerebrovascular malformation. J Neurosurg 48:292–296, 1978
16. **Goto K, Takahashi M, Tamakawa Y:** Duplication of the straight sinus. Radiology 120:117–119, 1976
17. **Gray H:** Anatomy of the Human Body, 20th ed, pp 687–703. Philadelphia, Lea & Febiger, 1966
17A. **Gürsoy G, Tolun R, Bahar S:** Aneurysmal dilatation of torcula. Neuroradiology 18:285–288, 1979
18. **Hacker H:** Superficial supratentorial veins and dural sinuses. In Newton TH, Potts DG (eds): Radiology of the Skull and Brain, Vol 2, pp 1851–1902. St. Louis, CV Mosby, 1974
19. **Harwood-Nash DC, Fitz CR:** Neuroradiology in Infants and Children, pp 957–959. St. Louis, CV Mosby, 1976
20. **Heinz ER:** Pathology involving the supratentorial veins and dural sinuses. In Newton TH, Potts DG (eds): Radiology of the Skull and Brain, Vol 2, pp 1878–1902. St. Louis, CV Mosby, 1974
21. **Hooshmand I, Rosenbaum AE, Stein RL:** Radiographic anatomy of the normal cerebral deep medullary veins: criteria for distinguishing them from their abnormal counterparts. Neuroradiology 7:75–84, 1974
22. **Huang YP, Wolf BS:** Veins of the white matter of the cerebral hemispheres (the medullary veins). Am J Roentgenol 92:739–755, 1964
23. **Huang YP, Wolf BS:** The basal cerebral vein and its tributaries. In Newton TH, Potts DG (eds): Radiology of the Skull and Brain, Vol. 2, pp 2111–2154. St. Louis, CV Mosby, 1974
24. **Kaplan HA, Browder J:** Atresia of the rostral superior sagittal sinus. Substitute parasagittal venous channels. J Neurosurg 38:602–607, 1973
25. **Kaplan HA, Browder J:** Importance of veins in partial cerebral lobectomy. J Neurosurg 41:360–366, 1974
26. **Kaplan HA, Browder A, Browder J:** Narrow and atretic transverse dural sinuses: clinical significance. Ann Otol Rhinol Laryngol 82:351–354, 1973
27. **Kaplan HA, Browder J, Krieger AJ:** Venous channels within the intracranial dural partitions. Radiology 115:641–645, 1975
28. **Kiihner A, Krastel A, Stoll W:** Arteriovenous malformations of the transverse dural sinus. J Neurosurg 45:12–19, 1976
29. **Lemire RJ, Loeser JD, Leech RW et al:** Normal and Abnormal Development of the Human Nervous System. Hagerstown, Harper & Row, 1975
30. **Liliequist B:** Angiography in intracerebral hemangioma. Neuroradiology 9:69–72, 1975
31. **Lloyd TV, Aman MV, Johnson JC:** Aberrant jugular bulb presenting as a middle ear mass. Radiology 131:139–141, 1979
32. **Mani RL, Hedgcock MW, Mass SI et al:** Radiographic diagnosis of mengingioma of the lateral ventricle. J Neurosurg 49:249–255, 1978
33. **McCord GM, Goree GA, Jimenez JP:** Venous drainage to the inferior sagittal sinus. Radiology 105:583–589, 1972
33A. **Naidich TP, Pudlowski RM, Naidich JB et al:**

Computed tomographic signs of the Chiari II Malformation. Part I: Skull and dural partitions. Radiology 134:65–71, 1980

33B. **Naidich TP, Pudlowski RM, Naidich JB:** Computed tomographic signs of Chiari II malformation. II: Midbrain and cerebellum. Radiology 134:391–398, 1980

33C. **Naidich TP, Pudlowski RM, Naidich JB:** Computed tomographic signs of the Chiari II malformation. III: Ventricles and cisterns. Radiology 134:657–663, 1980

34. **Newton HE, Gooding CA:** Compression of superior sagittal sinus by neonatal calvarial molding. Radiology 115:635–639, 1975

35. **Nixon GW, Ravin CE:** Malposition of the attached portion of the falx cerebri and the superior sagittal sinus. Am J Roentgenol 122:44–51, 1974

36. **O'Brien MS, Schechter MM:** Arteriovenous malformations involving the galenic system. Am J Roentgenol 110:50–55, 1970

37. **Osaka K, Sato N, Yamasaki S, Fujita K, Matsumoto S, Kodama S:** Dysgenesis of the deep venous system as a diagnostic criterion for holoprosencephaly. Neuroradiology 13:231–238, 1977

37A. **Osborn AG:** The craniofacial venous plexuses: An angiographic study. Presented at the 18th annual meeting of the American Society of Neuroradiology, March, 16–21, 1980, Los Angeles.

38. **Paff GH:** Anatomy of the Head and Neck. Philadelphia, WB Saunders, 1978

39. **Roberson GB, Kase CS, Walpow ER:** Telangiectasis and cavernous angiomas of the brainstem: 'cryptic' vascular malformations. Neuroradiology 8:83–89, 1974

40. **Rosenbaum AE, Stein RL:** Abnormal supratentorial deep cerebral veins. In Newton TH, Potts DG (eds): Radiology of the Skull and Brain, Vol 2, pp 1999–2110. St. Louis, CV Mosby, 1974

41. **Sarwar M, McCormick WF:** Intracerebral venous angioma. Arch Neurol 35:323–335, 1978

42. **Scotti LN, Goldman RL, Hardman DR et al:** Venous thrombosis in infants and children. Radiology 112:393–399, 1974

42A. **Spallone A:** Computed tomography in aneurysms of the vein of Galen. J Comp Asst Tomogr 3:779–782, 1979

43. **Stebbens WB:** Pathology of the Cerebral Blood Vessels, pp 38–47. St. Louis, CV Mosby, 1972

44. **Stein RL, Rosenbaum AE:** Normal deep cerebral venous system. In Newton TH, Potts DG (eds): Radiology of the Skull and Brain, Vol 2, pp 1904–1998. St. Louis, CV Mosby, 1974

45. **Stephens RB, Stilwell DB:** Arteries and Veins of the Human Brain, pp 124–167. Springfield, IL, CC Thomas, 1969

45A. **Stern J, Goldenberg M:** Jugular bulb diverticula in medial petrous bone. Am J Neuroradiol 1:153–155, 1980

46. **Waga S, Handa H:** Scalp veins as collateral pathway with parasagittal meningiomas occluding the superior sagittal sinus. Neuroradiology 11:199–204, 1976

46A. **Welch K, Maheedy MH, Abroms IF et al:** Computed tomography of Sturge-Weber syndrome in infants. J Comp Asst Tomogr 4:33–36, 1980

47. **Wendling LR, Moore JS Jr, Kieffer SA et al:** Intracerebral venous angioma. Radiology 119:141–147, 1976

48. **Wilner HI, Crockett J, Gilroy J:** The galenic venous system: a selective radiographic study. Am J Roentgenol 115:1–13, 1972

49. **Wolf BS, Huang YP:** The insula and deep middle cerebral venous drainage system: normal anatomy and angiography. Am J Roentgenol 90:472–489, 1963

50. **Wolf BS, Huang YP:** The subependymal veins of the lateral ventricles. Am J Roentgenol 91:406–426, 1964

51. **Wolf BS, Huang YP, Newman CM:** The superficial sylvian venous drainage system. Am J Roentgenol 89:398–410, 1963

52. **Wolpert SM:** Dural sinus configuration: measure of congenital disease. Radiology 92:1511–1516, 1969

53. **Zimmer AE, Annes GP:** The septal vein. Radiology 87:813–823, 1966

54. **Zimmerman RD, Breckbill D, Dennis MW et al:** Cranial CT findings in patients with myelomeningocele. Am J Roentgenol 132:623–629, 1979

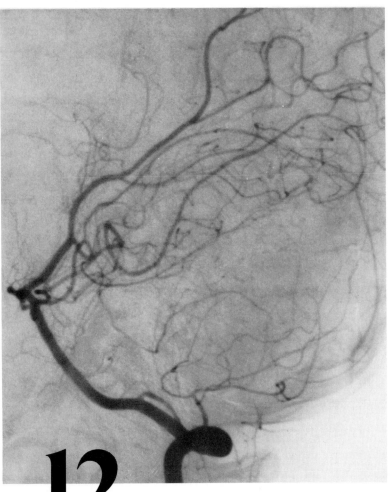

12 Arteries and Veins of the Posterior Fossa

With the advent of cranial computed tomography (CT), arteriography is no longer used as the primary screening examination for suspected posterior fossa lesions. Instead, vertebral angiography is now used mainly to evaluate patients with known lesions. This invasive procedure is best reserved to answer specific questions—defining the presence of vascular disease, determining the exact location of a neoplasm, delineating its vascular supply, or excluding lesions such as aneurysm or arteriovenous malformation that have been included in the initial differential diagnosis.[8, 17, 43, 60, 64, 65] This study of cerebral angiography will be concluded by examining the arteries and veins of the posterior fossa, reviewing their normal gross and radiographic anatomy, and illustrating the alterations in these structures seen in a variety of disease processes.

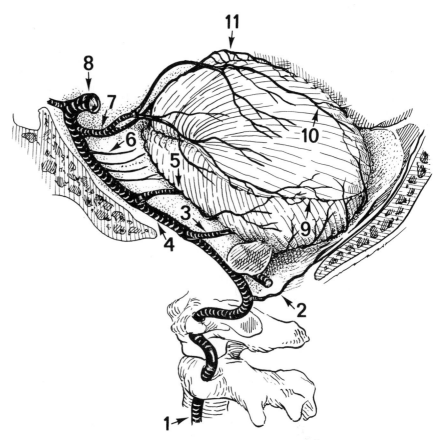

Fig. 12-1. Anatomic diagram of the vertebrobasilar system and its major branches (lateral view). The left half of the calvarium and the tentorium have been removed. **1.** Left vertebral artery. **2.** Posterior meningeal artery. **3.** Posterior inferior cerebellar artery. **4.** Basilar artery. **5.** Anterior inferior cerebellar artery. **6.** Pontine arteries. **7.** Superior cerebellar artery (main trunk). **8.** Posterior cerebral artery (cut off). **9.** Branches of the SCA and AICA in the great horizontal fissure. **10.** SCA hemispheric branches. **11.** Superior vermian branches of the SCA.

NORMAL GROSS ARTERIAL ANATOMY

Vertebral Artery

Normally the vertebral artery (VA) arises as the first branch of the subclavian artery, coursing superiorly and medially to enter the transverse foramen of C6 (see Figs. 2-1, 2-2). The VA pursues an almost vertical course as it ascends through the transverse foramina of C3-6. It then turns superolaterally to pass through the C2 foramen. After it emerges from this foramen, the VA courses upward through the transverse foramen of the atlas. It then curves backward around the atlanto-occipital joint and lies in a horizontal groove along the posterior arch of C1 (Fig. 12-1). As the VA approaches the midline it abruptly bends cephalad to enter the skull through the foramen magnum. Anterior to the upper medulla, the two vertebral arteries unite to form the basilar artery (Fig. 12-2, arrow 5).

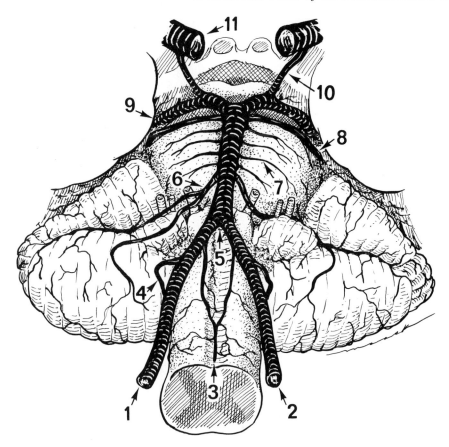

Fig. 12-2. Anatomic diagram of the vertebrobasilar system and its major branches (anterior view) **1.** Right vertebral artery. **2.** Left vertebral artery. **3.** Anterior spinal artery. **4.** Posterior inferior cerebellar artery. **5.** Basilar artery. **6.** Anterior inferior cerebellar artery. **7.** Pontine arteries. **8.** Superior cerebellar artery. **9.** Posterior cerebral artery. **10.** Posterior communicating artery. **11.** Internal carotid artery.

Extracranial Branches of the Vertebral Artery

Throughout its intraspinal course each VA gives rise to segmental branches that supply the vertebrae and supplement the spinal circulation. Each also has deep muscular rami that have numerous anastomoses with muscular branches of ECA, primarily the occipital artery. These may normally be quite prominent.[45, 45A, 61] Anastomotic channels also exist between segmental branches of the cervical VA and the ascending pharyngeal artery.[44, 45A]

Intracranial Branches of the Vertebral Artery

Intracranial VA rami include the posterior meningeal artery, direct bulbar branches to the medulla, the anterior spinal artery, the posterior inferior cerebellar artery, small basal meningeal branches, and, occasionally, the posterior spinal artery.[44, 61]

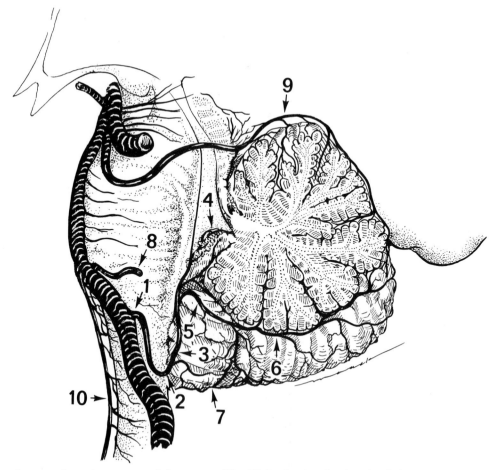

The **posterior meningeal artery** originates from the VA at or just below the foramen magnum (Fig. 12-1, arrow 2). It follows a relatively straight superomedial course to supply the falx cerebelli. It is often represented by one or two relatively small branches instead of a single large trunk.

The **posterior spinal artery** arises from the distal VA or posterior inferior cerebellar artery. It descends along the dorsal surface of the medulla and spinal cord. Together with the VA and other spinal radicular branches it forms a vascular network that continues inferiorly along the cord to the cauda equina.[76]

The **anterior spinal artery** also arises from the distal VA. In approximately 50% of cases it courses inferiorly and medially to unite with its counterpart from the opposite side. The anterior spinal artery then runs caudad in the anteromedian sulcus of the spinal cord (Fig. 12-2, arrow 3).

Fig. 12-3. Anatomic sketch of the vertebrobasilar system. The left cerebellar hemisphere has been removed to show the relationship of the posterior inferior cerebellar artery (PICA) to the tonsil and vermis. **1.** Anterior medullary segment of PICA. **2.** Lateral medullary segment (caudal loop) of PICA. **3.** Posterior medullary segment of PICA. **4.** Choroidal branches of PICA. **5.** Supratonsillar segment of PICA. **6.** Hemispheric and vermian branches of PICA. **7.** Tonsillar branches of PICA. **8.** Anterior inferior cerebellar artery (cut off). **9.** Superior vermian branches of the superior cerebellar artery. **10.** Anterior spinal artery.

PICA

ant. med.
↓
lat. med (caudal loop)
↓
post. med.
↓
supratonsillar

these 2 segments are displaced w/ brainstem masses.

The **posterior inferior cerebellar artery** (PICA) is both the largest and most variable branch of the VA. It normally arises from the VA about one or two cm below the basilar artery origin (Figs. 12-1, arrow 3; 12-2, arrow 4). In 18% of arteriograms, the PICA originates below the level of the foramen magnum.[52]

The first segment of the PICA courses laterally around the medulla and is called the anterior medullary segment (Fig. 12-3, arrow 1).[92] The PICA then forms a distinct caudal loop along the side of the medulla. This portion of the PICA is termed the lateral medullary segment (Fig. 12-2, arrow 2). When it reaches the posterior limit of the medulla, the PICA curves superiorly, completing its caudal loop and initiating a cranial loop (Fig. 12-3, arrow 3). At the apex of its cranial loop, the PICA then courses over or across the cerebellar tonsil, sending small branches to the choroid plexus of the fourth ventricle (Fig. 12-3, arrow 4) and the tonsil itself (Fig. 12-3, arrow 7).[73, 81] The length of these choroidal branches is quite variable.[41] After it crosses the cerebellar tonsil, the PICA curves downward behind this structure (Fig. 12-3, arrow 5), giving off medial branches to the inferior vermis and lateral branches to the cerebellar hemispheres (Fig. 12-3, arrow 6).[31]

Both the size of the PICA and its territory of supply are related to that of the anterior inferior cerebellar artery and the opposite PICA. When one PICA is small the ipsilateral anterior inferior cerebellar artery and contralateral PICA are usually relatively large.[76]

The Basilar Artery

The basilar artery (BA) is formed by the union of the two vertebral arteries (Fig. 12-2, arrow 5). The BA originates adjacent to the lower border of the pons. It extends superiorly along the ventral surface of the pons, terminating in the interpeduncular cistern by dividing into the paired posterior cerebral arteries. It may run superiorly in the midline, or it may wander from side to side. During its course the BA gives rise to pontine arteries, internal auditory (labyrinthine) arteries, the anterior inferior cerebellar arteries, the superior cerebellar arteries, and the posterior cerebral arteries.[76]

Small pontine branches arise at right angles from the BA to supply the pons and adjacent portions of the cerebellum (Figs. 12-1, arrow 6; 12-2, arrow 7). The internal auditory (labyrinthine) artery has a variable origin, arising either from the BA or anterior inferior cerebellar artery. In 85% of cases, the internal auditory branch arises from the anterior inferior cerebellar artery. It accompanies the acoustic nerve through the internal auditory meatus and supplies the inner ear.[22, 58]

Anterior Inferior Cerebellar Artery (AICA). The AICA usually arises from the proximal portion of the BA (Fig. 12-1, arrow 5). It courses posteriorly, inferiorly, and laterally across the pons.[58] Within the cerebellopontine angle cistern, the AICA lies ventral and medial to the facial and acoustic nerves (Fig. 12-2, arrow 6). As the AICA approaches the porus acusticus it frequently makes a tight loop before it runs over the cerebellum. Branches of the AICA supply the anterior segments of the superior and inferior semilunar lobules, the flocculus, part of the quandrangular lobule, choroid plexus in the lateral recess of the fourth ventricle, and part of the middle cerebellar peduncle.[76]

The AICA is usually the smallest of the three cerebellar arteries. It has a reciprocal relationship with the PICA and may share a common trunk with this vessel.

Superior Cerebellar Arteries (SCAs). The SCAs are the most constant and also the most rostral infratentorial branches of the basilar artery.[50] Most arise as a single trunk on each side of the BA although duplicate or even triplicate vessels have been identified.[24, 24A] From their origins near the pontomesencephalic junction, the SCAs course posterolaterally in the perimesencephalic cistern above the trigeminal nerve, encircling the brainstem in the groove between the pons and mesencephalon (Figs. 12-1, arrow 7; 12-2, arrow 8). In their proximal segments, the SCAs are separated from the posterior cerebral arteries by the oculomotor nerves. Distally, these vessels are separated by the tentorium cerebelli.

Each SCA has two main branches. A lateral branch supplies the superolateral aspects of the cerebellar hemispheres, the superior cerebellar peduncle, the dentate nucleus, and part of the middle cerebellar peduncle (Fig. 12-1, arrow 10). The medial SCA branch supplies the superior surface of the cerebellar hemisphere and also supplies rami to the superior vermis (Figs. 12-1, arrow 11; and 12-3, arrow 9). The superior vermian branches of both SCAs anastomose with each other in the quadrigeminal cistern and then course posteriorly over the vermis close to the midline.[50]

Posterior Cerebral Arteries. Within the interpeduncular cistern, the BA bifurcates into its two terminal branches — the posterior cerebral arteries (Fig. 12-2, arrow 9). These vessels are discussed in Chapter 10.

NORMAL RADIOGRAPHIC ANATOMY OF THE VERTEBROBASILAR SYSTEM AND ITS BRANCHES

The Vertebral Artery

In the majority of cases, the left VA is the dominant vessel (see Chapter 2). After the VA enters the foramina transversaria it follows a nearly straight vertical course until it turns superolaterally to exit from the C2 foramen. The VA then curves slightly anteriorly to pass upward through the transverse foramen of the atlas. Its course through C2 and C1 has the appearance of a half square as seen on the AP view (Fig. 12-4B). On the lateral view, the VA has a slight anteriorly convex curve as it runs through the C1 transverse foramen. After it exits from the spine, the VA curves backward on the dorsal arch of the atlas before it turns superomedially to enter the posterior fossa through the foramen magnum (Fig. 12-4A, arrow 1).

Extracranial Branches of the VA. The cervical portion of the VA gives rise to segmental muscular and radiculomedullary branches that can frequently be identified angiographically.[45A]

Intracranial Branches of the VA. The **posterior meningeal artery** arises from the VA at or just below the foramen magnum. It is seen in 30 to 40% of normal vertebral angiograms. The posterior meningeal artery initially follows a slightly undulating posteromedial course. The intracranial portion is relatively straight, coursing superiorly and paralleling the inner table of the skull. It lies in or adjacent to the midline (Fig. 12-4A, arrow 2). On the AP view, the posterior meningeal artery can be confused with vermian branches of the PICA. However, its comparatively straight course and characteristic location in the lateral projection distinguish it from the PICA.[92]

An anterior spinal branch arises from the distal VA and passes inferomedially toward the midline where it unites with its counterpart from the opposite side to form the **anterior spinal artery** (Fig. 12-4A, arrow 3). This vessel is best seen in the lateral projection, but is only occasionally identified on AP views. The **posterior spinal arteries** are seldom seen on normal angiograms.[61]

The **posterior inferior cerebellar artery** (PICA) follows a complex course. Its anterior medullary segment passes around the inferolateral aspect of the medulla (Fig. 12-4A, arrow 4). On the lateral view, a distinct caudal loop along the side of the medulla represents its lateral medullary segment (Fig. 12-4A, arrow 5). The posterior medullary segment then curves superomedially on the dorsal surface of the brain stem and forms a cranial loop that courses over or across the cerebellar tonsil (Figure 12-4A, arrow 6).

The choroidal artery to the fourth ventricle is a small vessel that usually arises from the cephalic loop or from supratonsillar PICA branches (Fig. 12-4A, arrow 7).[23] Angiotomography is helpful in depicting the choroidal artery.[41] Recent studies have identified the choroid plexus of the lateral ventricle in 35% of normal vertebral angiograms.[10]

After supplying its choroidal branches, the cranial PICA loop curves across the cerebellar tonsil and then runs inferiorly along its dorsal surface for a variable distance before dividing into tonsillar, hemispheric, and vermian branches. The vermian branch of the PICA follows a relatively constant course, demarcating the inferior and posterior vermian lobules as seen on the lateral view (Fig. 12-4A, arrow 8). The tonsillohemispheric branches descend along the posteromedial aspect of the tonsil. The tonsillar branches then course anteriorly while the hemispheric branches run posterolaterally to supply the inferior surface of the cerebellar hemispheres (Fig. 12-4A, arrow 9). The tonsillohemispheric branches are well visualized on both lateral vertebral angiograms and 0° AP studies. The medullary segments of PICA can be distinguished on AP Towne views; they overlap somewhat on the 0° projection (Fig. 12-4C).

A variety of normal measurements have been devised to localize the choroidal point of the PICA since the choroidal vasculature is in constant position regardless of the variable course of the PICA (Fig. 12-16).[52, 68, 88] The choroidal point is a helpful angiographic marker in the evaluation of posterior fossa masses.

The Basilar Artery and its Branches

The **basilar artery** (BA) is quite variable in its course, size, and length. In the lateral view it either appears relatively straight or exhibits a slight anterior convexity (Fig. 12-4A, arrow 10). It usually lies several millimeters behind the clivus. On the AP view, the BA may hug the midline (Fig. 12-4B, arrow 3), appear remarkably tortuous, or deviate to one side or the other.[80]

The small pontine BA branches and the internal auditory artery are infrequently visualized on vertebral angiograms.

On AP Towne views each **anterior inferior cerebellar artery** arises from the proximal BA and courses laterally into the cerebellopontine angle cistern (Fig. 12-4B, arrow 5). The AICA usually curves into an outward loop at the internal auditory canal (Fig. 12-5B, arrow 2) and continues somwhat farther laterally before dividing into terminal branches.

The radiographic appearance of the distal AICA branches is quite variable. They may terminate at the pons or continue laterally to supply the posteroinferior aspect of the cerebellar hemisphere. If the ipsilateral PICA is small, the caudomeatal branch of the AICA may give rise to an inferior accessory artery that supplements the usual PICA distribution. On lateral views the AICAs arise from the BA at variable levels and course across the pons. Adjacent to CN VII and CN VIII, the AICA has a characteristic single or double curve as it loops into the porus acusticus. This double curve often resembles an "N" or "M" as seen on the lateral view (Fig. 12-5A).[58]

The **superior cerebellar arteries** (SCAs) are seen well on both AP Towne and lateral vertebral angiograms. The initial segments of the SCAs tend to parallel the course of the posterior cerebral arteries and are separated from them by only a few millimeters (Fig. 12-4A, arrow 12). As the SCAs sweep behind the brainstem they approximate each other in the quadrigeminal plate cistern, as seen on the AP view (Fig. 12-5B, arrow 3). Their superior vermian branches continue posteriorly, following a somewhat straighter course (Fig. 12-4B, arrow 12). In the lateral projection, the superior vermian branches often lie a few millimeters above the proximal posterior cerebral artery branches since the vermis is a midline structure and lies just under the tentorial apex (Fig. 12-4A, arrow 14). The PCA branches are more lateral and are initially more inferiorly located.

Hemispheric branches of the SCA and PICA ramify over the cerebellum (Fig. 12-5B, arrow 5). They can be identified in the lateral view by their typical stepladder-like pattern (Fig. 12-5A, outlined arrows).[50] Occasionally, prominent marginal branches of the SCA course into the great horizontal fissure of the cerebellum, rendering it angiographically visible.[75, 80] Branches of the AICA may also course into this fissure (Fig. 12-6).

The radiographic anatomy of the **posterior cerebral arteries** is discussed in Chapter 10.

(Text continued on p. 389)

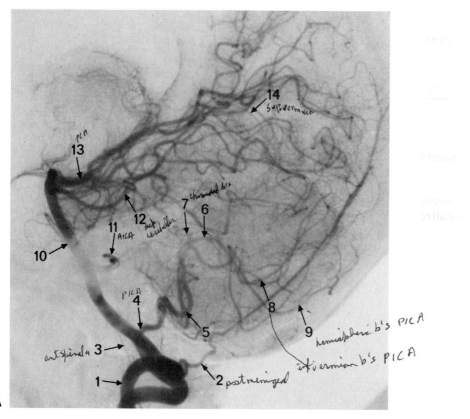

A

Fig. 12-4A. Normal left vertebral angiogram (arterial phase, lateral view). **1.** Left vertebral artery. **2.** Posterior meningeal artery. **3.** Anterior spinal artery. **4.** Posterior inferior cerebellar artery (anterior medullary segment). **5.** Caudal loop of PICA. **6.** Cranial loop of PICA. **7.** Choroidal branches of PICA with faint vascular blush in the choroid plexus. **8.** Inferior vermian branches of PICA. **9.** Hemispheric branches of PICA. **10.** Basilar artery. **11.** Anterior inferior cerebellar artery. **12.** Superior cerebellar artery. **13.** Posterior cerebral artery. **14.** Superior vermian arteries.

Fig. 12-4B. Normal left vertebral angiogram (arterial phase, AP Towne view). **1.** Vertebral artery in the transverse foramen of C1. **3.** Basilar artery. **4.** Posterior inferior cerebellar artery. **5.** Anterior inferior cerebellar artery. **6.** Superior cerebellar artery. **7.** Superior vermian branches of the SCAs.

Fig. 12-4C. Normal left vertebral angiogram (arterial phase, 0° AP view). The medullary segments of the two PICAs are clearly seen **(large arrow).** The AICAs are indicated **(small arrows).**

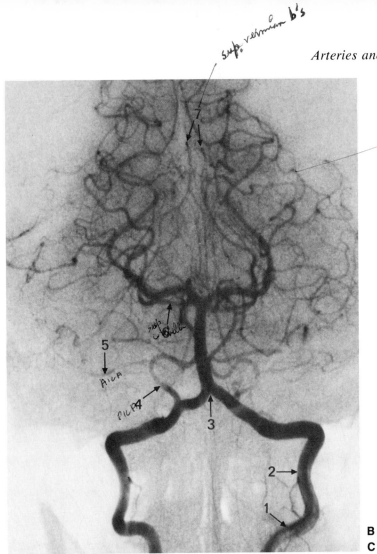

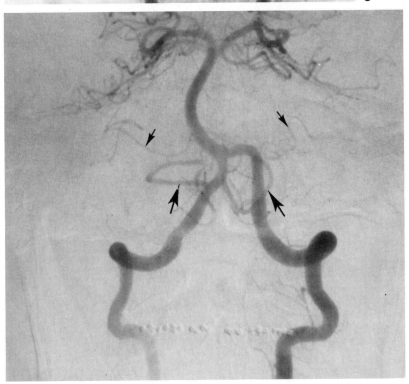

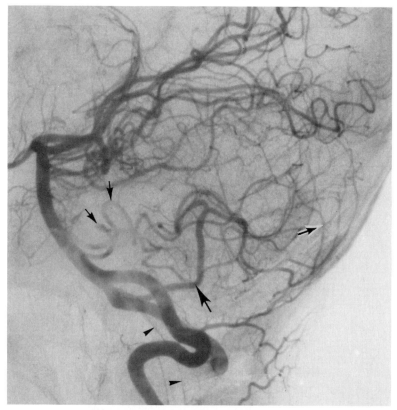

A

B

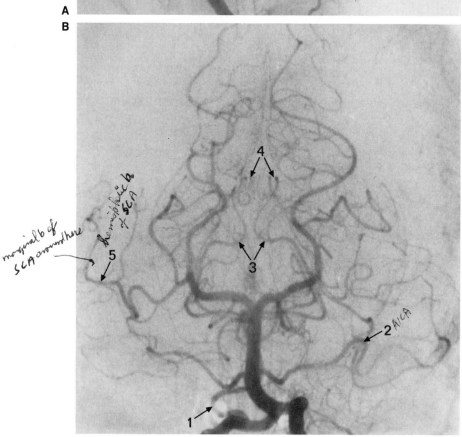

◀ **Fig. 12-5.** Normal left vertebral angiogram (**A,** arterial phase, lateral view). A single large PICA **(large arrow)** and two prominent AICAs **(small arrows)** are present. Note the double curve of the AICA, forming a distinct "M". Hemispheric branches of the PICA are indicated **(outlined arrow).** The anterior spinal artery is also indicated **(arrowheads).** Normal left vertebral angiogram (**B,** arterial phase, AP Towne view). Same patient as 12-5A. **1.** PICA. **2.** AICA (arrow on loop at porus acusticus). **3.** SCAs behind the brainstem. **4.** Vermian branches of the SCAs. **5.** Hemispheric branch of the SCA.

NORMAL VARIATIONS AND ANOMALIES OF THE VERTEBROBASILAR SYSTEM AND ITS POSTERIOR FOSSA BRANCHES

Vertebral Artery

The vertebral artery may originate from the proximal subclavian artery or from the aortic arch (see Chapter 2). Other anomalous origins (*i.e.,* from the innominate, common, or external carotid arteries) are rare.[6, 69A] Bifid or duplicate origin of the VA has been reported.[77] One segment or the entire length of a VA may be hypoplastic (Fig. 12-6). A vertebral artery may terminate as a PICA (Fig. 12-7).

Persistent embryonic carotid-vertebrobasilar anastomoses are discussed in Chapter 6.

The Posterior Inferior Cerebellar Arteries

The course and distribution of the PICAs vary greatly. In 18% of cases, the PICA originates from the extracranial vertebral artery, coursing superiorly through the foramen magnum to supply the tonsil and inferior segments of the cerebellar hemisphere (Fig. 12-8). In 35% of cases, the PICA origin is normal, but its caudal loop extends below the level of the foramen magnum (Fig. 12-9). In such instances, the lower segment of the loop does not delineate the inferior margin of the cerebellar tonsil.[73] One PICA may supply both inferior cerebellar hemispheres. A single trunk may take the place of both the AICA and

PICA or the latter vessel may be hypoplastic and its territory supplied by branches of the AICA.[52] If a trigeminal artery is present, the PICA may, occasionally, arise directly from this anomalous vessel.[13]

The Basilar Artery

The basilar artery may be duplicated or fenestrated.[80] The vertebro-basilar artery may become quite elongated and tortuous coursing into the cerebellopontine angle cistern or extending superiorly as far as the posterior third ventricle (Figs. 12-10 and 12-11).

The Anterior Inferior Cerebellar Artery

Infrequently, the AICA may arise from the VA or from the cavernous ICA.[26] The AICA may also originate from the PICA or from a single trunk common to both vessels. An accessory artery may supplement or replace part of the normal AICA distribution and has been identified in 20% of anatomic specimens.[58] The PICA may supply the usual AICA distribution.

The Superior Cerebellar Artery

Duplicate SCAs have been identified in eight percent of anatomic specimens, and triplicate SCAs in 2% of cases.[24, 50] Origin of an SCA arising from the ICA, posterior cerebral artery, or proximal basilar artery has also been reported.[24, 83]

(Text continued on p. 394)

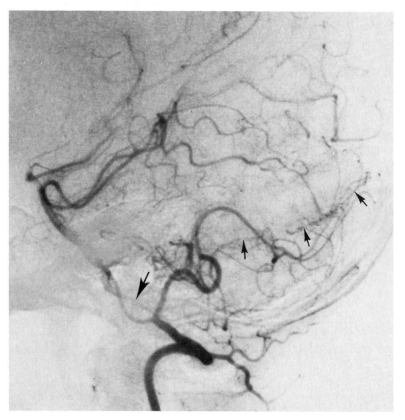

Fig. 12-6. Left vertebral angiogram (arterial phase, lateral view). Part of the VA is hypoplastic **(large arrow).** Branches of the AICA and SCA delineate the great horizontal fissure of the cerebellum **(small arrows).**

Fig. 12-7. Left vertebral angiogram **(lateral view).** The small VA terminates in its PICA branch.

Fig. 12-8. Left vertebral angiogram (arterial phase, lateral view). A large PICA **(arrow)** originates from the right VA below the foramen magnum.

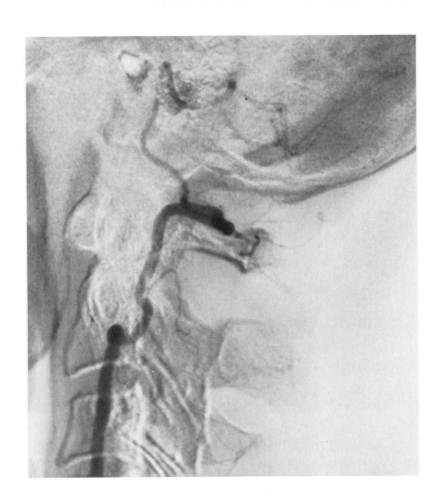

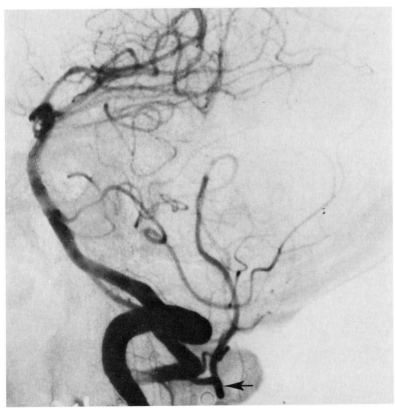

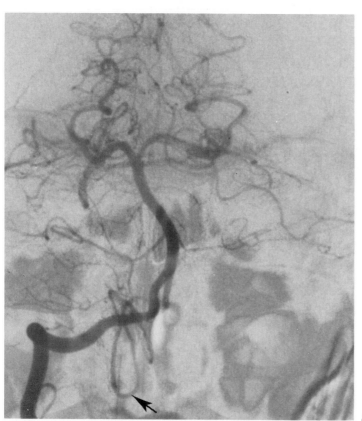

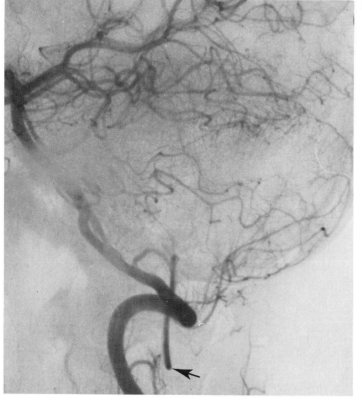

Fig. 12-9. Normal right vertebral angiogram (arterial phase). The caudal loop of PICA **(arrows)** extends below the foramen magnum. A (**A,** 0° view). Lateral **(B)** view.

A
B

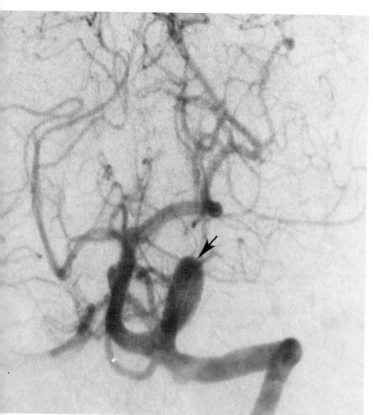

Fig. 12-10. Left vertebral angiogram (arterial phase, AP Towne view). Note the redundant vertebrobasilar artery loop **(arrow).**

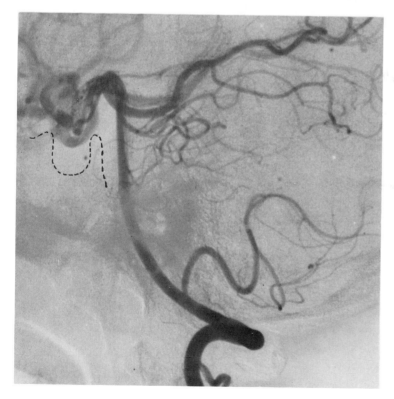

Fig. 12-11. Left vertebral angiogram (arterial phase, lateral view). The basilar artery is greatly elongated, extending several centimeters above the dorsum sellae.

VEINS OF THE POSTERIOR FOSSA: NORMAL GROSS ANATOMY

Three major venous drainage systems have been identified in the posterior fossa: a superior or Galenic draining group, an anterior or petrosal draining group, and a posterior or tentorial draining group.[33, 78]

Superior (Galenic) Group

The superior group of posterior fossa veins includes the precentral cerebellar vein, the superior vermian vein, the posterior and lateral mesencephalic veins, and the anterior pontomesencephalic vein.

Fig. 12-12. Anatomic sketch of the major posterior fossa veins (lateral view). Colliculocentral point-**black asterisk.** Copular point-**large black dot. 1.** Vein of Galen. **2.** Straight sinus. **3.** Precentral cerebellar vein. **4.** Superior vermian vein. **5.** Superior choroid vein. **6.** Internal cerebral vein. **7.** Superior thalamic vein. **8.** Posterior mesencephalic vein. **9.** Lateral mesencephalic vein. **10.** Anterior pontomesencephalic vein. **11.** Transverse pontine vein. **12.** Anterior medullary vein. **13.** Stem of the petrosal vein. **14.** Tonsillar veins. **15.** Inferior vermian vein. **16.** Hemispheric vein.

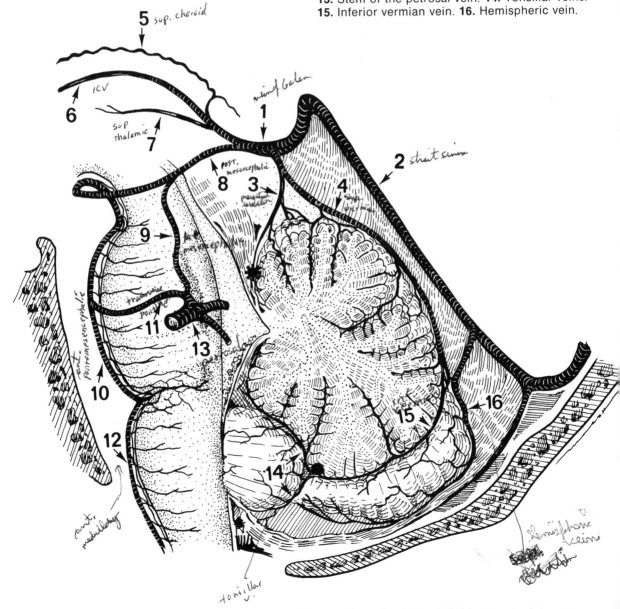

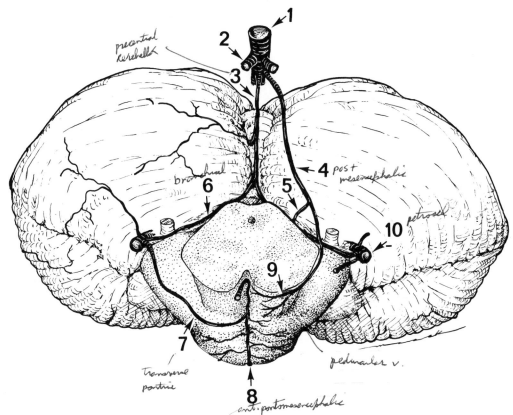

Fig. 12-13. Anatomic sketch of the major posterior fossa veins, anterosuperior view. **1.** Vein of Galen. **2.** Internal cerebral vein. **3.** Precentral cerebellar vein. **4.** Posterior mesencephalic vein. **5.** Lateral mesencephalic vein. **6.** Brachial vein. **7.** Transverse pontine vein. **8.** Anterior pontomesencephalic vein. **9.** Peduncular veins. **10.** Petrosal vein.

The **precentral cerebellar vein** (PCV) is a single midline vessel that originates in the fissure between the lingula and central lobule of the vermis (Figs. 12-12, arrow 3; and 12-13, arrow 3). Formed by brachial veins that course medially over the brachium pontis, the PCV courses superiorly and parallels the roof of the fourth ventricle.[25, 30, 91] It curves upward behind the inferior colliculi and precentral lobule of the vermis to terminate in the vein of Galen.

The **superior vermian vein** (SVV) usually originates near the declive of the vermis, curving anteriorly along the superior surface of the culmen (Fig. 12-12, arrow 4). Its tributaries often outline the vermian folia.[71] The SVV arcs slightly inferiorly in front of the vermis, then courses superiorly to enter the vein of Galen with or just anterior to the PCV. The distance between the SVV and straight sinus represents the width of the supracerebellar cistern.[78]

The **posterior mesencephalic vein** (PMV) arises from the lateral aspect of the cerebral peduncle and sweeps around the brain stem in the ambient cistern (Figs. 12-12, arrow 8, and 12-13, arrow 4). The PMV follows a course almost identical to the posterior segment of the basal vein of Rosenthal. It is usually smaller than the BVR though it may be quite prominent if the BVR is anomalous or incomplete. The PMV often receives the **lateral mesencephalic vein,** a vessel that courses superiorly along the mesencephalon (Figs. 12-12, arrow 9, and 12-13, arrow 5). The position of the lateral mesencephalic vein demarcates the junction of the tegmentum and cerebral peduncle.[29]

Numerous small veins in the pons and mesencephalon course anteriorly through the brain stem to empty into larger channels closely applied to its surface.[20] The **anterior pontomesencephalic vein** (APMV) is a vessel or plexus of longitudinal veins that courses superiorly along the surface of the pons and mesencephalon receiving numerous small tributaries (Figs. 12-12, arrow 10, and 12-13, arrow 8). It often curves into the interpeduncular fossa, demarcating the undersurface of the cerebral peduncles. The APMV usually drains into the basal vein of Rosenthal or the PMV. However, it may also join the petrosal vein or course inferiorly and become continuous with the anterior medullary veins.[9]

Anterior (Petrosal) Draining Group

Multiple venous channels drain the anterior portions of the cerebellum, pons, and medulla. These tributaries often unite to form a single prominent trunk, the petrosal vein.

The **petrosal vein** is a short trunk that originates in the cerebellopontine angle cistern (Figs. 12-12, arrow 13, and 12-13, arrow 10). It receives numerous tributaries from the pons, cerebellar hemispheres, brain stem, and fourth ventricle. The petrosal vein courses anterolaterally below the fifth cranial nerve and drains into the superior petrosal sinus just above the porus acusticus.[78] The **brachial vein** usually drains into the PCV (Fig. 12-13, arrow 6). However, it may also extend laterally over the brachium pontis to drain into the petrosal vein.

Posterior Group — inf vermian / inf hemispheric

These vessels drain posteriorly or laterally into the torcular Herophili and adjacent dural sinuses. The **inferior vermian veins** (IVVs) are paired paramedian vessels formed near the pyramidal lobule by numerous tributaries from the cerebellar tonsils (Fig. 12-12, arrow 15). The IVVs then curve posterosuperiorly along the inferior surface of the vermis, receiving hemispheric veins and terminating either in sinuses within the tentorium or in the

straight or transverse sinus adjacent to the torcular Herophili.[11] The **inferior hemispheric veins** drain the posteroinferior cerebellar hemispheres (Fig. 12-12, arrow 16). They usually empty into the IVVs but may also drain directly into the transverse sinuses.

VEINS OF THE POSTERIOR FOSSA: NORMAL ANGIOGRAPHIC APPEARANCE

Superior (Galenic) Draining Group

The **precentral cerebellar vein** (PCV) is best seen in the lateral projection of venous phase vertebral angiograms. As it ascends in front of the central lobule and culmen of the vermis it has an anteriorly convex curve (Fig. 12-14, arrow 5). The most distal portion of the PCV may have a slight anterior concavity just before it terminates in the vein of Galen. The PCV can occasionally be identified on AP views as it courses superiorly toward the vein of Galen. Occasionally its brachial tributaries are visualized, giving the PCV an inverted "Y" appearance (Fig. 12-15, arrows 5 and 6).

The "colliculocentral point," representing the anterior curve of the PCV as it exits from the precentral cerebellar fissure (as seen on the lateral view) should lie about halfway along a point drawn from the tuberculum sellae to the torcular. This line is called Twining's line (Fig. 12-16).

The **superior vermian vein** is usually well seen only on the lateral view (Fig. 12-14, arrow 12). It delineates the top of the vermis. Occasionally, small tributaries arising within the fissures of the culmen can be seen entering the SVV at right angles.[71]

On AP Towne projections, the paired **posterior mesencephalic veins** outline the superolateral aspects of the peduncles, forming an inverted "V" (Fig. 12-15, arrow 7).[25] Occasionally, small peduncular tributaries also outline the anterior surface of the peduncles. The distance between the PMVs represents the width of the upper brain stem. On lateral views, the PMVs follow a course similar to the basal vein of Rosenthal (Fig. 12-

14, arrow 7). The **lateral mesencephalic vein** courses perpendicularly to the BVR or posterior mesencephalic vein. It often connects these veins with tributaries of the petrosal vein (Figs. 12-14, arrow 8, and 12-15, arrow 8).

On lateral views, the **anterior pontomesencephalic vein** (prepontine vein) outlines the cerebral peduncles, interpeduncular fossa, and pons (Fig. 12-14, arrow 10). If it is continuous with the anterior medullary vein, the entire brain stem and medulla may be strikingly delineated (Fig. 12-14, arrow 14). On nonmagnified films, the APMV should lie several millimeters behind the clivus. The APMV is poorly seen on the AP projection (Fig. 12-15, arrow 13).

Anterior Group

The **petrosal vein,** the most prominent of this group, is a short trunk that courses inferolaterally just above and approximately perpendicular to the petrous ridge on the AP view (Fig. 12-15, arrow 9). Its position and course are quite variable.[12, 48] Occasionally, transverse pontine veins and hemispheric tributaries can be identified. In these cases, the anterior aspects of the midpons and cerebellum are outlined angiographically on the AP Towne view (Fig. 12-15, arrow 12). When the **brachial veins** of both sides are opacified, a typical inverted "V" appearance is seen (Fig. 12-15, arrow 6).

Posterior Draining Group

On AP Towne views, the paired **inferior vermian veins** run posterosuperiorly in the paravermian sulci (Fig. 12-15, arrow 11). On the lateral view they follow the inferior surface of the vermis (Fig. 12-14, arrow 11). Tonsillar tributaries unite near the pyramis to form the IVVs. The so-called "copular point" is a variable angiographic landmark, although some authors have attempted to define measurements that delineate its normal location (Fig. 12-16).[33, 34, 88] As a general rule of thumb the IVVs should lie at least several millimeters

away from the inner table of the skull (as seen on the lateral view). The overlying **inferior hemispheric veins** (Fig. 12-15, arrow 17) course much closer to the calvarium and should not be mistaken for the IVVs.

Supratentorial Group

Several supratentorial veins are routinely visualized on vertebral angiograms. These include the posterior segment of the BVR and also superior choroidal veins that are located in the floor of the body and trigone of the lateral ventricle (Fig. 12-14, arrow 1). Segments of the internal cerebral vein are also occasionally seen (Fig. 12-14, arrow 2). Superior and anterior thalamic veins draining the antero- and posteromedial aspects of the thalami are also frequently visualized on these studies (Fig. 12-14, arrow 3).

ABNORMALITIES OF THE VERTEBROBASILAR SYSTEM

The Abnormal Vertebral Artery

A variety of lesions may involve the extra- or intracranial segments of the VA.

Aneurysms. Extracranial aneurysms of the VA are uncommon and usually secondary to head and neck trauma. Most aneurysms involving the VA are intracranial, arise from the PICA (see below), and are atherosclerotic or congenital lesions.[36] The rare extracranial VA aneurysm may cause localized enlargement of the intervertebral foramina. This radiographic finding has also been observed in association with neurofibromatosis as well as focal tortuosity or anomalies of the VA.[72]

Arteriovenous Malformations. Branches of the VA may contribute to cervical, spinal, or intracranial AVMs.

Stenosis and Occlusion. Atherosclerotic disease commonly affects the VA at its origin (see Chapter 2). Intracranial stenosis is identified less frequently (Fig. 12-17). Trauma,

(Text continued on p. 403)

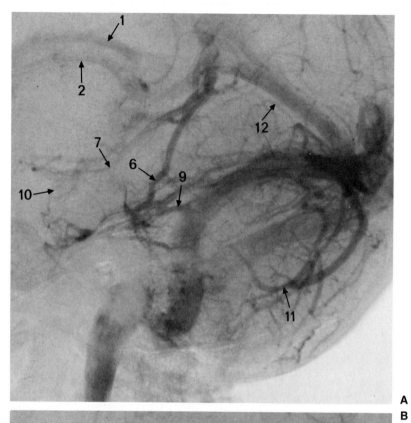

A

B

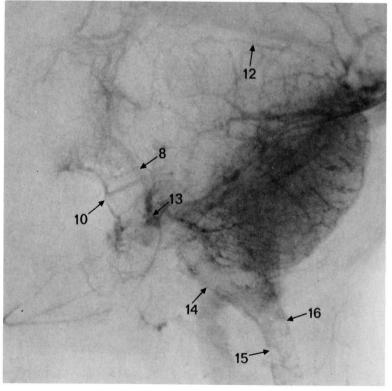

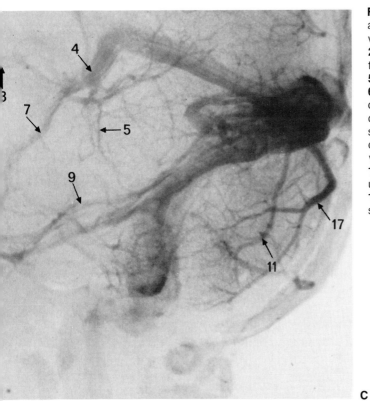

Fig. 12-14. Normal left vertebral angiograms (venous phase, lateral view). **1.** Superior choroid vein. **2.** Internal cerebral vein. **3.** Superior thalamic vein. **4.** Vein of Galen. **5.** Precentral cerebellar vein. **6.** Brachial vein. **7.** Posterior mesencephalic vein. **8.** Lateral mesencephalic vein. **9.** Superior petrosal sinus. **10.** Anterior pontomesencephalic vein. **11.** Inferior vermian vein. **12.** Superior vermian vein. **13.** Petrosal vein. **15.** Anterior medullary vein. **15.** Anterior spinal vein. **16.** Posterior spinal vein. **17.** Hemispheric vein.

C
D

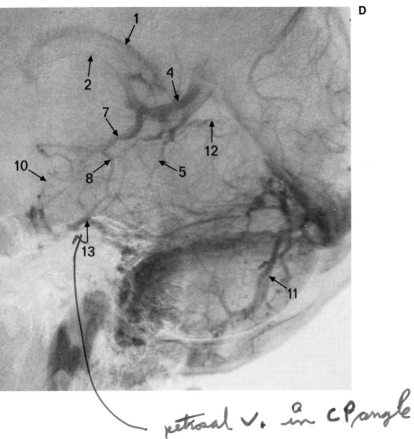

petrosal v. in CP angle

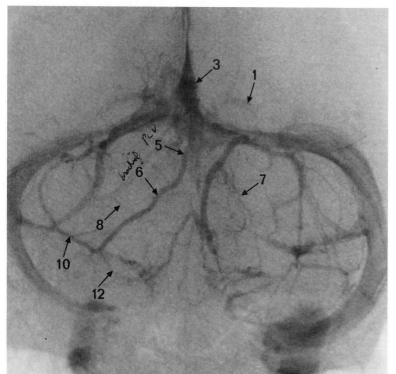

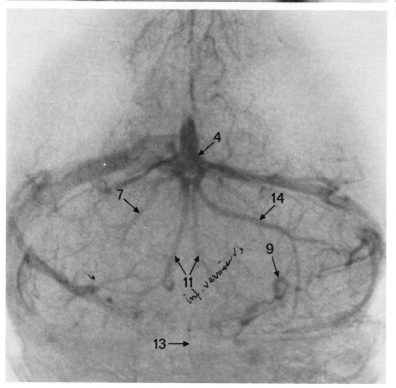

Fig. 12-15. Normal left vertebral angiograms (venous phase, AP Towne view). **1.** Superior choroid vein. **2.** Vein of Galen. **3.** Straight sinus. **4.** Torcular herophili. **5.** Precentral cerebellar vein. **6.** Brachial vein. **7.** Posterior mesencephalic vein. **8.** Lateral mesencephalic vein. **9.** Petrosal vein. **10.** Superior petrosal sinus. **12.** Inferior vermian vein. **12.** Transverse pontine vein. **13.** Anterior pontomesencephalic vein. **14.** Hemispheric vein.

A

B

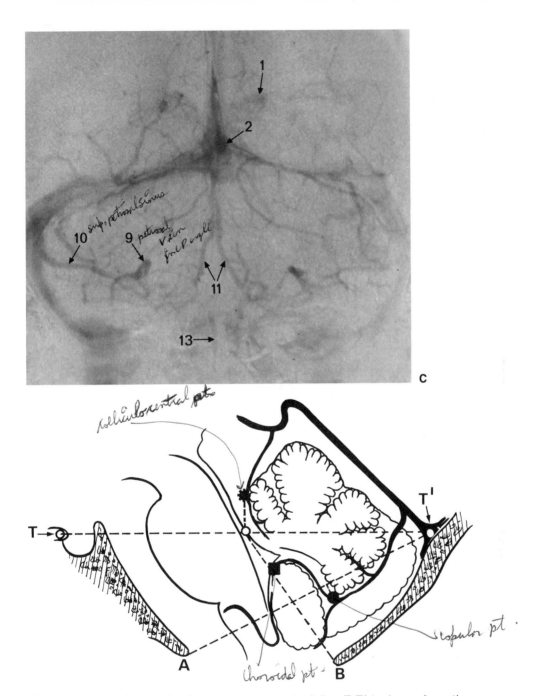

Fig.12-16. Normal posterior fossa measurements. A line **T-T**′ is drawn from the tuberculum sellae to the torcular Herophili (Twining's line). The "colliculocentral point" **(asterisk)**, representing the anterior curvature of the PCV, should normally lie about halfway along this line. The choroidal point **(black square)** should be about 2.5 cm down a line drawn from the midpoint of Twining's line to the posterior margin of the foramen magnum **(B)** on 2× magnification films.[52] The copular point **(black dot)**, representing the confluence of tonsillar veins to form the IVV near the pyramidal lobule of the vermis should lie a few millimeters below and slightly behind a point bisecting a line between the torcular **(T′)** and anterior margin of the foramen magnum **(A)**.

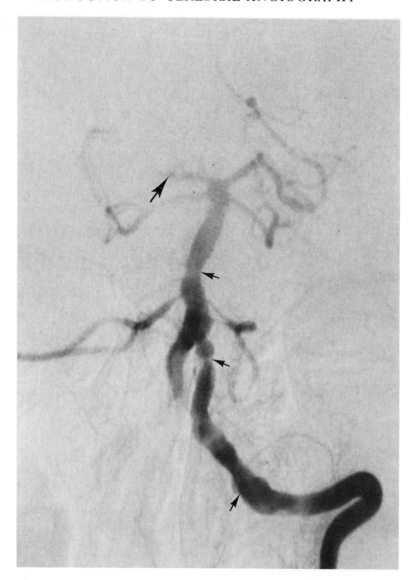

Fig. 12-17. Left vertebral angiogram (arterial phase, AP view) of severe atherosclerotic disease involving the vertebrobasilar system and its branches **(small arrows).** The right posterior cerebral artery is occluded **(large arrow).**

Fig. 12-18. Left vertebral angiogram (arterial phase, AP view) of a basilar tip aneurysm **(large arrow)** and subarachnoid hemorrhage. Note multiple areas of segmental narrowing secondary to vascular spasm **(small arrows).**

fibromuscular dysplasia, and spasm from sub-arachnoid hemorrhage may also narrow the VA (Fig. 12-18). Vertebrobasilar spasm has been reported as a significant cause of neuro-logical deficit in some patients with acute head injuries.[53]

Atherosclerotic elongation and tortuosity of the intracranial VA or its branches may cause hemifacial spasm or other neurologic ab-normalities (Fig. 12-10).[35, 40, 42] Large osteo-phytes can produce compression of the VA which is aggravated by certain head posi-tions.[61] Often basilar impression greatly dis-torts the VA. Rotational obstruction of the

VA will sometimes occur at the atlantoaxial joint.[5]

As with similar lesions elsewhere, the clini-cal manifestations of VA occlusive vascular disease vary according to the segment in-volved and the adequacy of collateral flow to the affected area. VA lesions can be partial or complete (Fig. 12-19). Total occlusion of the VA may be accompanied by vertigo, vomit-ing, and coarse nystagmus (usually toward the affected side). Ataxia and ipsilateral hypotonia with paralysis of the palate, pharynx, and larynx are common, as are facial pain and dysesthesias. Contralateral loss of pain and

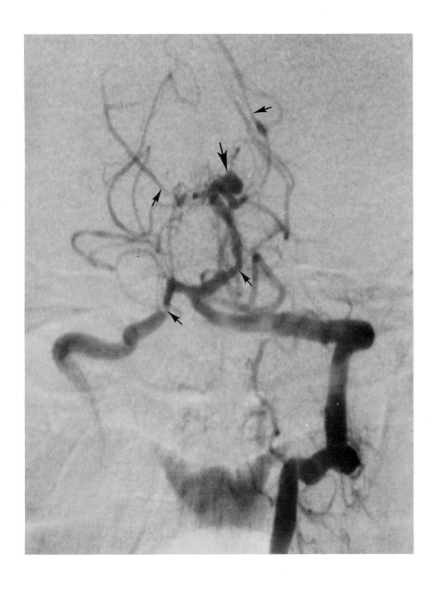

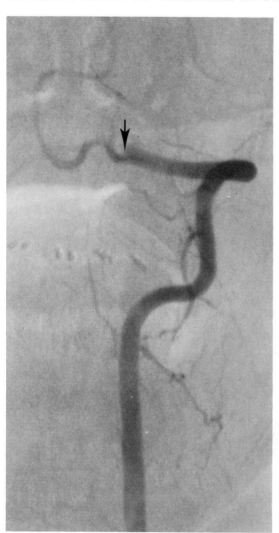

Fig. 12-19. Left vertebral angiogram (arterial phase, AP view). The vertebral artery is completely thrombosed distal to the PICA origin **(arrow)**.

Fig. 12-20. Left vertebral angiogram (arterial phase, lateral view) showing a large vascular mass **(arrows)** supplied by muscular and segmental branches of the cervical VA.

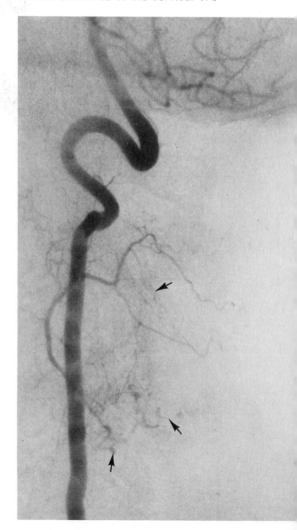

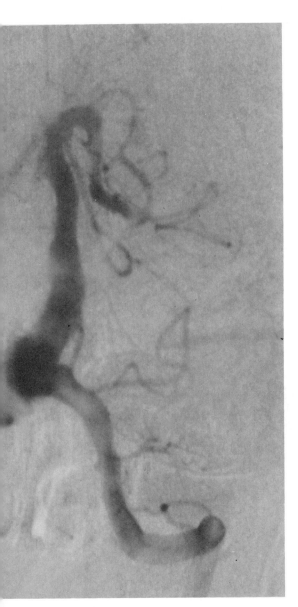

Fig. 12-21. Left vertebral angiogram (arterial phase, AP view) of severe BA ectasia.

temperature sensation on the trunk and extremities is evident with loss of proprioception and tactile discrimination. Consciousness is usually preserved. An ipsilateral Horner's syndrome may also be present.[18, 27]

Mass Lesions. Because of its location within the foramina transversaria, displacements of the extracranial VA are uncommon, although tumors arising from the clivus, foramen magnum, brain stem or cerebellum can displace the distal (*i.e.*, intracranial) VA.

Some extracranial vascular neoplasms may derive significant blood supply from the VA and its branches (Fig. 12-20). Meticulous angiography can be extremely helpful in demonstrating the relationship between major cervical vascular channels and the lesion; CT provides additional information in defining the relationship between the tumor, spinal canal, and adjacent soft tissue structures.[55] Meningioma, neurofibroma, paraganglioma, and hemangioblastoma of the cerebellum or spinal cord may derive supply from muscular, radicular, or meningeal branches of the VA. Astrocytomas of the brain stem and spinal cord are usually avascular.

The Abnormal Basilar Artery

Aneurysms of the posterior fossa itself represent less than 5% of all intracranial aneurysms, although some series report up to 15% that involve the posterior circulation.[49, 52] Since 15 to 20% of intracranial aneurysms are multiple, most authors recommend evaluation of the vertebrobasilar circulation even if aneurysms of the anterior circulation have already been identified.[49, 93]

Most saccular vertebrobasilar aneurysms occur at the BA bifurcation (Fig. 12-18).[92 A] Some aneurysms occur in the PICA. AICA aneurysms are rare.[37] Fusiform aneurysm or ectasia of the BA (sometimes inaccurately termed the "megadolichobasilar anomaly") may mimic an intracranial mass producing cranial nerve defects or presenting as a mass lesion within the cerebellopontine angle cistern or posterior third ventricle (Fig. 12-21).[4, 17 A, 19, 56, 66, 67] Rarely a tortuous BA mimics an intra-axial posterior fossa mass on CT.[19, 54, 86]

Arteriovenous Malformations. The BA may become enlarged and elongated if its branches supply a large vascular malformation.[15]

Occlusions and Stenosis. Occlusion of the intradural vertebrobasilar artery occurs approximately one-fourth as often as occlusion of the carotid artery. Atherosclerotic thrombosis is the most common cause.[85]

Other causes of BA narrowing include spasm secondary to trauma or subarachnoid hemorrhage (Fig. 12-18), fibromuscular dysplasia, encasement by tumor (see Fig. 10-15), or inflammatory disease.

The clinical manifestations of BA occlusion vary.[18A, 57] Gradual onset of symptoms or a fluctuating course may be present, but the symptoms often appear precipitously and death may occur within a short period of time.[37A] Bilateral cranial nerve and long tract deficits develop. Total BA occlusion produces either quadriplegia or hemiplegia on one side with partial paralysis on the other. This is accompanied by involvement of the bulbar nuclei and ascending sensory pathways. Severe dysphagia, dysarthria, disturbance of both deep and superficial sensation, and respiratory and circulatory abnormalities are common. Vertigo, vomiting, confusion, and loss of consciousness usually result. Death is usually attributed to complete BA occlusion. Isolated thrombosis of small BA pontine branches can be compatible with life but may produce severe neurologic impairment.[18]

Displacement of the Basilar Artery. Posterior displacement of the BA is most commonly caused by prepontine extra-axial masses. Tumors arising from the skull base, clivus, sella turcica, anterior tentorial incisura, posterior third ventricle, and cerebellopontine angle may displace part of or the entire BA posteriorly. Clivus chordoma or meningioma, large ICA or thrombosed BA aneurysms, sellar or suprasellar masses (such as craniopharyngioma, pituitary adenoma, suprasel-

lar arachnoid cyst) and destructive nasopharyngeal tumors are some typical causes of posterior BA displacement (see Fig. 10-13). Occasionally, exophytic brain stem masses may envelop the BA and produce seemingly paradoxical posterior displacement of this vessel (see Fig. 10-15).

Anterior displacement is more difficult to assess since the BA may normally lie only 2 to 3 mm dorsal to the clivus. Large pontine or cerebellar masses compress the BA against the clivus (Fig. 12-22).

Since the BA can normally wander from side to side as it ascends in the prepontine cistern, lateral displacement is also difficult to evaluate. Large cerebellopontine angle masses, exophytic pontine gliomas (see Fig. 10-15A), and tentorial meningiomas may rotate or displace the BA laterally (see Fig. 10-13).

Inferior displacement of the BA is uncommon. However, it can occasionally occur in severe hydrocephalus, descending transtentorial herniation, or secondary to large suprasellar or third ventricular mass lesions (Fig. 12-23).[70]

Fig. 12-22. Left vertebral angiogram (arterial phase, lateral view). A huge fourth ventricular mass displaces the BA anteriorly, compressing it against the clivus and displacing SCA branches posteriorly **(small arrows).** Tonsillar herniation is manifested by posteroinferior displacement of PICA and its branches into the foramen magnum **(large arrow).** Marked stretching of the thalamoperforating arteries indicates the presence of severe obstructive hydrocephalus.

Fig. 12-23. Left vertebral angiogram (arterial phase, lateral view). Severe obstructive hydrocephalus secondary to a large avascular mass in the posterior third ventricle is present. The BA is displaced somewhat inferiorly **(large arrow).** The proximal SCAs also appear depressed **(small arrows).**

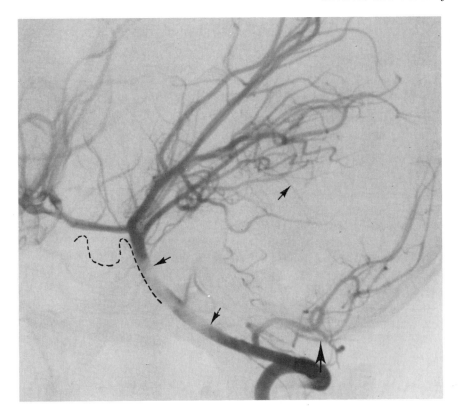

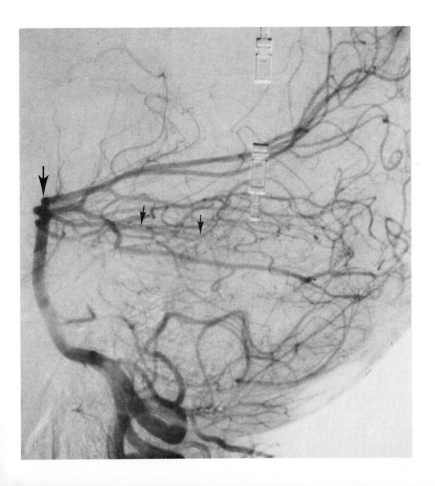

The Abnormal Posterior Inferior Cerebellar Artery

Congenital Anomalies. The most common anomaly involving the cerebellum is the Arnold-Chiari malformation.[70] The vermis is elongated and usually herniated through the foramen magnum, lying over a dorsally kinked medulla and upper cervical spinal cord (Fig. 12-24). The cerebellum grows upward through a malformed tentorial incisura.[59A-C] The cerebellar tonsils are frequently impacted in the foramen magnum.[47] The marked deformity caused by the underlying cerebellar malformation and its associated distorted vasculature occasionally makes accurate identification of the individual PICA branches difficult.[21] Caudal dislocation of the pons may be helpful in the angiographic diagnosis of the Chiari malformation.[90]

Aneurysms. PICA aneurysms represent less than one percent of all intracranial aneurysms. Most are located at or near the origin of the PICA. Distal lesions are uncommon. In cases of subarachnoid hemorrhage it is important to visualize both PICAs since aneurysms of this vessel might be overlooked if bilateral carotid and unilateral vertebral angiography has been performed and the contralateral VA was not refluxed. Often magnification and subtraction techniques, in addition to special views, are necessary for adequate delineation of PICA aneurysms.[69] A giant PICA aneurysm has been reported as a cause of foramen magnum syndrome.[38]

Occlusion. Most PICA occlusions occur at or near its origin from the VA. PICA thrombosis results in Wallenberg's (lateral medullary) syndrome, although VA occlusion may produce similar clinical manifestations.[18]

Mass Lesions. A variety of posterior fossa masses produce characteristic distortions of the PICA and its branches.

Sufficiently large-extra-axial masses may displace the PICA. Cerebello-pontine angle

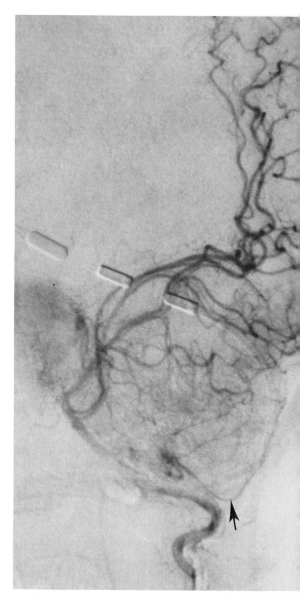

Fig. 12-24. Left vertebral angiogram (late arterial phase, lateral view) of an Arnold-Chiari malformation. Note the exceptionally small size of the posterior fossa. The inferior vermis and cerebellar tonsils are impacted into the foramen magnum **(arrow).**

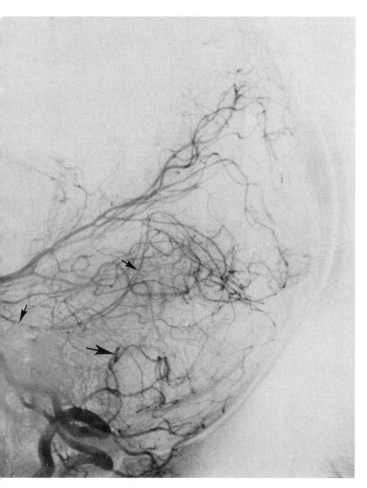

Fig. 12-25. Left vertebral angiogram (arterial phase, lateral view). A huge upper pontine glioma displaces the PICA backward **(large arrow)** and stretches the SCAs inferolaterally **(small arrows).**

and prepontine tumors often displace it posteroinferiorly. Lesions in or adjacent to the foramen magnum may cause upward displacement of the PICA.

Brain stem tumors usually displace the posterior medullary segment, cranial loop, and choroid point of PICA posteriorly as seen on the lateral view (Fig. 12-25).[32, 41, 52, 74] The distance between the posterior medullary and retrotonsillar segments may be diminished.[32] Pontine glioma is the most common brain stem tumor.

Fourth ventricular masses displace the tonsillar PICA branches laterally as seen on the AP view (Fig. 12-26). The choroidal point as well as the posterior medullary and supratonsillar PICA segments are often displaced lat-

erally and backward (Fig. 12-22).[63, 87] The PICA is usually not displaced inferiorly with these lesions unless they are unusually large. Invasive medulloblastomas, ependymomas, and subependymal gliomas are the most common fourth ventricular neoplasms.[52] Epidermoid tumors, meningioma, and choroid plexus papillomas do occur but are uncommon in this location.

Masses within the cerebellum produce focal stretching and displacement of hemispheric PICA branches. These vessels may appear displaced across the midline as seen in the AP projection. If the mass is sufficiently large the PICA may also be displaced anteriorly or inferiorly. Lesions in the cerebellar hemispheres are usually astrocytomas, metastatic tumors

(Text continued on p. 412)

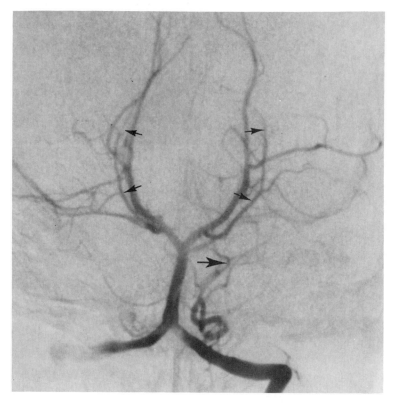

Fig. 12-26. Left vertebral angiogram (arterial phase, AP view) of a large fourth ventricular tumor. The SCAs are displaced laterally around the mass **(small arrows).** Note lateral displacement of the tonsillar and retrotonsillar PICA branches **(large arrow).**

Fig. 12-27. Left vertebral angiogram (**A,** arterial phrase, 0° AP view) and (**B,** lateral view). A cerebellar hemangioblastoma with a small vascular nidus **(large black arrow)** and large cystic component **(small black arrows)** has produced marked stretching and bowing of the adjacent hemispheric arteries. The PICA is displaced anteroinferiorly **(outlined arrow)** on the lateral view. On the 0° AP view, both PICAs **(outlined arrows)** are herniated through the foramen magnum **(dotted lines).**

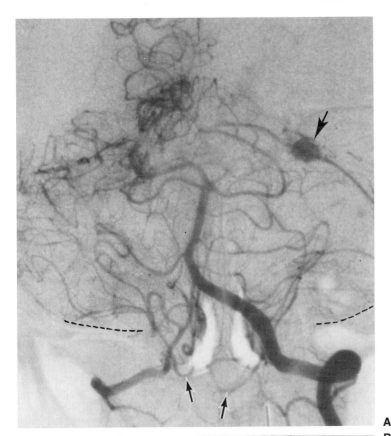

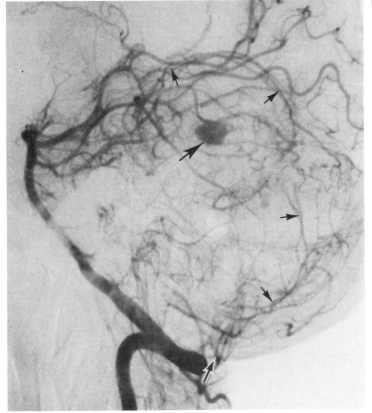

A
B

or hemangioblastomas (Fig. 12-27). Since hemangioblastomas may be cystic, solid, or mixed, vertebral angiography and CT are good complementary studies.[1, 14] Cerebellar hemangioblastomas may be solitary or multiple. They may also occur as part of von Hippel-Lindau disease, an autosomal dominant disorder characterized by retinal angiomas, cerebellar, medullary, and spinal hemangioblastomas, renal carcinoma, cysts, and angiomatous tumors of several visceral organs.[51]

Gliomas and medulloblastomas are the most common vermian neoplasms. On the AP view, the vermian branches of PICA may be spread apart. In the lateral projection, the PICA and its branches often appear displaced antero-inferiorly (Fig. 12-28).

Tonsillar herniation of PICA secondary to large posterior fossa or supratentorial masses can sometimes by determined angiographically. However, the caudal PICA loop may course below the foramen magnum in normal cases, making this an unreliable sign of tonsillar herniation. Identification of inferiorly displaced tonsillar PICA branches or stretching of hemispheric branches that are pulled down to or across the foramen magnum are more reliable indicators (Fig. 12-29).[51] Caudal displacement of the PICAs and their tonsillar branches can sometimes be identified on 0° AP views (Fig. 12-27A).

The Abnormal Anterior Inferior Cerebellar Artery

Aneurysms of the AICA are rare. In most of the reported cases, the aneurysm arose from the AICA near the porus acusticus.[37]

Occlusions. Thrombosis of the AICA and its acoustic or labyrinthine branches produces a definite clinical syndrome but is seldom demonstrated angiographically.[18]

Mass Lesions. Vertebral angiography is an important adjunct to CT and posterior fossa cis-

Fig. 12-28. Left vertebral angiogram (arterial phase, lateral view). A large vermian astrocytoma stretches and bows the inferior vermian arteries anteroinferiorly **(arrows)**. Marked anterior displacement of both the PICA and AICA is present.

ternography in the radiographic investigation of patients presenting with cerebellopontine angle syndromes.[39] Precise angiographic delineation of the blood supply to acoustic neurinomas and other vascular tumors within the cerebellopontine angle is helpful in surgery of these lesions.

While some authors have recently described characteristic changes in the configuration of the AICA and its branches with intra-axial posterior fossa lesions (Fig. 12-28), their greatest application has been in the evaluation of extra-axial tumors.[59, 82]

Displacement of the AICA and its branches is a reliable angiographic finding in the diagnosis of cerebellopontine angle tumors.[79] The exact type of AICA displacement seen with acoustic neurinomas depends on the anatomic relationship of this vessel to CN VIII and is therefore variable. The AICA may be either elevated or depressed as seen on the AP view. Superior displacement is more common (Fig. 12-30).[79] In the lateral view, arcuate posteroinferior displacement of AICA branches or reversal of the normal curvature of the meatal loop is often identified (Fig. 12-31).[59] Submentovertex views may also be helpful in delineating AICA displacements.

Meningiomas in the cerebellopontine angle can displace the AICA as well as derive significant blood supply from its branches. It should be noted that branches of the ECA and ICA may provide the major source of blood supply to cerebellopontine angle meningiomas and acoustic neurinomas.[84]

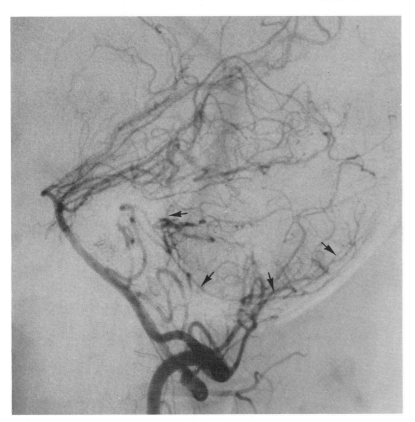

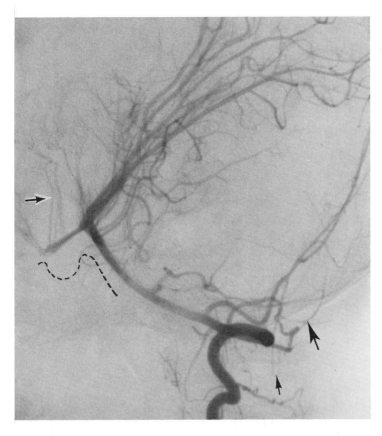

Fig. 12-29. Left vertebral angiogram (arterial phase, lateral view). A huge cerebellar astrocytoma displaces the BA anteriorly. Hemispheric **(large black arrow)** and tonsillar **(small black arrow)** branches of PICA are displaced through the foramen magnum, indicating pronounced tonsillar herniation. Marked stretching of the thalamoperforating arteries **(outlined arrow)** is caused by severe obstructive hydrocephalus.

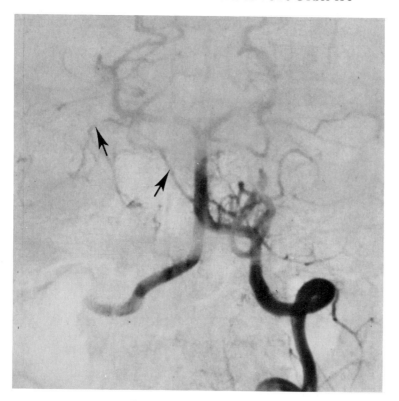

Fig. 12-30. Left vertebral angiogram (arterial phase, AP view). A large acoustic neuroma displaces the right AICA superiorly **(arrows).**

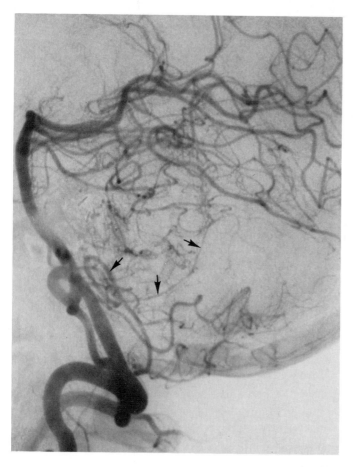

Fig. 12-31. Left vertebral angiogram (arterial phase, lateral view). A large recurrent acoustic neurinoma displaces the AICA anteroinferiorly **(arrows).**

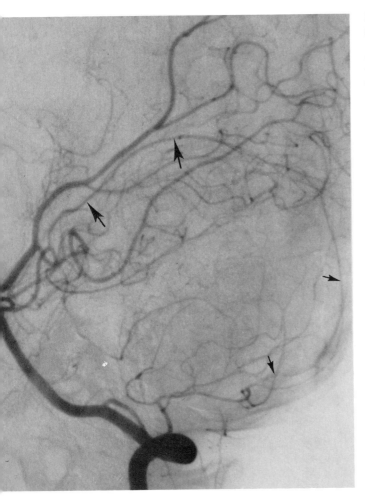

Fig. 12-32. Left vertebral angiogram (arterial phase, lateral view). A huge vermian astrocytoma has produced upward transtentorial herniation of the SCAs and their branches **(large arrows).** The inferior vermian branches of PICA are displaced posteriorly **(small arrows).**

Abnormalities of the Superior Cerebellar Arteries

Vascular Lesions. Aneurysms of the SCA are rare. Branches of the SCA supplying AVMs may become significantly enlarged. Occlusions of the SCA are rarely identified angiographically.[62] Tortuous SCAs have been reported as a cause of trigeminal neuralgia.[23A]

Mass Lesions. Expansile lesions within the superior vermis stretch the superior vermian SCA branches, displacing them laterally and superiorly. Upward herniation of these rami through the tentorial incisura may occur if the mass is sufficiently large (Fig. 12-32).

Cerebellar lesions may produce focal distor-

tion of the SCA hemispheric branches. The superior vermian arteries may be displaced away from their normal paramedian location as seen on the AP view.

Large mass lesions within the brain stem or fourth ventricle stretch and bow the perimesencephalic segments of the SCA laterally (Fig. 12-26). Extension of a midline supratentorial mass through the incisura can also produce this angiographic appearance (Fig. 12-33). Exceptionally large pontine gliomas occasionally displace the proximal SCAs inferiorly (Fig. 12-25). Large suprasellar, pineal, or posterior temporal masses may also depress the SCAs (Fig. 12-23). Medial and inferior displacement of the perimesencephalic SCA segments oc-

(Text continued on p. 418)

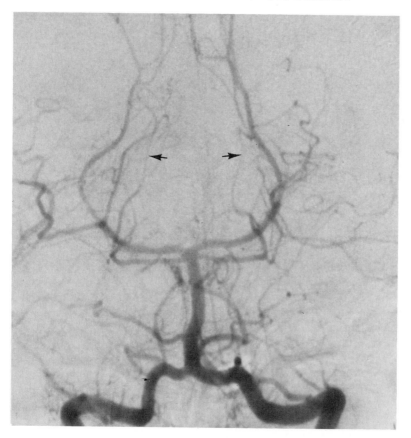

Fig. 12-33. Left vertebral angiogram (arterial phase, AP view). A large avascular pineal mass extends inferiorly through the incisura, splaying the posterior cerebral and superior cerebellar arteries laterally **(arrows)**.

Fig. 12-34. Left vertebral angiogram (arterial phase) of an infiltrating, fungating vascular neoplasm in the posterior temporal lobe (**A,** AP view; **B,** lateral view). The posterior cerebral arteries are displaced superolaterally; the SCAs are deviated inferomedially **(arrows)**. Separation of the peduncular segments of the PCA and SCA also typically occurs with tentorial meningiomas.

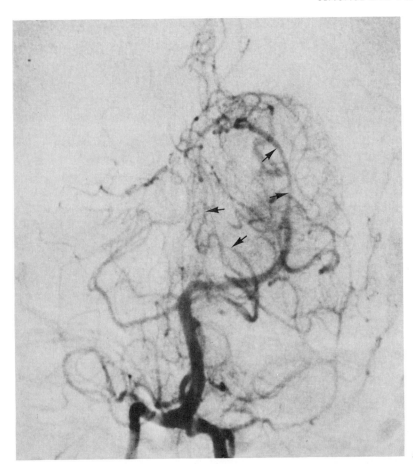

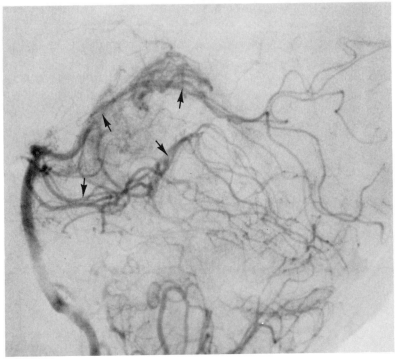

A
B

curs with descending transtentorial herniation (see Fig. 10-17).

Lesions in or adjacent to the tentorial incisura separate the peduncular segments of the SCA and posterior cerebral artery (Fig. 12-34). Superomedial SCA displacement can occur with extra-axial infratentorial masses or exophytic brain stem masses.

ABNORMALITIES OF THE POSTERIOR FOSSA VEINS

Congenital Anomalies and Malformations

The venous phase of vertebral angiograms is frequently helpful in defining congenital malformations of the posterior fossa.

In the **Arnold-Chiari malformation,** the inferiorly elongated, distorted vermis can sometimes by identified (Fig. 12-35). The anterior pontomesencephalic vein may indicate caudal dislocation of the pons. Veins around the brain stem sometimes delineate the low-lying medulla oblongata.[21, 90]

With a **Dandy-Walker cyst,** the torcular Herophili is elevated above the lambda and the transverse sinuses are steeply angled (see Chapter 11). Because the anterior portion of the cerebellum is everted over the colliculi and the caudal vermian lobules are absent, the superior cerebellar and anterior pontomesencephalic veins are displaced anterosuperiorly. The inferior vermian veins are absent.[25, 47]

Congenitally large cisternae magnae (the so-called "mega cisterna magna") and **posterior fossa arachnoid cysts** may bear some superficial resemblance to Dandy-Walker malformations on air studies or CT scans.[2, 3] While the transverse sinuses may be elevated, the torcular lies below the level of the lambda in both of these situations. The posterior fossa parenchymal veins show no evidence of mass effect in the presence of a large cisterna magna. Both the posterior fossa arteries and veins are normally formed, but displaced anteriorly with an arachnoid cyst.[25]

Pathological Veins and Circulatory Abnormalities

As occurs elsewhere, early draining posterior fossa veins can be associated with vascular malformations and neoplasms. The irregularity, dilatation, and bizarre appearance often associated with malignant supratentorial tumors seems to be less prominent with intratentorial lesions.[46]

Enlargement of the posterior fossa veins and dural sinuses can become marked with vascular malformations. The parenchymal veins may also become prominent when they serve as collateral venous drainage pathways in dural sinus occlusions.[28]

Distortions of the Posterior Fossa Veins with Mass Lesions

The angiographic diagnosis of infratentorial masses has been greatly simplified by dividing the posterior fossa into anterior and posterior compartments, as seen on the lateral phlebographic phase of vertebral angiograms.[16] The anterior compartment lies in front of the PCV and choroidal point of PICA. The posterior compartment contains all the structures lying behind these angiographic markers. The anterior compartment includes the brain stem, much of the fourth ventricle, and the subarachnoid spaces anterior to this dividing line. The posterior compartment contains the vermis, cerebellar hemispheres and posterolateral subarachnoid spaces.

Fig. 12-35. Left vertebral angiogram (venous phase, lateral view) of an Arnold-Chiari malformation. The vermis is elongated inferiorly **(arrows).**

Fig. 12-36. Left vertebral angiogram (venous phase, lateral view). The brainstem is displaced posteriorly by a large recurrent anterior tentorial and clivus meningioma (same case as Figure 10-13). Note the marked backward displacement of the anterior pontomesencephalic vein **(arrow)** and precentral cerebellar vein **(arrowhead).**

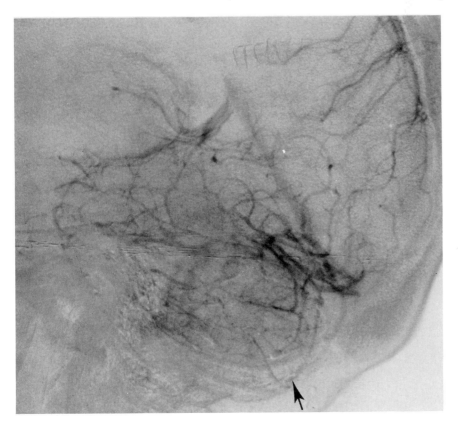

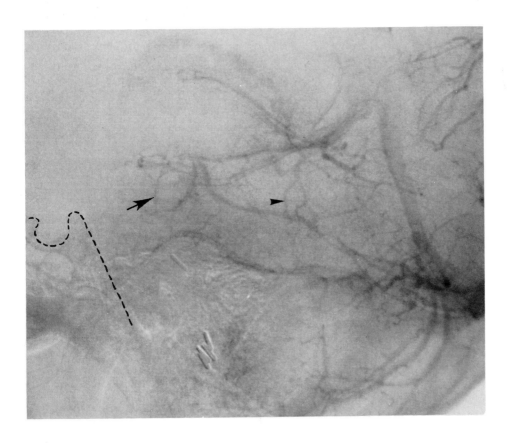

Posterior displacement of the APMV indicates an anterior extra-axial mass. Anterior displacement of the APMV coupled with posterior displacement of the PCV is characteristic of a brain stem lesion. Anterior displacement of both these vessels is indicative of a mass in the posterior compartment. Lateralization can be determined by assessing the position of normal midline markers (*i.e.*, the vermian arteries and veins) on the AP view.

Since different infratentorial masses often produce characteristic, identifiable distortions of the posterior fossa veins, the text will conclude with considering specific lesions in somewhat greater detail.

Extra-axial masses anterior to the brain stem and pons displace the posterior fossa veins backward (Fig. 12-36). The AMPV and PCV are displaced posteriorly. If the mass is sufficiently large, the PMVs may also appear elevated.

Extra-axial masses located within the cerebellopontine angle cisterns occasionally produce marked stretching of the petrosal vein over the lesion. The PV may appear displaced laterally on the AP view.[12] While some authors have proposed that a convex upward course of the PV indicates a cerebellopontine angle tumor, this configuration occurs in only 25% of normal cases and is therefore an unreliable angiographic finding.[48] Tributaries draining into the PV or IVV (if the mass extends inferiorly) are often displaced posteriorly in an arcuate fashion as seen on the lateral view (Fig. 12-37). Occasionally, the ipsilateral veins are compressed by the tumor, producing poor filling of the PV and its tributaries (Fig. 12-38).[33]

Expansile brain stem lesions displace the AMPV and transverse pontine veins anteriorly. Since these vessels lie on the surface of the pons they are a more accurate indicator of a brain stem lesion than is BA displacement. Veins posterior to the brain stem (such as the PCV) are displaced posteriorly (Fig. 12-39). The PCV may lose its normal, anteriorly convex curve, appearing flattened and straightened. Occasionally its normal curve

Fig. 12-37. Left vertebral angiogram (venous phase, lateral view). A meningioma in the cerebellopontine angle has produced arcuate displacement of petrosal and inferior vermian tributaries **(arrows)**.

may actually become reversed. The distance between the PCV and lateral anastomotic mesencephalic vein increases.[7] On the AP view, the posterior mesencephalic vein and the brachial tributaries of the PCV may be bowed laterally.

Fourth ventricular tumors usually displace the AMPV anteriorly. The most inferior segments of the PCV are often displaced upward and angled posteriorly.[63] The venous copular point may be displaced backward.[87]

Superior vermian masses characteristically displace the PCV anterosuperiorly. The SVVs are elevated; hence, the distance between them and the straight sinus is consequently diminished.[89] The AMPV may be displaced anteriorly (Fig. 12-40). **Inferior vermain masses** displace the IVVs, postero-inferiorly. Masses behind the vermis, such as arachnoid cyst, meningioma of the torcular or posterior tentorium, or extra-axial fluid, displace the vermian veins anteriorly so they appear farther away from the calvarium and straight sinus on the lateral view (Fig. 12-41).

Cerebellar hemispheric masses may shift the PCV and IVVs away from the midline as well as produce focal displacement of their adjacent veins.

Sufficiently large **supratentorial mass lesions** may distort some of the posterior fossa veins. The interpeduncular segment of the APMV may become compressed and displaced inferiorly. Large tumors in the pineal or quadrigeminal plate region can extend inferiorly through the tentorial notch, displacing the PCV posteriorly (Fig. 12-42). Descending herniation of the uncus and hippocampus through the incisura may also produce inferomedial displacement of the posterior mesencephalic veins.

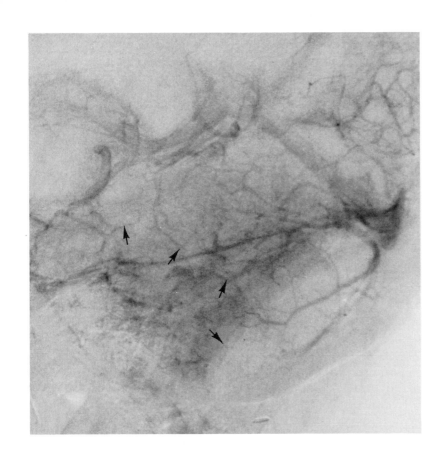

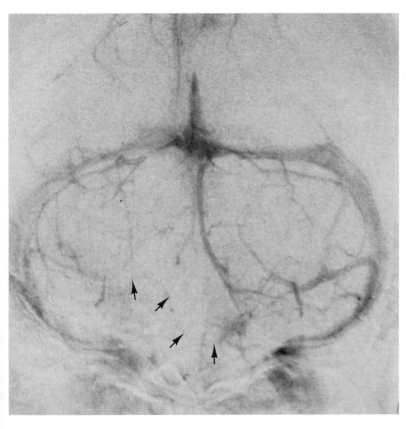

Fig. 12-38. Left vertebral angiogram (venous phase, AP Towne view). A large acoustic neurinoma has compressed tributaries of the right petrosal vein, producing poor filling of these vessels compared to the opposite side. The brainstem is rotated and one of the PV tributaries is displaced superiorly by the lesion **(arrows).**

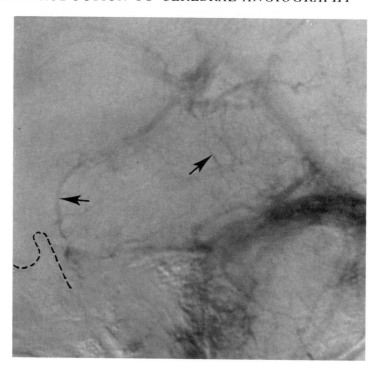

Fig. 12-39. Left vertebral angiogram (venous phase, lateral view). A huge brainstem glioma displaces the APMV anteriorly and the PCV posteriorly **(arrows).** These angiographic findings indicate an anterior compartment mass lesion.

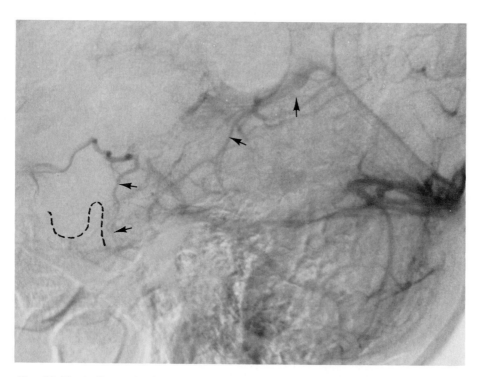

Fig. 12-40. Left vertebral angiogram (venous phase, lateral view). Hemorrhage in the superior vermis has produced anterior displacement of the APMV and PCV accompanied by superior displacement of the SVVs **(arrows).**

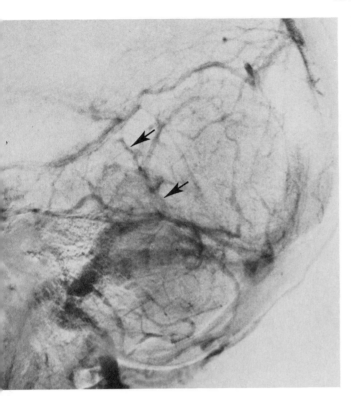

Fig. 12-41. Left vertebral angiogram (venous phase, lateral view) of a huge transtentorial meningioma (same case as Figure 10-12). The lesion has produced marked anterior dislocation of the vermis as indicated by the displaced SVVs **(arrows)**.

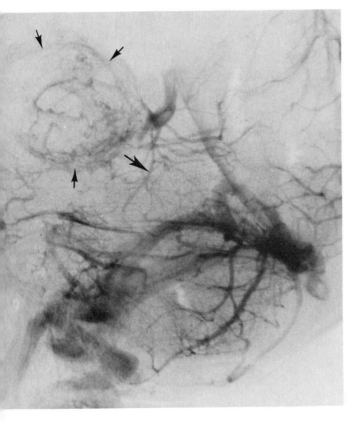

Fig. 12-42. Left vertebral angiogram (venous phase, lateral view). A large vascular pinealoma **(small arrows)** with infratentorial extension displaces the PCV backward, actually reversing its normal anteriorly convex curve **(large arrow)**.

REFERENCES

1. **Adair LB, Ropper AH, Davis KR:** Cerebellar hemangioblastoma: computed tomography, angiographic and clinical correlation in seven cases. CT: J Comp Tomogr 2:281–294, 1978
2. **Adam R, Greenberg JO:** The mega cisterna magna. J Neurosurg 48:190–192, 1978
3. **Archer CR, Darwish H, Smith K Jr:** Enlarged cisternae magnae and posterior fossa cysts simulating Dandy-Walker syndrome on computed tomography. Radiol 127:681–686, 1978
4. **Azar-Kia B, Palacios E, Spak M:** The megadolichobasilar artery anomaly and expansion of the internal auditory meatus. Neuroradiology 11:109–111, 1976
5. **Barton JW, Margolis MT:** Rotational obstruction of the vertebral artery at the atlantoaxial joint. Neuroradiology 9:117–120, 1975
6. **Bernardi L, Dettori P:** Angiographic study of a rare anomalous origin of the vertebral artery. Neuroradiology 9:121–123, 1975
7. **Billewicz O:** The normal and pathological radioanatomy of the lateral mesencephalic vein. Neuroradiology 8:295–299, 1977
8. **du Boulay GH, Radu EW:** How should one investigate the posterior fossa? Neuroradiology 15:253–261, 1978
9. **Bradac GB:** The ponto-mesencephalic veins (radio-anatomical study). Neuroradiology 1:52–57, 1970
10. **Bradac GB, Simon RS, Fiegler W, Schneider H:** A radioanatomical study of the choroid plexus of the fourth ventricle. Neuroradiology 11:87–91, 1976
11. **Braun JP, Tournade A, Panisset JL, Straub P:** Anatomical and neuroradiological study of the veins of the tentorium and the floor of the middle cranial fossa, and their drainage to the dural sinuses. J Neuroradiol 5:113–132, 1978
12. **Bull J, Kozlowski P:** The angiographic pattern of the petrosal veins in the normal and pathological. Neuroradiology 1:20–26, 1970
13. **Chambers AA, Lukin R:** Trigeminal artery connected to the posterior inferior cerebellar arteries. Neuroradiology 9:121–123, 1975
14. **Cornell SH, Hibri NS, Menezes AH, Graf CJ:** The complementary nature of computed tomography and angiography in the diagnosis of cerebellar hemangioblastoma. Neuroradiology 17:201–205, 1979
15. **Danziger J, Bloch S, Podlas H:** The pathological basilar artery. Clin Radiol 27:309–316, 1976
16. **Davis DO, Roberson GH:** Angiographic diagnosis of posterior fossa mass lesions. Semin Roentgenol 6:89–102, 1971
17. **Davis KR, Poletti CE, Roberson GH, Tadmor R, Kjellberg RN:** Complementary role of computed tomography and other neuroradiological procedures. Surg Neurol 8:437–447, 1977

17A. **Deeb ZL, Jannetta PJ, Rosenbaum AE, Kerber CW, Drayer BP:** Tortuous vertebrobasilar arteries causing cranial nerve syndromes: screening by computed tomography. J Comp Asst Tomogr 3:774–778, 1979
18. **DeJong RN:** The Neurologic Examination. Hagerstown, Harper & Row, 1979
18A. **Fine M, Palacios E, Shannon M et al:** Angiographic demonstration of recanalization of the basilar artery. Neuroradiol 18:269–271, 1979
19. **Frasson F, Ferrari G, Fugazolla C, Fiaschi A:** Megadolichobasilar anomaly causing brainstem sydrome. Neuroradiology 3:279–281, 1977
20. **Gabrielsen TO, Amundsen P:** The pontomesencephalic veins. Radiology 92:889–896, 1969
21. **Gabrielsen TO, Seiger FJ, Amundsen P:** Some new angiographic observations in patients with Chiari Type I and II Malformations. Radiology 115:627–634, 1975
22. **Gray H:** Antomy of the Human Body. Philadelphia, Lea & Febiger, 1966
23. **Greitz T, Sjorgen SE:** The posterior inferior cerebellar artery. Acta Radiol [Diagn] (Stockh) 1:284–297, 1963
23A. **Haines SJ, Jannetta PJ, Zorub DS:** Microvascular relationships of the trigeminal nerve. J Neurosurg 52:381–386, 1980
24. **Hardy DG, Peace DA, Rhoton AL Jr:** Microsurgical anatomy of the superior cerebellar artery. Neurosurg 6:10–28, 1980
24A. **Hardy DG, Rhoton AL Jr:** Microsurgical relationships of the superior cerebellar artery and the trigeminal nerve. J Neurosurg 49:669–678, 1978
25. **Harwood-Nash DC, Fitz CR:** Neuroradiology in Infants and Children. St. Louis, CV Mosby, 1976
26. **Haughton VM, Rosenbaum AE, Pearce J:** Internal carotid artery origins of the inferior cerebellar arteries. Am J Roentgenol 130:1191–1192, 1978
27. **Haymaker W:** Bing's Local Diagnosis in Neurological Diseases. St. Louis, CV Mosby, 1956
28. **Houser OW, Campbell JK, Campbell RJ, Sundt TM Jr:** Arteriovenous malformation affecting the transverse dural venous sinus—an acquired lesion. Mayo Clin Proc 54:651–666, 1979
29. **Huang YP, Wolf BS:** Veins of the posterior fossa—superior or Galenic draining group. Am J Roentgenol 95:808–821, 1965
30. **Huang YP, Wolf BS:** Precentral cerebellar vein in angiography. Acta Radiol [Diagn] (Stockh) 5:250–262, 1966
31. **Huang YP, Wolf BS:** Angiographic features of fourth ventricle tumors with special reference

to the posterior inferior cerebellar artery. Am J Roentgenol 107:543–564, 1969

32. **Huang YP, Wolf BS:** Angiographic features of brainstem tumors and differential diagnosis from fourth ventricular tumors. Am J Roentgenol 110:1–30, 1970

33. **Huang YP, Wolf BS:** Veins of the posterior fossa. In Newton TH, Potts DG (eds): Radiology of the Skull and Brain, Vol 2, pp 2155–2219. St. Louis, CV Mosby, 1974

34. **Huang YP, Wolf BS, Okudera T:** Angiographic anatomy of the inferior vermian vein of the cerebellum. Acta Radiol [Diagn] (Stockh) 9:327–344, 1969

35. **Jannetta PJ, Abbasy M, Maroon JC et al:** Etiology and definitive neurosurgical treatment of hemifacial spasm. J Neurosurg 47:321–328, 1977

36. **Jewel KL:** Bilateral extracranial vertebral artery aneurysms. Am J Roentgenol 128:324–325, 1977

37. **Johnson JH Jr, Kline DG:** Anterior inferior cerebellar artery aneurysms. J Neurosurg 48:455–460, 1978

37A. **Jones HR Jr, Millikan CH, Sandok BA:** Temporal profile (clinical course) of acute vertebrobasilar system cerebral infarction. Stroke 11:173–177, 1980

38. **Judice D, Connolly ES:** Foramen magnum syndrome caused by a giant aneurysm of the posterior inferior cerebellar artery. J Neurosurg 48:639–641, 1978

39. **Kendall B, Symon L:** Investigation of patients presenting with cerebellopontine angle syndromes. Neuroradiology 13:65–84, 1977

40. **Kerber CW, Margolis MT, Newton TH:** Tortuous vertebrobasilar system: a cause of cranial nerve signs. Neuroradiology 4:74–77, 1972

41. **Kumar AJ, Naidich TP, George AE, Lin JP, Kricheff II:** The choroidal artery to the fourth ventricle and its radiological significance. Radiology 126:431–439, 1978

42. **Laha RK, Jannetta PJ:** Glossopharyngeal neuralgia. J Neurosurg 47:316–320, 1977

43. **Larsen EB, Omenn GS, Margolis MT, Loop JW:** Impact of computed tomography on utilization of cerebral angiograms. Am J Roentgenol 129:1–3, 1977

44. **Lasjaunias P, Moret J, Théron J:** The so-called anterior meningeal artery of the cervical vertebral artery. Neuroradiology 17:51–55, 1978

45. **Lasjaunias P, Théron J, Moret J:** The occipital artery. Neuroradiology 15:31–37, 1978

45A. **Lasjaunias P, Manelfe C:** Arterial supply for the upper cervical nerves and the cervicocarotid anastomotic channels. Neuroradiol 18:125–131, 1979

46. **Lehmann R:** The potential of vertebral phlebography for the diagnosis of tumors in the posterior cranial fossa. Neuroradiology 10:263–270, 1976

47. **Lemire RJ, Loeser JD, Leech RW, Alvord EC Jr:** Normal and Abnormal Development of the Human Nervous System. Hagerstown, Harper & Row, 1975

48. **Leonhard T, Lehmann R:** The petrosal vein and its demonstration in the normal vertebral angiogram. Neuroradiology 10:271–275, 1976

49. **Lin JP, Kricheff II:** Angiographic investigation of cerebral aneurysms. Radiology 105:69–76, 1972

50. **Mani RL, Newton TH, Glickman MG:** The superior cerebellar artery: an anatomicroentgenographic correlation. Radiology 91:1102–1108, 1968

51. **Margolis MT, Newton TH:** An angiographic sign of cerebellar tonsillar herniation. Neuroradiology 2:3–8, 1971

52. **Margolis MT, Newton TH:** The posterior inferior cerebellar artery. In Newton TH, Potts DG (eds): Radiology of the Skull and Brain, Vol 2, pp 1710–1774. St. Louis, CV Mosby, 1974

53. **Marshall LF, Bruce DA, Bruno L, Langfitt TW:** Vertebrobasilar spasm: a significant cause of neurological deficit in head injury. J Neurosurg 48:560–564, 1978

54. **Miller EM, Newton TH:** Extra-axial posterior fossa lesions simulating intra-axial lesions on computed tomography. Radiology 127:675–679, 1978

55. **Miller EM, Norman D:** The role of computed tomography in the evaluation of neck masses. Radiology 133:145–149, 1979

56. **Moseley IF, Holland IM:** Ectasia of the basilar artery: the breadth of the clinical spectrum and the diagnostic value of computed tomography. Neuroradiology 18:83–91, 1979

57. **Moscow NP, Newton TH:** Angiographic implications in diagnosis and prognosis of basilar artery occlusion. Am J Roentgenol 119:597–604, 1973

58. **Naidich TP, Kricheff II, George AE, Lin JP:** The normal anterior inferior cerebellar artery. Radiology 119:355–373, 1976

59. **Naidich TP, Kricheff II, George AE, Lin JP:** The anterior inferior cerebellar artery in mass lesions. Radiology 119:275–283, 1976

59A. **Naidich TP, Pudlowski RM, Naidich JB et al:** Computed tomographic signs of the Chiari II malformation. Part I: Skull and dural partitions. Radiology 134:65–71, 1980

59B. **Naidich TP, Pudlowski RM, Naidich JB:** Computed tomographic signs of Chiari II malformation II: Midbrain and cerebellum. Radiology 134:391–398, 1980

59C. **Naidich TP, Pudlowski RM, Naidich JB:** Computed tomographic signs of the Chiari II malformation III: Ventricles and cisterns. Radiology 134:657–663, 1980

60. **Naidich TP, Solomon S, Leeds NE:** Computerized tomography in neurological evaluations. JAMA 240:565–568, 1978

61. **Newton TH, Mani RL:** The vertebral artery. In Newton TH, Potts DG (eds): Radiology of the Skull and Brain, Vol 2, pp 1659–1709. St. Louis, CV Mosby, 1974

62. **Newton TH, Margolis MT:** Pathology involving the superior cerebellar artery. In Newton TH, Potts DG (eds): Radiology of the Skull and Brain, Vol 2, pp 1831–1848. St. Louis, CV Mosby, 1974

63. **Numaguchi Y, Kishikawa T, Fukui M et al:** Angiographic diagnosis of fourth ventricle tumors. Radiology 128:393–403, 1978

64. **Osborn AG:** Cranial computed tomography in neurological diagnosis. Annu Rev Med 30:189–198, 1979

65. **Owen CVK, Cornell SH, Jacoby CG:** Posterior fossa intra-axial tumors: a comparison of computed tomography with other imaging methods. CT: J Comp Tomogr 3:31–39, 1979

66. **Peterson NT, Duchesneau PM, Westbrook EL, Weinstein MA:** Basilar artery ectasia demonstrated by computed tomography. Radiology 122:713–715, 1977

67. **Pinto RS, Kricheff II, Butler AR, Murali R:** Correlation of computed tomographic, angiographic, and neuropathological changes in giant cerebral aneurysms. Radiology 132:89–92, 1979

68. **Ross P, du Boulay G, Keller B:** Normal measurements in angiography of the posterior fossa. Radiology 116:335–340, 1975

69. **Rothman SLG, Azar-Kia B, Kier EL, Schechter MM, Allen WE:** The angiography of posterior inferior cerebellar artery aneurysms. Neuroradiology 6:1–7, 1973

69A. **Sartor K, Freckmann, Böker D-K:** Related anomalies of origin of left vertebral and left inferior thyroid arteries. Neuroradiology 19:27–30, 1980

70. **Scatliff JH, Kier EL, Zingesser LH, Schechter MM:** Terminal basilar artery deformity secondary to suprasellar masses and third ventricular dilatation. Am J Roentgenol 101:61–67, 1967

71. **Schilling H, Lehmann R:** Topographic measurement of the superior vermian vein by lateral vertebral phlebography. Neuroradiology 11:53–56, 1976

72. **Schubiger O, Yasargil MG:** Extracranial vertebral aneurysm with neurofibromatosis. Neuroradiology 15:171–173, 1978

73. **Scialfa G, Bank W, Megret M, Corbaz JM, Salamon G:** The arteries of the roof of the fourth ventricle. Neuroradiology 11:67–71, 1976

74. **Seiger JF, Gabrielsen TO:** Angiography of eccentric brainstem tumors. Radiology 105:343–351, 1972

75. **Seiger JF, Hemmer JF, Quisling RG:** The great horizontal fissure of the cerebellum: angiographic appearance. Radiology 117:321–327, 1975

76. **Stevens RB, Stillwell DL:** Arteries and Veins of the Human Brain. Springfield, Il, CC Thomas, 1969

77. **Suzuki S, Kuwabara Y, Hatano R, Iwai T:** Duplicate origin of the left vertebral artery. Neuroradiology 15:27–29, 1978

78. **Takahashi M:** Atlas of Vertebral Angiography, pp 43–47. Baltimore, University Park Press, 1974

79. **Takahashi M:** The anterior inferior cerebellar artery. In Newton TH, Potts DG (eds): Radiology of the Skull and Brain, Vol 2, pp 1796–1808. St. Louis, CV Mosby, 1974

80. **Takahashi M:** The basilar artery. In Newton TH, Potts DG (eds): Radiology of the Skull and Brain, Vol 2, pp 1775–1795. St. Louis, CV Mosby, 1974

81. **Takahashi M, Okudera T, Fukui M, Kitamura K:** The choroidal and nodular branches of the posterior inferior cerebellar artery. Radiology 103:347–351, 1972

82. **Takahashi M, Wilson G, Hanafee W:** The anterior inferior cerebellar artery: its radiographic anatomy and significance in the diagnosis of extra-axial tumors of the posterior fossa. Radiology 90:281–287, 1968

83. **Teal JS, Rumbaugh CL, Bergeron RT et al:** Persistent carotid-superior cerebellar artery anastomosis: a variant persistent trigeminal artery. Radiology 103:335–341, 1972

84. **Theron J, Lasjaunias P:** Participation of the external and internal carotid arteries in the blood supply of acoustic neurinomas. Radiology 118:83–88, 1976

85. **Thompson JR, Simmons CR, Hasson AN, Hinshaw DB Jr:** Occlusion of the intradural vertebrobasilar artery. Neuroradiology 14:219–229, 1978

86. **Thron A, Bockenheimer S:** Giant aneurysms of the posterior fossa suspected as neoplasms on computed tomography. Neuroradiology 18:93–97, 1979

87. **van Damme W, Reolon M, Pereira N, Wackenheim C:** Arterial and venous signs of tumors within the fourth ventricle. Neuroradiology 13:209–214, 1977

88. **van Damme W, Sturtzer F, Dosch J, Ammerich H:** A new method to localize the choroid point of the PICA and the venous copular point on the lateral projection of vertebral angiography. Neuroradiology 12:249–251, 1977

89. **Wackenheim A, Braun JP, Tournade A et al:** The herniation of the superior cerebellar vermis. Neuroradiology 7:221–227, 1974

90. **Weinstein M, Newton TH:** Caudal dislocation of the pons in the adult Arnold-Chiari malformation: an angiographic diagnosis. Am J Roentgenol 126:798–801, 1976

91. **Wilner HI, Crockett J, Gilroy J:** The Galenic venous system: a selective radiographic study. Am J Roentgenol 115:1–13, 1972

92. **Wolf BS, Newman CM, Khilnani MT:** The posterior inferior cerebellar artery on vertebral angiography. Am J Roentgenol 87:322–337, 1962

92A. **Wright DC, Wilson CB:** Surgical treatment of basilar aneurysms. Neurosurg 5:325–333, 1979

93. **Zacks DJ:** Multiple intracranial aneurysms. Am J Roentgenol 130:180–182, 1978

Index